Video Atlas of Arthroscopic Rotator Cuff Repair

Uma Srikumaran MD, MBA, MPH
Associate Professor of Orthopaedic Surgery
Shoulder Fellowship Director
Johns Hopkins School of Medicine;
Chair, Orthopaedic Surgery
Howard County General Hospital
Columbia, Maryland, USA

234 Illustrations

Thieme
New York • Stuttgart • Delhi • Rio de Janeiro

Library of Congress Cataloging-in-Publication Data is available from the publisher.

Important note: Medicine is an ever-changing science undergoing continual development. Research and clinical experience are continually expanding our knowledge, in particular our knowledge of proper treatment and drug therapy. Insofar as this book mentions any dosage or application, readers may rest assured that the authors, editors, and publishers have made every effort to ensure that such references are in accordance with **the state of knowledge at the time of production of the book.**

Nevertheless, this does not involve, imply, or express any guarantee or responsibility on the part of the publishers in respect to any dosage instructions and forms of applications stated in the book. **Every user is requested to examine carefully** the manufacturers' leaflets accompanying each drug and to check, if necessary in consultation with a physician or specialist, whether the dosage schedules mentioned therein or the contraindications stated by the manufacturers differ from the statements made in the present book. Such examination is particularly important with drugs that are either rarely used or have been newly released on the market. Every dosage schedule or every form of application used is entirely at the user's own risk and responsibility. The authors and publishers request every user to report to the publishers any discrepancies or inaccuracies noticed. If errors in this work are found after publication, errata will be posted at www.thieme.com on the product description page.

Some of the product names, patents, and registered designs referred to in this book are in fact registered trademarks or proprietary names even though specific reference to this fact is not always made in the text. Therefore, the appearance of a name without designation as proprietary is not to be construed as a representation by the publisher that it is in the public domain.

Thieme Medical Publishers, Inc.
333 Seventh Avenue, 18th Floor
New York, NY 10001, USA
www.thieme.com
+1 800 782 3488, customerservice@thieme.com

Cover design: Thieme Publishing Group
Typesetting by TNQ Technologies, India

Printed in USA by King Printing Company, Inc.   5 4 3 2 1

ISBN 978-1-62623-712-4

Also available as an e-book:
eISBN 978-1-62623-713-1

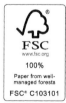

FSC
www.fsc.org
100%
Paper from well-managed forests
FSC® C103101

Dedicated to my wife Divya, and our daughters Nithya and Anshi

Contents

36 A Comparison of the Outcomes of Two Types of Synthetic Patches for Interpositional Graft Use in Irreparable Rotator Cuff Tears 258

Tom Morrison, Patrick H. Lam, and George A.C. Murrell

37 Dermal Augmentation for Challenging Large and Massive Rotator Cuff Tears 271

Devon T. Brameier and Paul M. Sethi

Videos

Preface

Video Atlas of Arthroscopic Rotator Cuff Repair presents diverse approaches to the surgical management of rotator cuff tears. The authors comprehensively review and detail various techniques covering direct repair as well as associated procedures such as biceps tenodesis, tendon transfers, and superior capsular reconstruction. Chapters are organized in a similar fashion to cover the surgical approach, from patient positioning to portal placement to surgical tips and tricks to pitfalls and complications. We present the information in a digestible format with direct links to the associated narrated videos. Although organized in a logical format for those interested in reading and viewing from beginning to end, the book can also serve as reference resource for a particular topic of interest. Accordingly, I hope this book will serve the student, orthopaedic surgeons-in-training, and those in practice looking to add to their surgical armamentarium.

Contributors

Joseph A. Abboud, MD
Professor of Shoulder and Elbow Surgery
The Sidney Kimmel Medical College
Thomas Jefferson University
Philadelphia, Pennsylvania, USA

Jeffrey S. Abrams, MD
Princeton Orthopaedic Associates, P.A.
Princeton, New Jersey, USA

Michael Bahk, MD
Southern California Orthopaedic Institute
Van Nuys, California, USA

Sevag Bastian, MD
Cedars-Sinai Kerlan-Jobe Institute
Los Angeles, Calfornia, USA

Michael Bender, MD
Methodist Sports Medicine
Indianapolis, USA

Kyle A. Borque, MD
Massachusetts General Hospital
Harvard Medical School
Boston, Massachusetts, USA

Devon T. Brameier, BSc
The ONS Foundation for Clinical Research
    and Education
Greenwich, Connecticut, USA

Aydin Budeyri, MD, FEBOT
The Shoulder Center
Baylor University Medical Center
Dallas, Texas, USA

Brandon C. Cabarcas, MD
Midwest Orthopaedics at Rush
Rush University Medical Center
Chicago, Illinois, USA

Hailey Casebolt, PA-C
Midwest Orthopaedics
Rush University Medical Center
Chicago, Illinois, USA

Frances Cuomo, MD
Montefiore Medical Center
Bronx, New York, USA

Ruth A. Delaney, FRCS
Dublin Shoulder Institute
Dublin, Ireland

Patrick J. Denard, MD
Southern Oregon Orthopedics
Medford, Oregon, USA

David M. Dines, MD
Sports Medicine & Shoulder Service
Hospital for Special Surgery
New York, New York, USA

Joshua S. Dines, MD
Sports Medicine & Shoulder Service
Hospital for Special Surgery
New York, New York, USA

Robert A. Duerr, MD
Jameson Crane Sports Medicine Institute
The Ohio State University Wexner Medical
    Center
Columbus, Ohio, USA

Bassem T. Elhassan, MD
Department of Orthopedic Surgery
Mayo Clinic
Rochester, Minnesota, USA

Ashleigh Elkins, MD
School of Medicine
The University of New South Wales
Sydney, New South Wales, Australia

Hussein Elkousy, MD
Texas Orthopedic Hospital
Houston, Texas, USA

Eric D. Field, MD
Mississippi Sports Medicine and Orthopaedic
    Center
Jackson, Mississippi, USA

Larry D. Field, MD
Mississippi Sports Medicine and Orthopaedic
  Center
Jackson, Mississippi, USA

Mark Frankle, MD
Department of Orthopaedics and Sports
  Medicine
University of South Florida Morsani College of
  Medicine
Florida Orthopedic Institute
Tampa, Florida, USA

Michael T. Freehill, MD
Stanford University School of Medicine
Palo Alto, California, USA

Michael C. Fu, MD
Sports Medicine & Shoulder Service
Hospital for Special Surgery
New York, New York, USA

Daniel B.L. Garcia MD
University of Saskatchewan
Saskatoon, Canada

Grant Garcia, MD
Midwest Orthopaedics
Rush University Medical Center
Chicago, Illinois, USA

Raffaele Garofalo, MD
Upper Limb Unit
F Miulli Hospital
Acquaviva delle Fonti-Ba, Italy

Anirudh K. Gowd, MD
Midwest Orthopaedics at Rush
Rush University Medical Center
Chicago, Illinois, USA

Konrad J. Gruson, MD
Montefiore Medical Center
Bronx, New York, USA

Laurence D. Higgins, MD, MBA
King Edward Memorial Hospital
Paget, Bermuda

J. Gabriel Horneff, MD
Rothman Institute
Thomas Jefferson University Hospitals
Bensalem, Pennsylvania, USA

J. Gabriel Horneff III, MD
Rothman Institute
Thomas Jefferson University Hospitals
Philadelphia, Pennsylvania, USA

Tyler J. Hunt, 2LT, MS-III
Lake Erie College of Osteopathic Medicine
Erie, Pennsylvania, USA

Chris Hyunchul Jo, MD
Department of Orthopedic Surgery
Seoul National University College of Medicine
SMG-SNU Boramae Medical Center
Seoul, Korea

John Itamura, MD
Cedars-Sinai Kerlan-Jobe Institute
Los Angeles, Calfornia, USA

Jean Kany, MD
Tolouse Shoulder Institute
Clinique de l'Union
Toulouse, France, Europe

Jack E. Kazanjian, DO, FAOAO
Premier Orthopedics and Sports Medicine
  Associates
Philadelphia College of Osteopathic Medicine
Havertown, Pennsylvania, USA

Paul Shinil Kim, MD
Department of Orthopedic Surgery
Seoul National University College of Medicine
SMG-SNU Boramae Medical Center
Seoul, Korea

Jacob M. Kirsch, MD
Boston Sports and Shoulder Center
Boston, Massachussets, USA

Pinkawas Kongmalai MD
Srinakarinwirot University
Ongkarak, Nakorn Nayok, Thailand

Sumant "Butch" Krishnan, MD
The Shoulder Center
Baylor University Medical Center
Dallas, Texas, USA

Patrick H. Lam, MD, PhD
Orthopaedic Research Institute
St George Hospital Campus
University of New South Wales
Sydney, Australia

Manesha Lankachandra, MD
Department of Orthopaedic Surgery
MedStar Union Memorial Hospital
Baltimore, Maryland, USA

Mark D. Lazarus, MD
Rothman Institute
Thomas Jefferson University Hospitals
Bensalem, Pennsylvania, USA

William N. Levine, MD
Columbia University Medical Center
New York, New York, USA

Joseph N. Liu, MD
Assistant Professor of Orthopedic Surgery
Department of Orthopedic Surgery
Loma Linda University Medical Center
Loma Linda, California, USA

Mark Mighell, MD
Department of Orthopaedics and Sports
  Medicine
University of South Florida Morsani College of
  Medicine
Florida Orthopedic Institute
Tampa, Florida, USA

Teruhisa Mihata, MD, PhD
Director
Shoulder and Elbow Surgery and Sports
  Medicine
Associate Professor
Department of Orthopedic Surgery
Osaka Medical College
Takatsuki, Osaka, Japan

Tom Morrison, MD
Orthopaedic Research Institute
St George Hospital Campus
University of New South Wales
Sydney, Australia

Colin P. Murphy, BA
Steadman Philippon Research Institute
Vail, Colorado, USA

George Murrell, MD, DPhil
Orthopaedic Research Institute
St George Hospital
Kogarah, New South Wales, Australia

George A.C. Murrell, MD, DPhil
Orthopaedic Research Institute
St George Hospital Campus
University of New South Wales
Sydney, Australia

Anand Murthi, MD
Department of Orthopaedic Surgery
MedStar Union Memorial Hospital
Baltimore, Maryland, USA

Matthew Noyes, MD
Department of Orthopaedic Surgery
Aultman Hospital
Canton, Ohio, USA

Michael J. O'Brien, MD
Department of Orthopaedics
Tulane University School of Medicine
New Orleans, Louisiana, USA

Ajay S. Padaki, MD
Columbia University Medical Center
New York, New York, USA

Matthew T. Provencher, CAPT, MD, MC, USNR
Steadman Philippon Research Institute
The Steadman Clinic
Vail, Colorado, USA

Hithem Rahmi, DO
Cedars-Sinai Kerlan-Jobe Institute
Los Angeles, California, USA

Catherine M. Rapp, MD
Beaumont Health
Royal Oak, Michigan, USA

Colin M. Robbins, BA
Steadman Philippon Research Institute
Vail, Colorado, USA

Anthony Romeo, MD
Midwest Orthopaedics
Rush University Medical Center
Chicago, Illinois, USA

Howard D. Routman, DO, FAOAO
Palm Beach Shoulder Service
Atlantis Orthopaedics
Palm Beach Gardens, Florida, USA

Anthony Sanchez, BS
Oregon Health & Science University
Portland, Oregon, USA

Joaquin Sanchez-Sotelo, MD, PhD
Department of Orthopedic Surgery
Mayo Clinic
Rochester, Minnesota, USA

Brett Sanders, MD
Center for Sports Medicine and Orthopaedics
Chattanooga, Tennessee, USA

Sriram Sankaranarayanan, MD
Clinical Assistant Professor of Orthopaedic
    Surgery
Department of Orthopaedic Surgery
NYU Orthopaedics
NYU Langone School of Medicine
New York, New York, USA

Felix H. Savoie, MD
Department of Orthopaedics
Tulane University School of Medicine
New Orleans, Louisiana, USA

Paul M. Sethi, MD
The ONS Foundation for Clinical Research
    and Education
Greenwich, Connecticut, USA

Jeremy Smalley, MD
Johns Hopkins University
Baltimore, Maryland, USA

Stephen Snyder, MD
Southern California Orthopaedic Institute
Van Nuys, California, USA

Daniel J. Song, MD
Evans Army Community Hospital
Colorado Springs, Colorado, USA

Uma Srikumaran MD, MBA, MPH
Associate Professor of Orthopaedic Surgery
Shoulder Fellowship Director
Johns Hopkins School of Medicine;
Chair, Orthopaedic Surgery
Howard County General Hospital
Columbia, Maryland, USA

Eric Tannenbaum, MD
Southern California Orthopaedic Institute
Van Nuys, California, USA

J. Ryan Taylor, MD, MPH
Physician
Orthopedic Surgery
Revere Health Orthopedics
Lehi, Utah, USA

Thomas "Quin" Throckmorton, MD
Campbell Clinic
University of Tennessee
Germantown, Tennessee, USA

Alexander Vara, MD
Orthopedic Specialists of South Florida
Miami, Florida, USA

Nikhil N. Verma, MD
Midwest Orthopaedics at Rush
Rush University Medical Center
Chicago, Illinois, USA

Tertuliano Vieira, MD
State Hospital of Urgency and Emergency
Vitoria, Brazil

Jon J.P. Warner, MD
Massachusetts General Hospital
Harvard Medical School
Boston, Massachusetts, USA

Brett P. Wiater, MD
Beaumont Health
Royal Oak, Michigan, USA

J. Michael Wiater, MD
Beaumont Health
Royal Oak, Michigan, USA

Mark R. Wilson, MD
Palmetto Bone and Joint
Chapin, South Carolina, USA

Mark R. Wilson, MD
Mississippi Sports Medicine and Orthopaedic
  Center
Jackson, Mississippi, USA

Jeong Yong Yoon, MD
Department of Orthopedic Surgery
Seoul National University College of Medicine
SMG-SNU Boramae Medical Center
Seoul, Korea

Connor G. Ziegler MD
Steadman Philippon Research Institute
The Steadman Clinic
Vail, Colorado, USA

1 Single-Row Rotator Cuff Repair Using Graft Augmentation and Bone Marrow Aspirate Concentrate Augmentation

Anand Murthi and Manesha Lankachandra

Summary

Large rotator cuff tears with poor tissue quality are a difficult surgical problem. Various biologic options are available that can reinforce the native tissue in a repair and potentially improve healing rates. The video describes our technique for use of a biofiber graft at the repair site and harvesting and use of bone marrow aspirate concentrate over the repair. This chapter highlights the available literature on the use of biologics in rotator cuff repair.

Keywords: biofiber graft, bone marrow aspirate concentrate (BMAC), rotator cuff tear, single row

1.1 Patient Positioning

- The patient is positioned in the beach chair, with care taken to support the medial edge of the scapula while still allowing for unencumbered shoulder extension. It often helps to make sure the patient's hips are moved far enough over toward the operative side to allow the arm to hang freely.
- We use a pneumatic arm holder on the operative side, which helps with glenohumeral distraction and arm positioning in general.
- Prior to placement in the arm holder, an examination under anesthesia is performed to evaluate for any stiffness.
- After the last drape is placed, strips of incise drapes are used to secure the edges of the drape to the patient circumferentially around the shoulder. Even with a sticky extremity drape, this step helps to keep the drapes from shifting intraoperatively.

1.2 Portal Placement

- The bony landmarks of the acromion, scapular spine, clavicle, and coracoid are palpated and drawn out.
- A standard posterior viewing portal is made 2–3 cm inferior and 1–2 cm medial to the posterolateral edge of the acromion. Entry into the glenohumeral joint can be made easier by palpating the bony edge of the glenoid with the tip of the trocar, "rolling over" the rounded edge to find the joint space. Gentle lateral traction on the humerus can also help to expand this space, making it easier to find. Aiming the trocar toward the previously marked coracoid is also helpful because it allows the trocar to fall over the posterior lip of the glenoid rim.
- Once the viewing portal is established, an anterior viewing portal is made with an outside-in technique. A spinal needle is placed lateral and superior to the coracoid, aiming for the rotator interval. After the needle is positioned appropriately superior to the subscapularis tendon and inferior to the long head of the biceps tendon, a

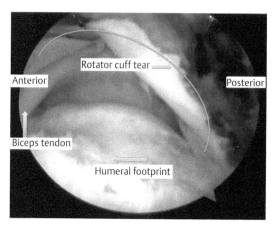

Fig. 1.1 Lateral arthroscopic view of massive rotator cuff tear.

portal is made and a cannula is placed. A common mistake is to direct the needle too laterally and superiorly. Instead, aim the needle toward the glenoid face and keep this trajectory in mind when placing the cannula.

- For subacromial work, an anterolateral portal is made, again using an outside-in technique with a spinal needle. For this portal, remember to consider the location and type of rotator cuff tear (▸ **Fig. 1.1**). Instruments should be able to access the most anterior and posterior parts of the tear as well as the footprint. It is helpful to think about placing this portal at a point equidistant to the anterior and posterior edges of the tear, but each tear is different.

1.3 Surgical Technique

- After a diagnostic glenohumeral shoulder arthroscopy is performed, a subacromial decompression is done. The same posterior portal is used, sliding the trocar under the inferior surface of the acromion until it reaches the coracoacromial ligament, which can be palpated with the tip of the trocar as an irregular surface just inferior to the anterior acromion.
- After the decompression, attention is turned to the rotator cuff. With large, chronic tears, the rotator cuff tendons are sometimes scarred down in a retracted position to the undersurface of the acromion and the underlying capsule. Releasing these adhesions allows the tendons to be mobilized back to the tuberosity more easily, facilitating a tension-free repair. However, there is a balance between performing adequate releases and damaging the already attenuated rotator cuff tissue.
- Any remaining soft tissue on the tuberosity is removed with electrocautery, and the tuberosity surface is prepared with a bur up to the edge of the articular cartilage. Preparing the footprint up to the edge of the articular surface allows placement of anchors as medially as possible, avoiding lateralization and unnecessary tension on the repair.
- At this point, the bone marrow aspirate is harvested from the humeral head. Using this site allows for relatively minimal donor site morbidity and saves the time and expense of prepping and draping a distant site. The amount of bone marrow aspirate and the equipment needed vary with the system used, but in general a Jamshidi needle is used to extract the required material, which is handed off the field for concentration.

- Turning to the rotator cuff repair, the goal in these larger tears is a tension-free repair with multiple sutures passing through the repair construct. Therefore, triple loaded anchors are generally chosen and are passed through the lateral portal. Remember that this portal must be large enough to allow for passage of multiple suture limbs and the graft, so an appropriately sized cannula must be chosen.
- First, one limb from the anterior anchor is passed through the anterior-most cuff, and its corresponding loop strand is parked outside of the anterior portal. Similarly, the posterior-most suture from the posterior anchor is passed through the posterior cuff and its loop strand is parked outside of the posterior portal. The middle four suture limbs are then passed through the middle portion of the tear, and these four suture "post" strands are brought outside the body and passed through the biofiber graft under direct visualization.
- The two graft sutures are tied and cut to begin reducing the tear, and the graft is then shuttled down the cannula into the subacromial space. The graft is placed on the edge of the rotator cuff using graspers and a probe. It is useful here to have assistance keeping the graft in position while the sutures are tied, sandwiching the rotator cuff tendon between the tuberosity and the graft. The graft acts as a scaffold at the tendon–bone interface.
- After the repair is complete, the fluid is suctioned out of the subacromial space and the bone marrow aspirate concentrate (BMAC) is injected over the repair and into the graft using a spinal needle.
- The portals are closed in standard fashion and the patient is placed in a sling and bolster.

1.4 Rehabilitation

- We do not change our rehabilitation protocol when using a graft or BMAC as an adjunct to rotator cuff repair.
- The patient is immobilized for 6 weeks (phase 1), coming out of the sling for non-weight-bearing waist-level activity (typing, writing, hygiene) and elbow and wrist range of motion.
- At 6 weeks, range of motion is started, focusing on supine overhead stretching (phase 2).
- At 12 weeks, a strengthening program can begin (phase 3).
- This program should be customized based on the abilities and motivation of the patient as well as the robustness of the repair.

1.5 Rationale and Evidence for Approach

- The use of biologics in orthopedics, and in shoulder surgery and rotator cuff repair, in particular, is relatively new. There is a paucity of human studies, and even fewer studies assess clinical outcomes even in the short term. However, there are some products and techniques that have come into widespread and accepted use.
- Neviaser initially described the use of graft material in rotator cuff repair in 1978.[1] In this report, freeze-dried graft of a rotator cuff was used to bridge an irreparable repair. In our practice, graft material is more commonly used to reinforce a repair with poor-quality tissue.
- There are multiple options for graft material, although allograft and synthetic materials are most commonly used.[2] In ▶ **Video 1.1**, we used a synthetic graft at the repair site. No studies directly compare different types of grafts with each other, so the choice of type of graft is generally surgeon-dependent.

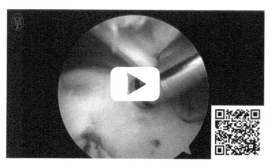

Video 1.1 Single-row rotator cuff repair using graft augmentation and bone marrow aspirate concentrate augmentation.

- Biomechanically, graft augmentation attempts to decrease rates of gap formation, facilitating better healing at the repair site. Biomechanical studies in cadavers using allografts and xenografts have shown decreased tendon gapping and load-to-failure.[3,4] In vivo studies are lacking.
- Histologic studies show evidence of increased cell adhesion and proliferation, depending on the graft type.[5]
- Clinical outcome studies for the GRAFTJACKET (Wright, Memphis, TN) showed higher American Shoulder and Elbow Surgeons scores at 2 years.[6]
- Mesenchymal stem cells from bone marrow have the potential to differentiate into tendon cells. However, the clinical significance of this application for rotator cuff repair is not clear. In animal studies, there is some evidence for increased cell differentiation into tenocytes, but it is unclear whether this improves rotator cuff healing.[7]
- Human studies are few, but the few available studies using BMAC, using a centrifuge to concentrate the mesenchymal stem cells in bone marrow aspirate, showed increased healing rate of the repaired rotator cuff.[8,9] The clinical relevance of these findings is unclear.

References

[1] Neviaser JS, Neviaser RJ, Neviaser TJ. The repair of chronic massive ruptures of the rotator cuff of the shoulder by use of a freeze-dried rotator cuff. J Bone Joint Surg Am. 1978; 60(5):681–684

[2] Gillespie RJ, Knapik DM, Akkus O. Biologic and synthetic grafts in the reconstruction of large to massive rotator cuff tears. J Am Acad Orthop Surg. 2016; 24(12):823–828

[3] Mc Carron JA, Milks RA, Mesiha M, et al. Reinforced fascia patch limits cyclic gapping of rotator cuff repairs in a human cadaveric model. J Shoulder Elbow Surg. 2012; 21(12):1680–1686

[4] Shea KP, Obopilwe E, Sperling JW, Iannotti JP. A biomechanical analysis of gap formation and failure mechanics of a xenograft-reinforced rotator cuff repair in a cadaveric model. J Shoulder Elbow Surg. 2012; 21(8):1072–1079

[5] Ricchetti ET, Aurora A, Iannotti JP, Derwin KA. Scaffold devices for rotator cuff repair. J Shoulder Elbow Surg. 2012; 21(2):251–265

[6] Barber FA, Burns JP, Deutsch A, Labbé MR, Litchfield RB. A prospective, randomized evaluation of acellular human dermal matrix augmentation for arthroscopic rotator cuff repair. Arthroscopy. 2012; 28(1):8–15

[7] Gulotta LV, Kovacevic D, Ehteshami JR, Dagher E, Packer JD, Rodeo SA. Application of bone marrow-derived mesenchymal stem cells in a rotator cuff repair model. Am J Sports Med. 2009; 37(11):2126–2133

[8] Hernigou P, FlouzatLachaniette CH, Delambre J, et al. Biologic augmentation of rotator cuff repair with mesenchymal stem cells during arthroscopy improves healing and prevents further tears: A case-controlled study. Int Orthop. 2014; 38(9):1811–1818

[9] Deprés-Tremblay G, Chevrier A, Snow M, Hurtig MB, Rodeo S, Buschmann MD. Rotator cuff repair: A review of surgical techniques, animal models, and new technologies under development. J Shoulder Elbow Surg. 2016; 25(12):2078–2085

Suggested Readings

Greenspoon JA, Petri M, Warth RJ, Millett PJ. Massive rotator cuff tears: Pathomechanics, current treatment options, and clinical outcomes. J Shoulder Elbow Surg. 2015; 24(9):1493–1505

Smith RD, Carr A, Dakin SG, Snelling SJ, Yapp C, Hakimi O. The response of tenocytes to commercial scaffolds used for rotator cuff repair. Eur Cell Mater. 2016; 31:107–118

2 SCOI Row Rotator Cuff Repair—A Medial Row, Tension-Free, Triple-Loaded, Crimson Duvet–Augmented Rotator Cuff Repair

Eric Tannenbaum, John Taylor, Stephen Snyder, and Michael Bahk

Summary

The Southern California Orthopedic Institute (SCOI) row rotator cuff repair technique involves a medial row, tension-free, triple-loaded, crimson duvet–augmented construct. This chapter describes a rotator cuff repair with a 95% healing rate for small-to-medium-sized rotator cuff tears and emphasizes the above key elements as part of the repair. This chapter highlights pertinent supportive literature. We also describe the lateral decubitus position, standard portals (posterior, anterior midglenoid, lateral, percutaneous anchor portals), tricks for bursectomy, how to perform the "perfect decompression," rotator cuff repair techniques and rehabilitation processes, and typical timeline.

Keywords: rotator cuff repair, rotator cuff tear, SCOI row, single row

2.1 Patient Positioning

- Following intubation, two pillows are placed between the legs and two between the down leg and the operative table to limit pressure on the bony prominences. All other bony prominences are well padded with foam padding.
- On anesthesia's count, the patient is rolled into the lateral decubitus position supported with a 3-foot-long Vacupak "beanbag" size 32 (Olympic Medical, Seattle, WA). The knees and hips are flexed to a comfortable position.
- A gel axillary roll is placed under the patient's lower axilla to prevent injury to the brachial plexus throughout the case.
- A foam head-and-neck support with a section cutout for the patient's ear is utilized by the anesthesiologist to place the head in a neutral position.
- Prior to suctioning, the bean bag is molded around the torso to maintain the patient in the lateral position with a 20° posterior tilt.
- Sequential compression devices are applied to bilateral lower extremities to mitigate risks of intraoperative deep vein thrombosis.
- The operating room table is rotated 45° posterior, allowing room for the surgeon to stand at the patient's head.
- Prior to placement in traction, the patient's shoulder is examined under anesthesia for range of motion and ligamentous laxity.
- A 3-point shoulder traction unit is attached to the inferior end of the operating room table on the contralateral side using a Clark rail attachment.
- The patient's hand/forearm is placed between two foam pads and wrapped with Coban.
- A stockinette is rolled over the foam padding. The distal end of the stockinet is the folded back onto the arm, leaving a 2-inch loop at the distal end of the extremity and then wrapped again with Coban.

- A metal S-hook or carabiner is used to connect the arm to the traction boom and 10–15 lb of traction is placed with the arm in approximately 70° of abduction and 10° of forward flexion (the glenohumeral position). Later in the case, the weights will be changed to the other cable when placing the arm into the bursoscopy position with 15° of abduction and 5° of forward flexion.
- The arm is then prepped in the usual sterile fashion with Chloraprep.
- A U-drape is placed around the shoulder starting from the neck. A rectangular drape is applied above the shoulder to connect legs of the U-drape and finally arthroscopy drapes are placed.
- A sterile green towel is wrapped around the arm paying careful attention not to touch the nonsterile extremity and contaminate the surgical field. This is wrapped with sterile Coban using the tubing of the Coban to create a quiver for the arthroscopic instruments (switching sticks, graspers, etc.).

2.2 Portal Placement

The bony landmarks are traced out along margins of the clavicle, acromion, and scapular spine. An orientation line is drawn from the posterior edge of the acromioclavicular (AC) joint extending laterally down the arm approximately 5 cm perpendicular to the lateral border of the acromion.

2.2.1 Posterior Midglenoid Portal (PMGP)

- The posterior shoulder anatomy is palpated and the humeral head is balloted, rocking it anterior to posterior to sense the location of the joint line. The posterior midglenoid portal is typically created 2–3 cm inferior and 1–2 cm medial from the posterolateral acromial edge.
- A small stab incision is made through the skin in this location using a #11 knife blade in the direction of the skin lines. Only the skin is incised.
- Insert the arthroscopic cannula with a tapered-tip obturator through the skin/muscle until the humeral head is palpated with the tip.
- Direct the cannula medial to the humeral head aiming to the center of the glenohumeral joint. The arthroscope is oriented with the glenoid inferior or parallel to floor.

2.2.2 Anterior Midglenoid Portal (AMGP)

- This may be done using an inside-out technique or an outside-in technique. For the purposes of this chapter, we utilized the outside-in technique for our anterior portal creation.
- Viewing with the arthroscope from the posterior portal, a spinal needle is placed approximately 3 cm inferior and 2 cm medial to the anterior edge of the acromion through the rotator interval and into the joint in the anterior triangle between the biceps and the subscapularis tendons. A #11 blade is used to make a stab incision through the skin along Langer's lines and insert an operating cannula such as a clear crystal cannula (Arthrex, Naples, FL) over a blunt trocar.

2.2.3 Midlateral Subacromial Portal (MLSP)

- This portal is created after lowering the arm into the bursoscopy position (15° of abduction; 5° of forward flexion) and following completion of the bursectomy providing visualization of the rotator cuff tear.
- A spinal needle is placed approximately 3 cm lateral to the edge of the acromion, typically anterior to the orientation line drawn when tracing the bony landmarks (▶ **Fig. 2.1**). It is important to locate the portal on the "50-yard line," a position directly in line with the center of the cuff tear (not the center of the acromion).
- Insert the smooth 6.25-mm clear cannula with a tapered obturator.
- A radiofrequency ablater can be placed in this portal to remove any soft tissue from the undersurface of the acromion, including the AC ligament and to define the borders of the acromion for the subacromial decompression (SAD).
- A bur or high-speed bone-cutting shaver can be the placed through the lateral portal to start the SAD. The scope is placed into the lateral portal and the bur is placed in the posterior portal to complete the SAD.

2.3 Surgical Technique

- 15-point arthroscopy of the shoulder is performed. The glenohumeral joint is viewed from the anterior and posterior portals while the subacromial position is evaluated with the arthroscope in the anterior, posterior, and lateral ports.
- In the glenohumeral position, debride the frayed edges of the cuff tendon on the articular side using a 4.0–5.5 mm shaver.
- Debride the footprint area on the articular side of the greater tuberosity from both the anterior and posterior portals.
- Lower the arm into the bursoscopy position.
- Insert the scope into the bursa via the PMGP and reposition the cannula in the AMGP to enter the subacromial space.
- Insert the shaver into the anterior portal to start the bursectomy and remove the anterior bursal curtain; then switch the scope and shaver to complete the bursectomy by shaving the remaining posterior bursa, especially the posterior bursal curtain.

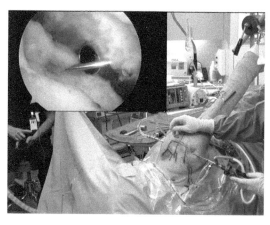

Fig. 2.1 The midlateral subacromial portal (MLSP) is identified with a spinal needle placed lateral to the acromial margin at the midpoint of the rotator cuff tear, not the midpoint of the acromion.

- Create the midlateral portal (outside-in) as described above.
- Place the radiofrequency ablater in the lateral portal to remove soft tissue from the undersurface of the acromion, followed by the bur to start the SAD. The anterolateral corner of the acromion and the lateral margin are typically burred at this point.
- Place the scope in the lateral portal and place the bur posteriorly to complete the SAD. The posterior AC joint marks the posteromedial corner of the resection. The medial acromial facet is carefully resected.
- The bone on the proximal humerus surface adjacent to the cartilage edge may require further shaving to remove any remaining soft tissue.
- The rotator cuff tissue is evaluated for quality and mobility. How well it can be brought laterally without undue tension is assessed with a grasper. The natural tension of the rotator cuff tissue is respected.
- We prefer medial row suture anchor placement to respect the tissue's natural tension and biology. This is adjacent to the humeral head cartilage or on the medial aspect of the greater tuberosity. Placing unnatural or excessive tension on the repair via lateralization may compromise the repair.
- Gentle releases may be performed, capsular or subacromial, to help mobilize the rotator cuff tears. Aggressive slides are typically avoided to preserve the quality and integrity of the already compromised rotator cuff tissue.
- A spinal needle is utilized to identify the location of the first suture anchor placement percutaneously. Multiple anchors may be placed with one well-chosen percutaneous position as confirmed by the spinal needle (▶ **Fig. 2.2**). The first triple-loaded suture anchor is placed posteriorly with subsequent suture anchors placed anteriorly.
- Once the appropriate location is identified with the spinal needle, just off the edge of the acromion, a small skin incision is made.
- A starter punch is placed in the chosen anchor position followed by placement of a triple-loaded suture anchor with the vertical orientation lines perpendicular to the cuff.
- The most posteromedial suture is retrieved through the anterior portal using a crochet hook. The chosen suture is retrieved medial to the other sutures. A Spectrum (ConMedLinvatec, Largo, FL) suture passer, often a medium crescent, is pierced through the posterior edge of the cuff tear and a #1 polydioxanone suture (PDS) is passed through the cuff and retrieved using a grasper from the anterior portal.

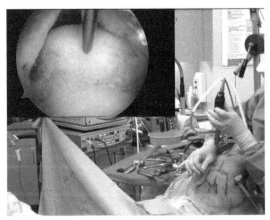

Fig. 2.2 A spinal needle is placed percutaneously near the lateral acromial border to identify the ideal location for percutaneous anchor placement; the spinal should easily access the medial greater tuberosity adjacent to the humeral head cartilage and, if well placed, can allow multiple suture anchors anteriorly and posteriorly.

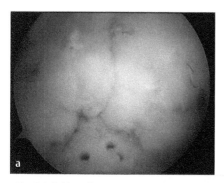
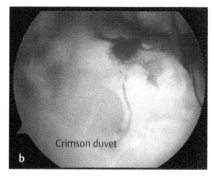

Crimson duvet

Fig. 2.3 (a,b) Final SCOI row rotator cuff repair that is biomechanically sound with triple-loaded suture anchors, medialized for a tension-free repair and biologically augmented by bone marrow vents.

- The PDS is tied around the previously retrieved suture or the Super Shuttle (ConMedLinvatec) is loaded in the anterior portal and passed back out the posterior portal.
- The partner suture limb is retrieved out of the posterior portal using the crochet hook. The suture may be tied now with the "tie-as-you-go" technique or it may be provisionally held in Suture Savers (ConMedLinvatec) and tied at the end to make sure no dog-ears or malreduction is performed. If the "tie-as-you-go" technique is used, careful templating of the suture anchors and suture placement in the rotator cuff must be performed prior to actual placement. The sutures are tied using an SMC sliding knot and backed up with three alternating half hitches on reversed posts.
- The remaining two sutures from the anchor are passed and tied in the same fashion using whichever curve of the Spectrum hook that makes passing the stitch easiest. Each suture should be situated equally apart with the center suture being directly in line with the center of the anchor.
- If needed, a second suture anchor is placed depending on the size of the tear. More than two anchors may be necessary if the tear is larger than 2 cm.
- A mini-Revo punch (ConMedLinvatec) is used to create bone marrow vents in the greater tuberosity lateral to the rotator cuff repair to allow the release of mesenchymal stem cells, platelets, growth factors, and cytokines to form a super clot over the footprint and repair site that will form the so-called "crimson duvet" (▶ **Fig. 2.3**).

2.4 Surgeon Tips and Tricks

- A triple-loaded suture anchor will ensure excellent and adequate biomechanical fixation of the rotator cuff repair.[1]
- Medialization of the suture anchor placement will ensure minimum tension on the rotator cuff repair.[2]
- Bone marrow vents optimize biologic healing.[3]
- The combination of the above three factors helps constitute the basis of the SCOI row repair, a very specific repair technique that does not fall within the typical single-row or double-row repair techniques described and which also has documented healing rates of 91% in medium-to-large rotator cuff tears.[4]

- An alternative method to the "tie-as-you-go" technique demonstrated in ▶ **Video 2.1** involves placing small plastic straws called suture savers around each pair of consecutively passed suture limbs to temporarily reduce the cuff to the footprint. These sutures are then retrieved out of the lateral portal (viewing from the anterior portal) and tied typically in an anterior-to-posterior manner.
- Suture anchors are always inserted near the medial edge of the anatomical neck a few mm away from the humeral head cartilage instead of the lateral placement on the greater tuberosity.
- Anchors are placed at a 45° or "tent peg" angle under the subchondral bone.
- Bone marrow vents are created throughout the tuberosity during the repair to allow healing bone marrow elements to flow out to cover and nourish the healing tendon, creating a "crimson duvet" or "superclot." This creates a dense, fibrous meshwork replete with mesenchymal stem cells, platelets, growth factors, and cytokines.
- The suture knot stack can be placed at the surgeon's discretion via control of the suture loop placement with the knot pusher or with a probe.

2.5 Pitfalls/Complications

- Proper portal placement is important to optimizing a successful surgery. The lateral portal in the subacromial space placed at the midpoint of the rotator cuff tear ensures good visualization of the rotator cuff repair.
- The medial suture limb (the limb that will pass through the rotator cuff) should be retrieved medially to the other retained sutures in the suture anchor via a crochet hook. Retrieving this suture laterally instead will cross the sutures and potentially prevent a sliding knot from being performed.
- The lateral limb of the suture should be retrieved lateral to the remaining other sutures in the suture anchor. This will also prevent sutures from crossing each other and not sliding.
- Before tying a sliding suture knot, slide both limbs of the sutures fully back and forth to make sure the soon-to-be-tied suture will slide.
- A looped or pincher grasper can also be used to untwist a set of sutures before tying by looping around the suture anchor strand.
- Hard greater tuberosity bone may require a bone tap in addition to a suture anchor awl.

2.6 Rehabilitation

- The first goal is to protect the repair during the first 4 to 8 weeks to allow the repaired tissue to heal. Immobilization using an abduction sling will help accomplish this goal by allowing tension-free healing. The sling is worn 23/24 hours a day with gentle daily passive stretching.
- After 4–8 weeks of immobilization, active range of motion (AROM) may be initiated with strengthening typically 2–4 months after surgery, depending on the size of the tear and tissue quality.
- Four phases of rehabilitation (note: larger tears may require slower progression):
  – Phase I (0–8 weeks): immobilization and gentle passive range of motion.
  – Phase II (4–8 weeks): active AROM (AAROM), followed by AROM.

– Phase III (8–12 weeks): progressive rotator cuff and scapular strengthening.
– Phase IV (12–16 weeks): advanced strengthening.
– Gradual return to sport is initiated after completion of phase IV.

2.7 Rationale and/or Evidence for Approach

- Arthroscopic single-row rotator cuff repairs demonstrated a failure of 17 out of 18 repairs to heal.[5]
- Double-row repair techniques were described to restore the native footprint and increase mechanical fixation to help improve healing rates.[6]
- Proponents of the double-row repair believe that a single-row repair only partially restores the native rotator cuff footprint and believe that the double-row technique provides improved tendon-to-bone contract area, mechanical properties, and increased fixation strength at time zero.
- However, multiple level I and II studies fail to demonstrate a difference in clinical outcomes and re-tear rates when comparing the two techniques.[7,8]
- One potential explanation for this is that the supraspinatus footprint has been shown to be significantly smaller than originally described in the cadaveric study published by Curtis et al in 2006.[9] A more recent anatomic study performed by Mochizuki et al found the supraspinatus footprint to be a much smaller, triangular area with the majority of the greater tuberosity covered by the infraspinatus tendon/footprint.[10]
- Furthermore, tears that typically occur in a hypovascular zone of the cuff requiring debridement of the degenerative nonviable edges of the cuff result in a shorter tendon to repair back to the footprint. A shorter tendon will thus require increased tension if pulled and repaired to the original length of the lateral border of the footprint as done with a double-row repair.
- Davidson and Rivenburgh published a study demonstrating that increased tension is detrimental to the repair and that functional outcome is inversely proportional to rotator cuff repair tension.[11]
- All the prospective randomized controlled trials comparing double- versus single-row repairs performed lateralized single-row repairs by pulling the tendon in a relatively tensioned position on the lateral edge of the tuberosity,[7,8] thereby placing similar increased tension with both techniques.
- Hersche and Gerber assessed passive tension in the supraspinatus and found a 45-N differential between the medial and lateral footprint.[12]
- A study was published by our group at SCOI looking at in vivo measurements comparing medial versus lateral footprint positions and demonstrated a 5.4-fold increase in tension when the tendon edge was reduced to the lateral as opposed to the medial footprint.[2]
- Based on the aforementioned studies, we strongly encourage a low-tension repair performed best with a single row of medial anchors as described in our "SCOI row" technique video. Triple-loaded suture anchors are always recommended based on multiple studies published by Alan Barber, demonstrating 100% increase in fixation over double-loaded single-row anchor fixation.[1]
- Furthermore, a study by the Hospital for Special Surgery demonstrated that increasing the number of sutures decreases cyclic gap formation and increases load to failure.[13] When the number of sutures is kept constant, single-row and double-row repair constructs are biomechanically equivalent.

- Bone marrow vents created in the greater tuberosity adjacent to the repair has been shown to be important for healing.[14] Bone marrow cells have been shown to infiltrate the rotator cuff using a green fluorescent protein marker in a rat model.[15] Milano published a prospective randomized trial comparing cuff repair with and without marrow vents and demonstrated better healing rates in the cuffs repaired with vents.[16]

References

[1] Barber FA, Herbert MA, Schroeder FA, Aziz-Jacobo J, Mays MM, Rapley JH. Biomechanical advantages of triple-loaded suture anchors compared with double-row rotator cuff repairs. Arthroscopy. 2010; 26(3): 316–323

[2] Dierckman BD, Wang DW, Bahk MS, Burns JP, Getelman MH. In vivo measurement of rotator cuff tear tension: Medial versus lateral footprint position. Am J Orthop. 2016; 45(3):E83–E90

[3] Jo CH, Shin JS, Park IW, Kim H, Lee SY. Multiple channeling improves the structural integrity of rotator cuff repair. Am J Sports Med. 2013; 41(11):2650–2657

[4] Dierckman BD, Ni JJ, Karzel RP, Getelman MH. Excellent healing rates and patient satisfaction after arthroscopic repair of medium to large rotator cuff tears with a single-row technique augmented with bone marrow vents. Knee Surg Sports TraumatolArthrosc. 2018; 26(1):136–145

[5] Galatz LM, Ball CM, Teefey SA, Middleton WD, Yamaguchi K. The outcome and repair integrity of completely arthroscopically repaired large and massive rotator cuff tears. J Bone Joint Surg Am. 2004; 86(2):219–224

[6] Lo IK, Burkhart SS. Double-row arthroscopic rotator cuff repair: Re-establishing the footprint of the rotator cuff. Arthroscopy. 2003; 19(9):1035–1042

[7] Burks RT, Crim J, Brown N, Fink B, Greis PE. A prospective randomized clinical trial comparing arthroscopic single- and double-row rotator cuff repair: Magnetic resonance imaging and early clinical evaluation. Am J Sports Med. 2009; 37(4):674–682

[8] Lapner PL, Sabri E, Rakhra K, et al. A multicenter randomized controlled trial comparing single-row with double-row fixation in arthroscopic rotator cuff repair. J Bone Joint Surg Am. 2012; 94(14):1249–1257

[9] Curtis AS, Burbank KM, Tierney JJ, Scheller AD, Curran AR. The insertional footprint of the rotator cuff: An anatomic study. Arthroscopy. 2006; 22(6):609.e1

[10] Mochizuki T, Sugaya H, Uomizu M, et al. Humeral insertion of the supraspinatus and infraspinatus. New anatomical findings regarding the footprint of the rotator cuff. J Bone Joint Surg Am. 2008; 90(5):962–969

[11] Davidson PA, Rivenburgh DW. Rotator cuff repair tension as a determinant of functional outcome. J Shoulder Elbow Surg. 2000; 9(6):502–506

[12] Hersche O, Gerber C. Passive tension in the supraspinatus musculotendinous unit after long-standing rupture of its tendon: A preliminary report. J Shoulder Elbow Surg. 1998; 7(4):393–396

[13] Jost PW, Khair MM, Chen DX, Wright TM, Kelly AM, Rodeo SA. Suture number determines strength of rotator cuff repair. J Bone Joint Surg Am. 2012; 94(14):e100

[14] Snyder S, Burns J. Rotator cuff healing and the bone marrow "crimson duvet." From clinical observations to science. Tech Shoulder Elbow Surg. 2009; 10:130–137

[15] Kida Y, Morihara T, Matsuda K, et al. Bone marrow-derived cells from the footprint infiltrate into the repaired rotator cuff. J Shoulder Elbow Surg. 2013; 22(2):197–205

[16] Milano G, Saccomanno MF, Careri S, Taccardo G, DeVitis R, Fabbriciani C. Efficacy of marrow-stimulating technique in arthroscopic rotator cuff repair: A prospective randomized study. Arthroscopy. 2013; 29(5): 802–810

3 Single-Row Undersurface All-Inside Rotator Cuff Repair

Ashleigh Elkins and George A.C. Murrell

Summary

We demonstrate an efficient approach to rotator cuff repair through a non-traditional intra-articular viewing approach. This undersurface technique is efficient, effective, and durable.

Keywords: single row, rotator cuff repair, all inside, undersurface

3.1 Patients Selected for Surgery

At our center, patients are referred for surgery if they have a symptomatic full thickness rotator cuff tear, or a partial thickness tear, which involves 50% or greater of the tendon's thickness. The dimensions and thickness of the tear are determined based on preoperative ultrasound results. The ultrasounds are performed by an experienced musculoskeletal sonographer.

3.2 Patient Positioning

Patients are placed into the beach chair position. Anesthesia is in the form of an interscalene block with light sedation.

3.3 Patient Preparation

- Prophylactic antibiotics are administered prior to the procedure.
- Drapes are applied across the patient's body.
- The shoulder, arm, and hand are prepared with an alcohol–iodine solution.
- A sterile drape sleeve is applied to the hand and forearm and secured with sterile bandaging.
- A sterile plastic drape is placed over the spider arm, and the forearm and hand are secured to the spider arm.
- Drapes are applied to cover the neck and torso regions.
- Iobans (3 M Australia, North Ryde, Australia) are applied over the shoulder region.

3.4 Posterior Portal Placement

- A sterile marking pen is used to mark the spine of the scapula, acromion, and acromioclavicular joint and the coracoid process.
- The posterolateral corner of the acromion is palpated and a line is drawn 1 cm inferior and 1 cm medial to this landmark.
- A scalpel is used (#11 blade) on the skin to create the posterior portal.
- The trocar is introduced, aimed toward the previously marked coracoid process.
- White balance is performed prior to introduction of the arthroscope.
- The arthroscope is introduced and the trocar is removed.

- Initial diagnostic arthroscopy is performed through this portal prior to the creation of the lateral portal (creation of this is described below).

3.5 Initial Diagnostic Shoulder Arthroscopy

- Via the posterior portal, initial diagnostic arthroscopy of the shoulder is performed (▶ **Fig. 3.1a**).
- The glenohumeral joint is inspected for concomitant shoulder pathologies.
- The glenoid labrum is evaluated for concomitant labral tears, including superior labrum anteroposterior tears, the glenoid and humeral head are inspected for bony Bankart lesions and Hill–Sachs lesions, the long head of biceps is evaluated for tears, and the capsule is assessed for evidence of adhesive capsulitis.
- Once the glenohumeral joint has been thoroughly assessed, the torn rotator cuff tendon is assessed from its undersurface.
- The head of the arthroscopic shaver is used as a reference point to measure the size of the tear, as there needs to be a minimum 5 mm defect in the supraspinatus tendon to permit passage of the shaver and sutures.

3.6 Creation of the Lateral Portal

- The position of the lateral portal is imperative to the success of the undersurface technique.
- The optimal position for the lateral portal for the undersurface technique is halfway between the anterior and posterior edges of the tear; this is so there is equal access to all aspects of the tendon.
- The position of the lateral portal is also important so that it allows the surgeon to place and deploy an anchor in the lateral part of the greater tuberosity (landing site).
- With the arthroscope remaining in the posterior portal, a spinal needle is inserted through the approximate position for the lateral portal, which is usually 1 cm inferior to the lateral margin of the acromion.
- The spinal needle is viewed using the arthroscope to determine whether the position is correct.
- The spinal needle needs to be angled in a way that sutures can be easily passed through the torn edges of the tendon, so that anchors can be placed perpendicular to the lateral margin of the supraspinatus footprint, and so that a shaver can debride the landing site.
- Once the appropriate position is identified with the spinal needle, a sterile surgical marker is used to mark the position of the portal and a #11 blade is used to create the portal. A cannula is not necessary when using the undersurface technique.
- The lateral portal is primarily used to insert the instruments necessary to perform the repair, as described below.

3.7 Preparation of the Tendon and Landing Site

- If the supraspinatus tear is of partial thickness, a #11 blade scalpel is introduced through the lateral portal and is used to convert the partial-thickness tear into a full-thickness tear.
- A 4.0- or 5.5-mm shaver (Stryker Endoscopy, San Jose, CA) is passed through the lateral portal and it is used to debride the torn edge of the tendon (▶ **Fig. 3.1b**). This is a light debridement as our aim is to retain the maximal amount of host tendon.

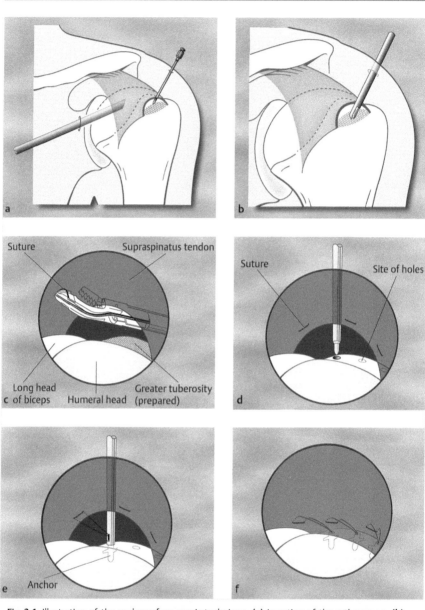

Fig. 3.1 Illustration of the undersurface repair technique. **(a)** Insertion of the arthroscope. **(b)** Preparation of the greater tuberosity landing site with an arthroscopic shaver. **(c)** Passing sutures through the edge of the torn tendon. **(d)** Use of a T-handled punch to prepare holes for the suture anchors. **(e)** Deployment of anchors into the holes on the greater tuberosity. **(f)** Completed repair with the torn tendon reattached to the greater tuberosity.

- After debridement of the tendon edge, the shaver is then used to debride the landing site of soft tissue. This process is also important for tendon-bone healing, as it induces bleeding.

3.8 Arthroscopic Suturing

- The Opus SmartStitch Suture Device (ArthroCare, Sydney, Australia) is used for suturing in the undersurface technique. This device assists placement of inverted mattress sutures.
- The SmartStitch Device is passed through the lateral portal. The edge of the torn tendon is grasped using the device and sutures are passed through the tendon (▶ **Fig. 3.1c**).
- If the tear is large enough to warrant a second suture, the second suture is usually placed posterior to the first suture.

3.9 Preparing and Deploying Suture Anchors

- A mallet is used to drive a T-handled punch into the landing site to create a hole for the suture anchor (▶ **Fig. 3.1d**).
- If more than one anchor is required to complete the repair, the first anchor site is placed laterally on the landing site and subsequent holes are created posteriorly, and often, more medially.
- After the creation of the holes for the anchors, sutures are then passed through the anchors (Opus Magnum, ArthroCare), which are then inserted into the holes (▶ **Fig. 3.1e**).
- The sutures are then tightened using the TensionLock winding mechanism on the Opus gun.
- The first suture is not tightened completely to allow for more room to visualize the insertion site for the second anchor. An early issue with the technique arose when the first suture was completely tightened, which made visualization of the next anchor difficult, and sometimes required conversion to a bursal-sided technique.
- Once all suture anchors are deployed, the sutures are tightened (▶ **Video 3.1**).

3.10 Closing

- Prior to closing the portals, the integrity of the repair is assessed arthroscopically by viewing the torn tendon from the undersurface while gently manipulating the arm (▶ **Fig. 3.1f**).

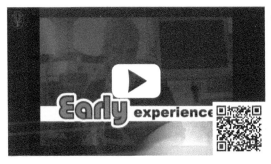

Video 3.1 Introduction and Rationale for the single-row undersurface all-inside rotator cuff repair.

- The arthroscope is removed, and the portals are closed using interrupted nylon sutures and Steri strips.
- Dressings are applied to the shoulder and the operated arm is placed in a sling with an abduction pillow (UltraSling, DJO Global, Dallas, TX).

3.11 Rehabilitation

- All patients who undergo an undersurface rotator cuff repair undergo a standardized rehabilitation protocol in the first 6 months postsurgery.
- Overhead activities are not permitted in the first 3 months postsurgery except for performing the prescribed exercises.
- The week prior to surgery, all patients attend a group education session conducted by a physiotherapist.
- For the first 6 weeks postsurgery, patients are instructed to wear a sling with a small abduction pillow to help reduce the tension on the repair.
- The rehabilitation protocol in the first 6 weeks consists of a number of gentle, passive range-of-motion exercises, including elbow flexion and extension range-of-motion exercises, grip-strengthening exercises, scapula-strengthening exercises, and pendulum exercises. No lifting is permitted in the first 6 weeks following surgery.
- From day 8 postoperatively, stick exercises are introduced to help improve range of motion in external and internal rotation, and shoulder flexion and extension.
- After the first 6 weeks, the patients are then reviewed by a physical therapist who then initiates isometric strengthening exercises in flexion, extension, adduction, and external rotation. Some further range-of-motion exercises are added, including flexion stretches using a wall, active supported external rotation, and towel stretches. At this stage, patients are permitted to lift up to 1 kg to chest height.
- The patients then undergo a review by the same physical therapist at 3 months postsurgery. At this stage, patients are permitted to perform overhead activities of less than 15 minutes duration. Active resistance exercises are introduced at this stage, which utilize therabands and light weights. Patients are permitted to lift between 2 and 5 kg.

3.12 Six-Month Review

- At 6 months, the patients are again reviewed by the surgeon. A comprehensive physical examination is performed to assess strength and range of motion.
- Patients also complete the L'Insalata questionnaire to determine patient-rated functionality and pain associated with the shoulder.
- An experienced musculoskeletal sonographer performs an ultrasound assessment to determine the integrity of the repair.
- If the repair is found to be intact on this assessment, the patient is usually encouraged to return to their pre-injury duties and activities.

3.13 Rationale for the Technique

- Rotator cuff tears are a common cause of shoulder pain and dysfunction, and re-tear is a common complication of rotator cuff repair.
- Most arthroscopic repair techniques include initial diagnostic arthroscopy of the glenohumeral joint to identify the torn rotator cuff and other concomitant shoulder pathologies. In standard rotator cuff repair techniques, the arthroscope

is then repositioned in the subacromial space, and the tendon is approached from its bursal surface. This requires dissection or removal of the subacromial bursa to visualize the torn tendon and, often, concomitant acromioplasty. Because of the presence of the subacromial bursa, it can be difficult to visualize the torn tendon.

- Acromioplasty has long been performed routinely with rotator cuff repair. This is related to the theory of extrinsic subacromial impingement, which links the anatomical shape of the acromion to impingement and compression from the bursal side leading to abrasion and tearing of the rotator cuff. Recent studies suggest that there is little, if any, clinical benefit to performing an acromioplasty concurrently with rotator cuff repair; and performing an acromioplasty induces bleeding, which can further impair visualization.

- All arthroscopic rotator cuff repair methods are technically demanding, which is a key drawback. The technical difficulty of many arthroscopic repair methods is reflected by their long surgical duration. In 2006, rotator cuff repair had the longest operative time of all upper limb day procedures performed in the United States, at 73 minutes. Reported mean operative time for arthroscopic repair techniques range from 32 minutes to 113 minutes. Longer operating times are associated with higher economic costs, and potentially adverse clinical outcomes. Long operative times may be associated with infection and thromboembolic complications, and as suggested by some studies, possible increased risk of re-tear.

- Given these limitations of standard rotator cuff repair techniques, in 2008 we described an arthroscopic rotator cuff repair technique in which the entire repair was performed from within the glenohumeral joint. The torn tendon was repaired using a single row, tension band inverted mattress suture technique using knotless Opus Magnum suture anchors (ArthroCare). The technique utilizes advances in arthroscopic suture devices, such as the Opus SmartStitch Device and the Perfect Passer System (ArthroCare). These devices allow the surgeon to deploy sutures through the edge of the torn tendon in an inverted mattress configuration. The technique could be carried out while visualizing the tear from within the glenohumeral joint, without the need to perform an acromioplasty or dissect the subacromial bursa.

- Biomechanical studies of the undersurface repair technique showed that the technique produced good repair strength and good footprint compression.

- Our preliminary results in small cohorts of patients with this technique has been promising, with a markedly reduced operative time compared to the bursal-sided technique, and lower re-tear rates achieved with the technique (▶ Video 3.2).

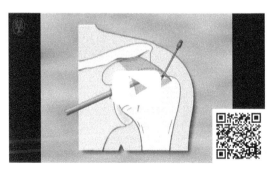

Video 3.2 Demonstration of complete technique for the single-row undersurface all-inside rotator cuff repair.

3.14 Advantages of the Technique

- One of the key advantages of the undersurface technique compared to other techniques that approach the torn tendon from the bursal surface is its fast operative time. Results from a recent study of 1,000 cases found that the mean operative time for the undersurface technique is 16 minutes (unpublished data). Previous studies from our institute have shown that, on average, undersurface repairs are between 12 and 32 minutes faster to perform than bursal-sided repairs when using the same suture anchors. The reason why the undersurface repair is faster is because there is no need to perform a bursectomy or acromioplasty. Subacromial bursectomy and acromioplasty are time-consuming procedures. They also induce bleeding, which impairs visualization of the torn tendon and other structures within the glenohumeral joint. Shorter operative times are beneficial from an economic perspective as they result in lower operating room costs (▶ **Video 3.3**).
- Viewing from beneath the rotator cuff is also beneficial because it prevents inadvertent suturing of the long head of the biceps tendon, which may occur if viewing the rotator cuff tendon from its bursal surface.
- The re-tear rate for patients who have undergone an undersurface rotator cuff repair is low. A recent study performed at our institution analyzed 1,000 patients who underwent an undersurface repair, which revealed a re-tear rate of 8.5% (unpublished data). This is favorable given that re-tear rates quoted in the literature range between 15% and 90%. The re-tear rate for the undersurface repair is lower than the re-tear rate for the bursal-sided technique, with a study at our institution finding that the re-tear rate for the bursal-sided repair was 21%.
- Visualization of the torn tendon is optimized by the undersurface technique. Approaching the tendon from within the glenohumeral joint allows for greater visualization of the torn tendon and other shoulder structures, such as the long head of biceps tendon, the labrum, and the capsule, as the view is not obscured by the subacromial bursa.
- The undersurface technique is also relatively easy to perform. It is fairly easy to debride the tendon edge and the landing site with the arthroscope remaining in the glenohumeral joint and passing the arthroscopic shaver through a lateral portal. With the development of advanced suture-passing devices, such as the Opus Magnum SmartStitch Device and the Perfect Passer System (both from ArthroCare), it is also relatively straightforward to pass sutures through the edge of the torn tendon in an inverted mattress configuration. This suture configuration compresses the tendon onto the landing site in a tension band configuration and a greater time zero strength compared with simple sutures.

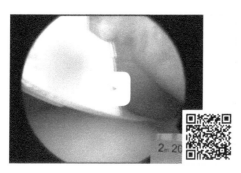

Video 3.3 Unedited 4-minute repair using the single-row undersurface all-inside technique.

- There is no need to perform an acromioplasty or subacromial decompression when the undersurface technique is performed. Although traditionally performed concomitantly with rotator cuff repair, recent evidence suggests that acromioplasty confers no additional benefit to the management of rotator cuff disease. Gartsman and O'Connor performed a randomized control trial comparing a group of patients that underwent only rotator cuff repair, and a second group that underwent rotator cuff repair and subacromial decompression. At 1-year follow-up, there was no difference in the American Shoulder and Elbow Surgeon's score between the two groups. A meta-analysis found no statistically significant difference between patients undergoing isolated rotator cuff repair and those who undergo concomitant rotator cuff repair and subacromial decompression with respect to functional outcomes and rates of reoperation. However, acromioplasty may still be indicated in the management of patients with a type 3 acromion.
- Patient-reported outcomes following undersurface rotator cuff repair have also been promising. Patients have reported a reduced frequency and magnitude of shoulder pain, improvement in shoulder stiffness, improvement in overhead activities, as well as improved shoulder function at 6 months postsurgery. In this study, these parameters also demonstrated similar improvements in patients who underwent bursal-sided repairs. The key difference in terms of self-reported outcomes between the bursal-sided and undersurface repair groups were that patients who underwent bursal-sided repairs had more frequent pain during activity and more difficulty reaching behind the back than patients who underwent undersurface repair.

3.15 Disadvantages

- The main disadvantage of the undersurface rotator cuff repair technique is that occasionally it is necessary to complete the repair from the bursal side of the tendon. This is because it can be difficult to visualize the tendon landing site during placement of the final suture anchors toward the end of the repair. This is particularly a problem for larger tears requiring more suture anchors.
- With increasing experience with the technique, we have developed a method to avoid conversion to a bursal-sided repair. For larger tears, we often do not completely tighten the first anchor prior to deployment of the second anchor. The first anchor is subsequently tightened at the end of the repair. Subjectively, this has reduced the number of cases in which conversion to a bursal-sided repair is required. The main disadvantage of converting to a bursal-sided repair is inconvenience.
- The undersurface technique does not allow double-row fixation.
- Initially, we had concerns about the level of footprint contact achieved with the undersurface technique, especially with the arm in the abducted position. A biomechanical study of the technique demonstrated that there was good contact pressure at the footprint and that there was good repair strength.

3.16 Conclusion

The all-inside undersurface arthroscopic rotator cuff repair technique is a novel, fast, safe, and effective surgical technique that has produced promising results with respect to both surgical duration and the re-tear rate.

Suggested Readings

Cummins CA, Murrell GA. Mode of failure for rotator cuff repair with suture anchors identified at revision surgery. J Shoulder Elbow Surg. 2003; 12(2):128–133

Fehringer EV, Sun J, VanOeveren LS, Keller BK, Matsen FA, III. Full-thickness rotator cuff tear prevalence and correlation with function and co-morbidities in patients sixty-five years and older. J Shoulder Elbow Surg. 2008; 17(6): 881–885

Le BTN, Wu XL, Lam, PH, Murrell GAC. Factors predicting rotator cuff retears: An analysis of 1000 consecutive rotator cuff repairs. Am J Sports Med. 2014; 42(5):1134–1142

Matsen FA, III. Clinical practice. Rotator-cuff failure. N Engl J Med. 2008; 358(20):2138–2147

Walton JR, Murrell GAC. A two-year clinical outcomes study of 400 patients, comparing open surgery and arthroscopy for rotator cuff repair. Bone Joint Res. 2012; 1(9):210–217

Millar NL, Wu X, Tantau R, Silverstone E, Murrell GA. Open versus two forms of arthroscopic rotator cuff repair. Clin Orthop Relat Res. 2009; 467(4):966–978

Murrell GAC. Advances in rotator cuff repair - Undersurface repair. Tech Shoulder Elbow Surg. 2012; 13(1):28–31

Singh C, Lam PH, Murrell GAC. Is acromioplasty of benefit for rotator cuff repair? Tech Shoulder Elbow Surg. 2015; 16(1):32–37

Wu XL, Baldwick C, Briggs L, Murrell GAC. Arthroscopic undersurface rotator cuff repair. Tech Shoulder Elbow Surg. 2009; 10(3):112–118

Gartsman GM, O'Connor DP. Arthroscopic rotator cuff repair with and without arthroscopic subacromial decompression: A prospective, randomized study of one-year outcomes. J Shoulder Elbow Surg. 2004; 13(4):424–426

Milano G, Grasso A, Salvatore M, Zarelli D, Deriu L, Fabbriciani C. Arthroscopic rotator cuff repair with and without subacromial decompression: A prospective randomized study. Arthroscopy. 2007; 23(1):81–88

Mac Donald P, McRae S, Leiter J, Mascarenhas R, Lapner P. Arthroscopic rotator cuff repair with and without acromioplasty in the treatment of full-thickness rotator cuff tears: A multicenter, randomized controlled trial. J Bone Joint Surg Am. 2011; 93(21):1953–1960

Shin SJ, Oh JH, Chung SW, Song MH. The efficacy of acromioplasty in the arthroscopic repair of small- to medium-sized rotator cuff tears without acromial spur: Prospective comparative study. Arthroscopy. 2012; 28(5):628–635

Abrams GD, Gupta AK, Hussey KE, et al. Arthroscopic repair of full-thickness rotator cuff tears with and without acromioplasty: Randomized prospective trial with 2-year follow-up. Am J Sports Med. 2014; 42(6):1296–1303

Chahal J, Mall N, MacDonald PB, et al. The role of subacromial decompression in patients undergoing arthroscopic repair of full-thickness tears of the rotator cuff: A systematic review and meta-analysis. Arthroscopy. 2012; 28 (5):720–727

Jain NB, Higgins LD, Losina E, Collins J, Blazar, PE, Katz JN. Epidemiology of musculoskeletal upper extremity ambulatory surgery in the United States. BMC Musculoskelet Disord. 2014; 15(4):4

Churchill RS, Ghorai JK. Total cost and operating room time comparison of rotator cuff repair techniques at low, intermediate, and high volume centers: Mini-open versus all-arthroscopic. J Shoulder Elbow Surg. 2010; 19(5): 716–721

Walton JR, Murrell GA. Effects of operative time on outcomes of rotator cuff repair. Tech Should Surg. 2012; 13(1): 23–27

Rubenis I, Lam PH, Murrell GA. Arthroscopic rotator cuff repair using the undersurface technique: A 2-year comparative study in 257 patients. Orthop J Sports Med. 2015; 3(10):2325967115605801

Andres BM, Lam PH, Murrell GA. Tension, abduction, and surgical technique affect footprint compression after rotator cuff repair in an ovine model. J Shoulder Elbow Surg. 2010; 19(7):1018–1027

Frank JM, Chahal J, Frank RM, Cole BJ, Verma NN, Romeo AA. The role of acromioplasty for rotator cuff problems. Orthop Clin North Am. 2014; 45(2):219–224

4 Double-Row Repair with Biceps Tendon Augmentation

Jeffrey S. Abrams and Tertuliano Vieira

Summary

Double-row repair techniques to address rotator cuff tears have increased the healing rate to the greater tuberosity. The biceps tendon is considered a pain generator when rotator cuff tears extend toward the rotator interval, and tenodesis or tenotomy has been popularized. Attempts at improving greater tuberosity coverage are often made at the expense of muscular tendinous tension, placing this functional unit at risk. Incorporating the long head of the biceps into the repair can graft the injured tendon with autogenous tissue, and reduce risk of postoperative pain emanating from the biceps because of tenodesis. The authors will demonstrate a technique that will assist the biological healing of the rotator cuff retracted tear and combine biceps tenodesis to augment the cuff repair.

Keywords: biceps augmentation cuff repair, biceps tenodesis, grafts, rotator cuff tears

4.1 Examination under Anesthesia

- Supine patient with passive shoulder motion evaluated in flexion, abducted external rotation, and abducted internal rotation.
- Any restriction as a result of soft tissue adhesions is gently manipulated to create a full range of motion prior to surgical repair.

4.2 Positioning

- Can be performed in lateral decubitus or beach chair.
- Appropriate padding of pelvis and lower extremities.
- Protective support to head and neck to neutralize cervical positioning.

4.3 Portal Placement

- Standard posterior viewing portal, 2 cm lateral to the junction of the spine of the scapula and posterior acromion edge.
- Anterior portal inferior to the acromioclavicular joint.
- Lateral portal 3 cm lateral to the edge of the acromion.
- Accessory portals for suture anchor placement along the margin of the anterior acromion and midlateral margin.

4.4 Surgical Technique

- Articular exam, debridement, and capsulotomy of posterior and inferior capsule adjacent to the labrum.

- Evaluate tear margins and delaminations using anterior and posterior articular viewing portals.[1,2]
- Bursectomy to develop anterior, lateral, and posterior margins, and define margins of the rotator cuff tear.
- Subacromial decompression using both posterior and lateral viewing portals. Additional clavicle spur excision is performed when prominent.
- Prepare greater tuberosity with soft tissue debridement.
- Suture anchor placement. Triple-loaded anchor placed approximately 1 cm posterior to the biceps tendon, adjacent to the medial margin of the greater tuberosity (▶ **Fig. 4.1**).[3]
- Suture the leading margin of the supraspinatus with a mattress suture. Followed by a more medial simple suture (▶ **Fig. 4.1**).
- Coracohumeral ligament release to lateral margin of the coracoid provides additional flexibility in mobilizing the anterior retracted tear.
- Posterior suture anchor placed on the greater tuberosity adjacent to the posterior tear margin (▶ **Fig. 4.2**).[4,5]
- Posterior sutures retrieved through the posterior cuff as mattress sutures repairing delaminations and reconstructing the posterior cable (▶ **Fig. 4.2**).
- Posterior mattress sutures are tied first but are not cut and are retrieved out of the insertion portal to help manage sutures.
- Biceps tendon is viewed from the posterior articular portal.
- The rotator interval is opened lateral to the coracoacromial ligament and a suture is placed through biceps and retrieved out through the anterior portal. The biceps are tenotomized adjacent to the labrum junction and retrieved through the anterior window (▶ **Fig. 4.3**).
- Remove bursal tissue to permit a clear pathway for the biceps.
- Tie anterior rotator cuff sutures, mattress first, then simple suture.
- Use the third stitch from the anchor and place one arm through the biceps stump approximately 2 cm from the cut edge.

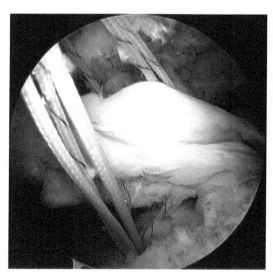

Fig. 4.1 Anterior suture anchor and suture placement. Anchor is located 1 cm posterior to the biceps tendon and sutures passed with mattress and crossing simple suture configuration.

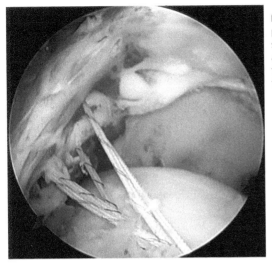

Fig. 4.2 Posterior suture anchor is placed at the supraspinatus–infraspinatus junction. Sutures retrieved as mattress sutures to allow repositioning of the multiple layers of tendon.

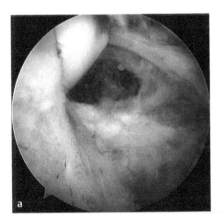
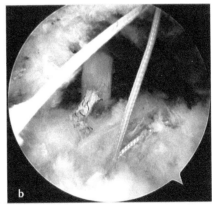

Fig. 4.3 The tenotomized biceps tendon is retrieved through an opening in the rotator interval and pulled into the subdeltoid space. A traction stitch is clamped to avoid retraction. **(a)** Articular view of divided biceps exiting through the opened interval. **(b)** Bursal view of biceps positioned and retracted with subdeltoid bursae.

- As the biceps suture is tied, gentle partial release of traction suture will permit biceps to wrap over the anterior supraspinatus margin (▶ **Fig. 4.4**).
- The free edge of the biceps can be directed posterior, medial, or obliquely to reinforce thin tissue. The previously placed biceps suture is used to pierce the posterior cuff, and the suture is retrieved and tied (▶ **Fig. 4.5**).
- If the supraspinatus stump is unable to reach greater tuberosity, it can be sewn to the traversing biceps tendon.
- A set of posterior mattress sutures, combined with supraspinatus biceps sutures, can be combined to a knotless anchor for additional reinforcement (▶ **Fig. 4.6**, ▶ **Video 4.1**).

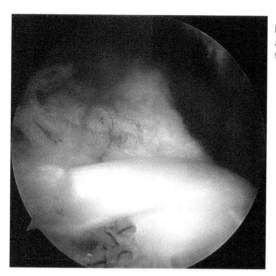

Fig. 4.4 The biceps are fixed to the anterior suture anchor, overlapping the anterior repair.

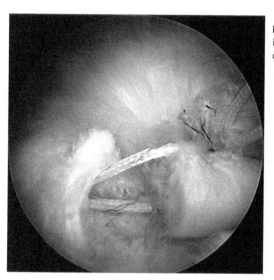

Fig. 4.5 The free edge of the biceps is sewn into the infraspinatus tendon using the biceps sutures.

4.5 Surgical Benefits

- Anterior reinforcement of supraspinatus attachment with overlapping biceps tendon[6] will maximize the strength of the anterior rotator cuff cable attachment.[7]
- Biceps tenodesis to the suture anchor removes the articular portion of the biceps and stabilizes the biceps above the groove.
- Supraspinatus tendon extension using biceps as a graft. Creating additional fixation for humeral head coverage will help stabilize the glenohumeral joint and reduce superior migration.[8,9]

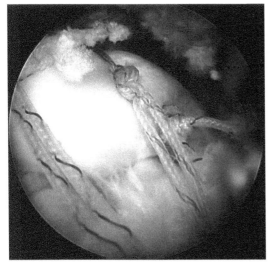

Fig. 4.6 A midanchor can be added to reinforce the posterior sutures creating a double row. Biceps and supraspinatus crescent sutures are secured covering the greater tuberosity footprint.

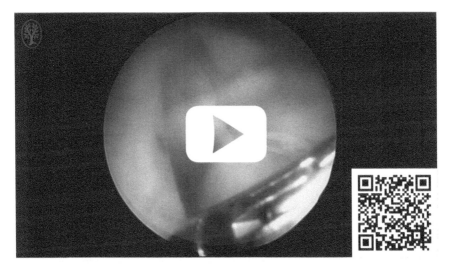

Video 4.1 Demonstration of a rotator cuff tear with additional strain on the supraspinatus portion of the repair and repair with our described augmentation technique. The tenotomized biceps tendon can be used as a bridge to increase the greater tuberosity coverage and reduce the tension of the repair. The anterior portion of the repair is reinforced with the anchor tenodesis and the posterior cable is reinforced with the free edge of the biceps fixed to the infraspinatus. The posterior unit is further secured with a double row transosseous equivalent fixation.

- Posterior cuff reinforcement with delamination repair to suture the anchor and biceps cable attachment provides stability to the posterior cable and creates an extra articular suspension bridge.[10]
- Add collagen to assist humeral head depression and spacing below the acromion.[11]

4.6 Avoid Pitfalls and Complications

- Loss of biceps fixation during retrieval and suture anchor fixation. Careful partial release of traction on the suture holding the cut biceps tendon allows for repositioning of this tendon on top of the biceps.
- Anterior adhesions can be created if biceps passage captures tissue during the passage out of the articular region. The tendon is passed lateral, not through the coracoacromial ligament.
- Biceps should reach to the infraspinatus–supraspinatus junction posteriorly to benefit this area if reinforcement is desired.
- Supraspinatus leading edge closure after release of coracohumeral ligament from the posterior margin of the coracoid.
- Subscapularis tears and repairs performed prior to the posterosuperior repair.

4.7 Rehabilitation

- Standard protection with neutralized brace. Add a 4-inch Ace wrap to support the biceps muscular area for comfort.
- Early pendulum exercises, biceps flexion, and extension.
- Assisted external shoulder rotation at 1 week.
- Table slides beginning at 1 week.
- Sling removal and supine assist elevation after 5 weeks. Increase assisted external rotation.
- Independent active elevation and begin resistive exercises between 8 and 12 weeks.

4.8 Rationale and Benefits

- Autogenous tissue graft to thicken compromised thin tendon repair.[11]
- Biceps tenodesis to reduce risk of continued or new pain.[3]
- Recreated extraarticular rotator cuff cable with reinforced anterior and posterior fixation.[10]
- Lower expense because of autogenous tissue graft and reduced number of suture anchors.
- Tendon extension with added collagen from the graft, creating additional coverage of greater tuberosity and improved healing.[7,9,11]

References

[1] Gartsman GM, Drake G, Edwards TB, et al. Ultrasound evaluation of arthroscopic full-thickness supraspinatus rotator cuff repair: Single-row versus double-row suture bridge (transosseous equivalent) fixation. Results of a prospective, randomized study. J Shoulder Elbow Surg. 2013; 22(11):1480–1487

[2] Lapner PL, Sabri E, Rakhra K, et al. A multicenter randomized controlled trial comparing single-row with double-row fixation in arthroscopic rotator cuff repair. J Bone Joint Surg Am. 2012; 94(14):1249–1257

[3] Checchia SL, Doneux PS, Miyazaki AN, et al. Biceps tenodesis associated with arthroscopic repair of rotator cuff tears. J Shoulder Elbow Surg. 2005; 14(2):138–144

[4] Gimbel JA, VanKleunen JP, Lake SP, Williams GR, Soslowsky LJ. The role of repair tension on tendon to bone healing in an animal model of chronic rotator cuff tears. J Biomech. 2007; 40(3):561–568

[5] Barber FA, Herbert MA, Coons DA. Tendon augmentation grafts: Biomechanical failure loads and failure patterns. Arthroscopy. 2006; 22(5):534–538

[6] Castagna A, Conti M, Mouhsine E, Bungaro P, Garofalo R. Arthroscopic biceps tendon tenodesis: The anchorage technical note. Knee Surg Sports Traumatol Arthrosc. 2006; 14(6):581–585

[7] Abrams JS. Biceps tenodesis augmenting repair. In: Gumina S, ed. Rotator Cuff Tear: Pathogenesis Evaluation and Treatment. Rome, Italy: Springer;2017:339–344

[8] Mihata T, Mc Garry MH, Pirolo JM, Kinoshita M, Lee TQ. Superior capsule reconstruction to restore superior stability in irreparable rotator cuff tears: A biomechanical cadaveric study. Am J Sports Med. 2012; 40(10):2248–2255

[9] Mihata T, Lee TQ, Watanabe C, et al. Clinical results of arthroscopic superior capsule reconstruction for irreparable rotator cuff tears. Arthroscopy. 2013; 29(3):459–470

[10] Burkhart SS, Esch JC, Jolson RS. The rotator crescent and rotator cable: An anatomic description of the shoulder's "suspension bridge." Arthroscopy. 1993; 9(6):611–616

[11] Barber FA, Burns JP, Deutsch A, Labbé MR, Litchfield RB. A prospective, randomized evaluation of acellular human dermal matrix augmentation for arthroscopic rotator cuff repair. Arthroscopy. 2012; 28(1):8–15

5 Double Row with "Rip-Stop" Rotator Cuff Repair

Mark R. Wilson, Eric D. Field, and Larry D. Field

Summary

Double-row repairs as well as rip-stop configurations have been proposed to limit failures found after arthroscopic rotator cuff repairs. A type II rotator cuff repair failure is encountered when the rotator cuff tendon detaches from the medial fixation row, which is often located at the musculotendinous junction. Rip-stop techniques have been shown to effectively reduce suture tendon pullout when compared to traditional transosseous double-row repairs in biomechanical studies. If an additional horizontal "rip-stop" suture can be added to previously described techniques designed to restore a secure tendon–bone interface, a higher incidence of rotator cuff healing can potentially be achieved. This technique is commonly employed by the authors to secure rotator cuff tears and allows not only for double-row fixation but also an interlocking double-row suture construct that improves security and fixation strength.

Keywords: double-row repair, interlocking double-row suture construct, rip-stop, rotator cuff repair, suture tendon pullout

5.1 Patient Positioning

Beach chair or lateral decubitus positions are both acceptable.

5.2 Portal Placement

- Standard posterior portal placed initially for diagnostic arthroscopic evaluation.
- Anterior and lateral portals placed for working portals.
- Anterolateral and posterolateral subacromial accessory portals as needed.

5.3 Surgical Technique

- The surgical technique described is indicated for large, multitendon tears with adequate rotator cuff tendon mobility to allow for near anatomic reduction to the tuberosity footprint (▶ **Fig. 5.1**, ▶ **Fig. 5.2**).
- With the patient positioned in the beach chair position and following induction of anesthesia, the operative arm is prepped and draped in sterile fashion.
- A diagnostic arthroscopy using a 30° arthroscope is performed using a standard posterior portal.
- In the video provided (▶ **Video 5.1**), a partial subscapularis tendon tear is identified and repaired prior to introduction of the arthroscope into the subacromial space. Once all glenohumeral joint pathology is adequately addressed, the arthroscope is introduced into the subacromial space.
- In the video provided (▶ **Video 5.1**), one can see a large tear involving both the supraspinatus and infraspinatus tendons being reduced with aid of a grasper to their respective bony attachments prior to anchor placement.

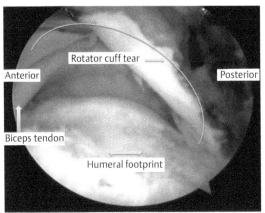

Fig. 5.1 A tear involving the rotator cuff can be seen from the lateral portal in a left shoulder in the beach chair position. Biceps tendon is in view anteriorly. The rotator tendon is elevated using a grasper showing the humeral footprint insertion.

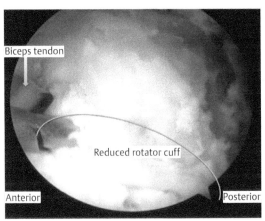

Fig. 5.2 The rotator cuff tear is reduced using a grasper as seen from the lateral portal in a left shoulder with beach chair positioning. The grasper seen is inserted using an accessory anterolateral portal. The biceps tendon may be seen crossing through the biceps interval.

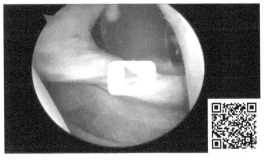

Video 5.1 Surgical demonstration of a double row with "Rip-Stop" Rotator Cuff Repair.

- Using the described technique, two double-loaded biocomposite anchors (Healicoil Regenesorb 5.5 mm, Smith & Nephew, Andover, MA) are placed at the most medial aspect of the rotator cuff footprint adjacent to the humeral head articular cartilage.
- As seen in the video and viewed through the lateral portal, each limb of alternating sutures from the anterior double-loaded anchor is passed through the rotator cuff

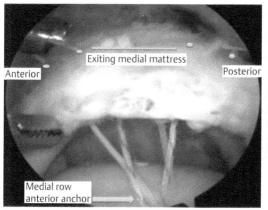

Fig. 5.3 The first anchor of two medial row anchors is viewed from the lateral portal in a left shoulder in the beach chair position. All four sutures have been passed in a horizontal mattress configuration through the cuff tissue. A grasper can be seen positioned through an accessory anterolateral portal, and an outflow cannula is positioned in the anterior portal.

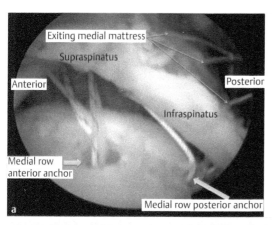

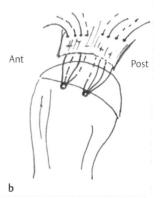

Fig. 5.4 **(a)** Two medial row anchors can be seen from the lateral portal in a left shoulder in the beach chair position. The four exiting suture limbs are marked with arrows passing through the tendon of the infraspinatus in horizontal mattress configuration. **(b)** An illustration of a left shoulder during the first step of the double-row, rip-stop technique includes the passing of two double-loaded medial anchors in the horizontal mattress configuration.

tendon in a horizontal mattress configuration (▶ **Fig. 5.3**) using a 60° retrograde suture passer through the anterior portal (IDEAL Suture Grasper, Mitek Sports Medicine, DePuy Synthes, Raynham, MA).

- The posterior anchor sutures are then passed and retrieved in a similar fashion, utilizing a posterior portal (▶ **Fig. 5.4a**). Of note, it is advisable that these sutures broadly incorporate all detached rotator cuff tissue to maximize the tendon–bone interface during the subsequent steps (▶ **Fig. 5.4b**).
- Once all medial row sutures have been passed, a third triple-loaded anchor (Healicoil Regenesorb) is placed into the lateral border of the greater tuberosity footprint. As seen in the video provided (▶ **Video 5.1**) and viewed through the lateral portal, each of the three lateral row sutures are passed and retrieved in a simple orientation medial to the medial row horizontal mattress sutures (▶ **Fig. 5.5a**).

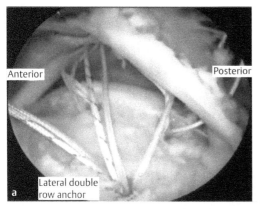
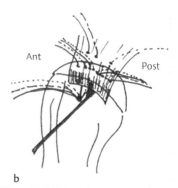

Fig. 5.5 **(a)** As viewed from the lateral portal in a left shoulder in the beach chair position, three limbs of each suture from the lateral row triple-loaded anchor have been passed through the cuff tissue medial to the rip-stop horizontal mattress sutures from both medial row anchors. A grasper is utilized through an accessory anterolateral portal to manipulate the rotator cuff tissue. **(b)** An illustration of a left shoulder during the second step of the double-row, rip-stop technique includes passing lateral double-row anchor sutures in simple fashion medial to horizontal mattress suture configuration of the medial anchors. A grasper is illustrated and is used to manipulate the rotator cuff tissue.

- ▶ **Fig. 5.5**b illustrates utilization of a grasper during this step to lateralize the rotator cuff tissue and facilitate placement of lateral row sutures.
- Following placement of all sutures, the medial row horizontal mattress sutures are securely tied prior to tying the lateral row anchor sutures so that the medial row sutures act as a "rip-stop" for these lateral row sutures and thus effectively increasing the strength of this double-row configuration (▶ **Fig. 5.6**).
- In the video provided, all lateral row sutures are tied in sequential order, creating the double-row repair (▶ **Fig. 5.7**a, b).
- After final arthroscopic photos are taken, a sterile dressing is applied, and the patient is placed in a shoulder abduction brace (▶ **Video 5.1**).

5.4 Surgeon Tips and Tricks

- Use the lateral or accessory lateral subacromial portal for visualization using the arthroscope. Visualizing from a lateral access site maximizes the opportunity to recognize the rotator cuff tear pattern and reducibility as well as better identify and incorporate lamination of rotator cuff tissue into the repair.
- Adequate mobilization of the rotator cuff tissue prior to anchor placement allows for better planning of medial and lateral row placement and reduces tension on this double-row repair construct and rotator cuff tissue.
- A grasper can be used through an accessory lateral portal to thoroughly assess the most anatomic and desirable position to reduce the rotator cuff to the tuberosity with the most appropriate degree of repair tension.

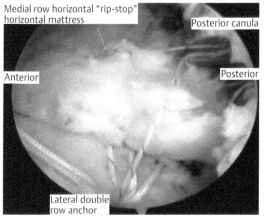

Fig. 5.6 As viewed from the lateral portal in a left shoulder in the beach chair position, three limbs of each suture from the lateral row triple-loaded anchor have been passed through the cuff tissue medial to the rip-stop horizontal mattress sutures from both medial row anchors. A medial row rip-stop suture is seen tied, reducing the rotator cuff tissue. A posterior cannula is seen with the one of the three limbs from the lateral anchor.

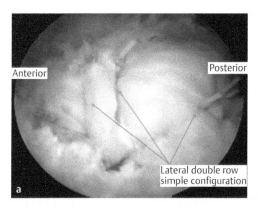

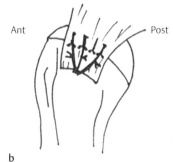

Fig. 5.7 **(a)** The double-row, rip-stop configuration as seen from the lateral portal in a left shoulder in the beach chair position. Note all three simple sutures of the lateral row anchor have been tied after securely tying the more medial rip-stop sutures. **(b)** An illustration of a left shoulder after the third step of the double-row, rip-stop technique includes the final construct.

- Place medial row anchors close to the articular edge as this represents the most medial aspect of the rotator cuff footprint.
- Pass all sutures from medial and lateral row anchors before tying any sutures.

5.5 Pitfalls/Complications

- Poor suture management makes rotator cuff repair more difficult; consider using a retrograde suture retriever advanced through the anterior and posterior portals for the sake of efficiency and to potentially improve the location of the sutures as they are retrieved through the rotator cuff tissue. Retrieving sutures from either of these two portal site locations allows for the arthroscope to be positioned in a lateral subacromial portal thus improving visualization of the rotator cuff tissue while retrieving and tying sutures.

5.6 Rehabilitation

- All patients undergo a formal postoperative therapy regimen consisting of 4–6 weeks of immobilization followed by passive and active assisted range-of-motion protocol for 4–6 weeks.
- By weeks 10–12, patients are placed in a strengthening program, and immobilization is discontinued.

5.7 Rationale and/or Evidence for Approach

- Rip-stop techniques have been shown to adequately reduce suture tendon pullout when compared to traditional transosseous double-row repairs in biomechanical studies.[1,2]
- Data also suggest that the rip-stop technique reduces cinching found with more complicated stitch patterns while reducing the risk of suture cutout.[3]
- Finally, investigators have demonstrated that tendon anchor gapping is best reduced with multiple anchors in a double-row configuration.[4,5]

References

[1] Lee BG, Cho NS, Rhee YG. Modified Mason–Allen suture bridge technique: A new suture bridge technique with improved tissue holding by the modified Mason–Allen stitch. Clin Orthop Surg. 2012; 4(3):242–245

[2] Barber FA, Herbert MA, Schroeder FA, Aziz-Jacobo J, Mays MM, Rapley JH. Biomechanical advantages of triple-loaded suture anchors compared with double-row rotator cuff repairs. Arthroscopy. 2010; 26(3):316–323

[3] Denard PJ, Burkhart SS. A load-sharing rip-stop fixation construct for arthroscopic rotator cuff repair. Arthrosc Tech. 2012; 1(1):e37–e42

[4] Kim DH, Elattrache NS, Tibone JE, et al. Biomechanical comparison of a single-row versus double-row suture anchor technique for rotator cuff repair. Am J Sports Med. 2006; 34(3):407–414

[5] Ma CB, Comerford L, Wilson J, Puttlitz CM. Biomechanical evaluation of arthroscopic rotator cuff repairs: Double-row compared with single-row fixation. J Bone Joint Surg Am. 2006; 88(2):403–410

6 SpeedBridge Repair of Massive Rotator Cuff Tears Using Provisional Traction Suture Reducing Anchor and Bioinductive Bovine Augment Patch

Hithem Rahmi, Sevag Bastian, and John Itamura

Summary

Massive rotator cuff tears can be a challenge to repair and to heal. Factors that play into whether a massive tear is repairable or not include the degree of mobilization to return the tendon to the footprint, tissue quality, and size of the tear. We propose basic tendon releases and the use of multiple traction sutures placed in the tendon in a luggage tag fashion for increased mobilization of the tendon. The traction sutures placed at the anterior leading edge of the supraspinatus tendon are then placed into an anchor laterally for provisional reduction of the anterior leading edge of the tear. This subsequently reduces the size of the tear to be repaired and a simple double-row SpeedBridge technique is then applied posterior to the reducing anchor allowing for a more tension-free repair. A bioinductive bovine augment patch is arthroscopically placed to aid in enhanced healing of tendon to bone.

Keywords: bioinductive, bovine patch, double-row repair, massive rotator cuff tear, tendon healing

6.1 Positioning

6.1.1 Lateral Decubitus Position

- The patient is placed in the lateral decubitus position.
- A sandbag is used to aid in positioning.
- Care is taken to pad all bony prominences.
- An axillary roll is placed underneath the axilla for padded protection.
- Surgical preparation is done with chlorhexidine solution.
- The surgical extremity is placed in a padded lateral arm positioner (▶ **Fig. 6.1**a,b).

6.2 Portal Placement

6.2.1 Standard Portals

- A standard posterior viewing portal is made (▶ **Fig. 6.2**).
- An anterior portal is then made through the rotator interval using a spinal needle to determine angle and position of the portal under direct visualization prior to incision.
- A midlateral portal is made for subacromial access, two digits from the lateral edge of the acromion in a horizontal fashion.
- A posterolateral portal (portal of Wilmington) is made for viewing the subacromial space during rotator cuff repair. This frees up the posterior portal for suture management.

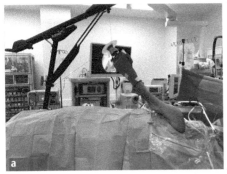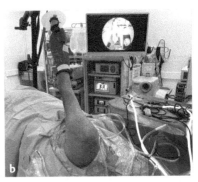

Fig. 6.1 (a) Lateral positioning of a left shoulder using an arm holder in 45° of abduction and 20–30° of forward flexion. (b) View from where the main surgeon stands. Notice where we like to place our instruments on the Mayo stand and the monitor.

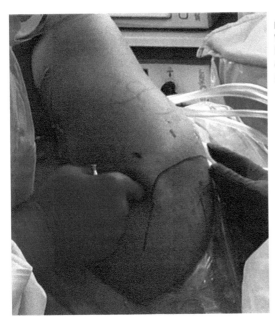

Fig. 6.2 Marking of our usual portals. We generally go about two finger-breadths off the acromion for both our midlateral and posterolateral portals.

6.3 Surgical Technique

6.3.1 Initial Portal Placement

- A standard posterior viewing portal is made.
- Thorough assessment of intraarticular pathology is performed.
- A standard anterior viewing portal is made, and a 7-mm instrument cannula is placed (Arthrex, Naples, FL) under visualization.
- Debridement, synovectomy, removal of loose bodies, labral repair, and/or biceps tenotomy are made at this time as needed. We perform a biceps tenodesis if the patient has preoperative clinical bicipital symptoms.

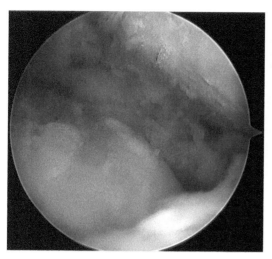

Fig. 6.3 A view of the subacromial space from the posterior portal showing the extent of our rotator cuff tear.

6.3.2 Subacromial Access/Assessment

- Access the subacromial space from the posterior portal.
- Develop the lateral portal, a two-finger breadth width from the lateral edge of the acromion. This is midlateral.
- Perform a meticulous subacromial bursectomy. We do not routinely perform a subacromial decompression.
  - Complete rotator cuff exposure is key. This is performed with both shaver and electrocautery.
- Assess the rotator cuff for tear pattern and size (▶ **Fig. 6.3**).
- For access to the posterior rotator cuff, develop a posterolateral working portal with the aid of a spinal needle.
  - Maintain adequate spacing between the lateral portal and posterior portal (▶ **Fig. 6.4**).

6.3.3 Preparation of the Rotator Cuff Footprint

- Place a PassPort Cannula (Arthrex) in the lateral portal for suture shuttling and an instrument cannula in the posterolateral portal.
- Debride any remnant cuff tissue from the footprint using an arthroscopic wand and shaver.
- Use a bur instrument to gently decorticate the bone.
- An assistant should internally and externally rotate the arm posteriorly and anteriorly, respectively (▶ **Fig. 6.4**).

6.3.4 Perform Soft Tissue Releases

Use a soft tissue elevator to release adhered rotator cuff tissue from the superior glenoid neck as well as above the rotator cuff in the subacromial space.

6.3.5 Traction Sutures

- Place a FiberLink suture (Arthrex) in a luggage tag fashion in the rotator cuff at the anterior leading edge of the supraspinatus. If the posterior aspect of the

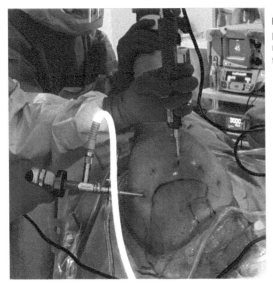

Fig. 6.4 Position of our posterior portal for the arthroscope and the midlateral working portal while in the subacromial space.

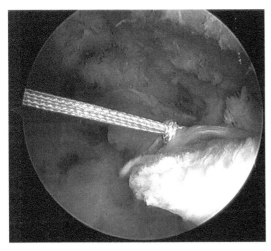

Fig. 6.5 FiberLink (Arthrex, Naples, FL) used in a luggage tag fashion placed in the anterior leading edge of the cuff tear.

tendon tear also needs to be tagged, an additional suture may be needed (▶ **Fig. 6.5**).
- Assess the rotator cuff excursion by pulling the traction sutures laterally from the lateral portal and assess the relationship of the tendon to the footprint.
- If there is poor cuff excursion, perform more soft tissue releases as needed.

6.3.6 Placement of Provisional Traction Suture Reducing Anchor

- Remove the traction sutures except for the one at the anterior leading edge of the supraspinatus.

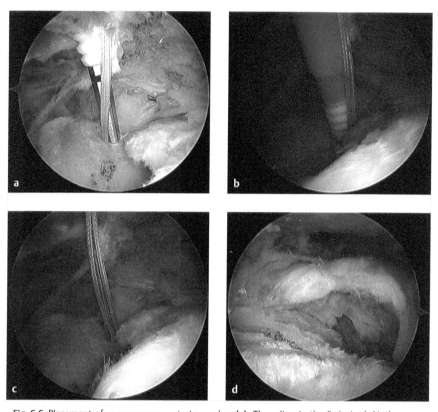

Fig. 6.6 Placement of our accessory anterior anchor **(a)**. Threading in the SwiveLock (Arthrex, Naples, FL) **(b)**, anchor is placed **(c)**, and view of the cuff tear from the lateral portal once the accessory anterior anchor has been placed **(d)**.

- Reduce the cuff to the footprint with the traction suture using a 4.75-mm SwiveLock anchor (Arthrex) as far lateral as possible.
- This helps convert a large retracted L-shaped tear, into a more manageable U-shaped tear (► **Fig. 6.6**a–d).

6.3.7 Perform a Repair Using the SpeedBridge (Arthrex) with the Medial Seal Technique (► Fig. 6.7)

- Perform the SpeedBridge technique for the remaining supraspinatus and posterior cuff (► **Fig. 6.8**).
- We incorporate a medial seal stitch to the SpeedBridge construct (see ► **Video 6.1** and pitfalls section below).

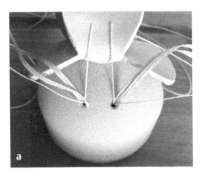
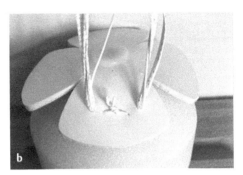
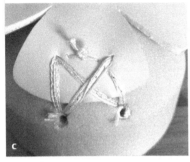

Fig. 6.7 Technique of the Speed-Bridge with medial seal technique. It is broken down into three steps, a-c. The left side of the image is anterior, and the right side is posterior. This is modeled as though we are looking through the lateral portal. (a) The medial row suture limbs from the two medial row anchors have been passed in a 3:1:1:3 fashion from anterior to posterior in the cuff. The first 3 sutures that consist of 2 FiberTape (Arthrex, Naples, FL) sutures and 1 strand of FiberWire (Arthrex, Naples, FL) suture can be passed all together in one pass using a SutureLink (Arthrex, Naples, FL) shuttling stitch. The second limb of the FiberWire stitch is then passed separately. This is then repeated in reverse order for the posterior anchor. (b) The medial seal stitch has been tied and laid on top of the cuff with the superior limbs cut. (c) Completion of the Speed-Bridge construct.

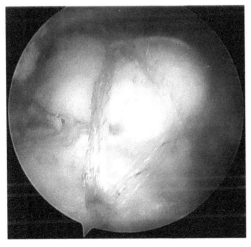

Fig. 6.8 Completion of the SpeedBridge double-row repair viewed from the lateral portal.

41

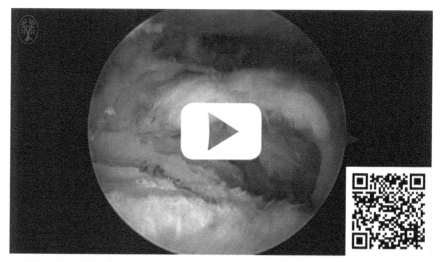

Video 6.1 Arthroscopic view from the posterolateral portal of a large to massive tear. After extensive subacromial bursectomy and rotator cuff tissue releases, an anterior leading edge traction suture is placed in a luggage tag fashion. This is then reduced down to the footprint with a 4.75 Swivel Lock (Arthrex) anchor. A smaller U-shape tear is now visualized. The medial row anchors of the speed bridge repair are placed. The suture limbs are passed through the cuff with a medial seal stitch performed with use of the sliding fiberwire sutures. Once the medial seal stitch is fixated down to the rotator cuff tissue, the lateral row anchors are placed completing the speed bridge repair. The bioinductive patch is then inserted subacromially with the delivery device. The medial end of the patch is fixated to the rotator cuff tissue with use of bioabsorbable staples. It is then fixated laterally with bone staples completing the procedure.

6.3.8 Placement of Bioinductive Bovine Augment Patch

- Remove the PassPort Cannula from the lateral portal for introduction of patch instrumentation (see ▶ **Video 6.1**).
- Adequately visualize the patch as it is laid flat onto the cuff.
- Assure adequate placement of the patch before placing staples and that the patch is not too far medial. Use the patch delivery instrument to hold the patch in an ideal position during stapling.
- Place bioabsorbable staples medially into the cuff tissue and bone staples laterally. Make sure to avoid the lateral row anchors of the speed bridge construct (▶ **Fig. 6.9**).

6.4 Surgeon Tips and Tricks

6.4.1 Visualization

- Adequate subacromial bursectomy to visualize the full extent of tear.
- Arthroscope placed through posterolateral portal (portal of Wilmington) for better cuff visualization both anteriorly and posteriorly. This allows usage of the posterior portal for suture management.

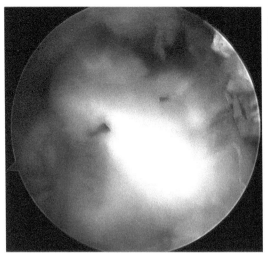

Fig. 6.9 View of the bioinductive patch augment from the lateral portal once fixed to the cuff repair site and greater tuberosity.

6.4.2 Traction Stitch

- On the anterior leading edge of tear through the lateral portal.
- Allows better access for suture passage.
- Aids in reducing the tear to footprint.
- Keeps tissue taut for easy release both superficial and deep to retracted tear.
- Use a blunt arthroscopic elevator and take care to avoid damage to the suprascapular nerve.
- Can use to provisionally assess ease of reduction and give access for suture passage into healthier medial tissue.
- If placing a provisional reducing anchor prior to the SpeedBridge technique, make sure this anchor is as anterior as possible. This will allow better reduction of cuff repair.

6.4.3 Medial Seal

- Once both medial row anchors are in place, tie the medial seal stitch through the lateral portal first. Take one limb from the sliding FiberWire (Arthrex) for this.
- Make sure knot is secured with at least five half hitches. It may require more.
- Check knot security by tightening from both superior and inferior limbs prior to delivering through the cannula (see ▶ **Video 6.1**).
- Pull on inside limbs to slide onto tissue, then cut outside limbs above the knot to aid in suture management. Inside limbs should be outside through opposite portals (limb from more anterior anchor through the anterior portal and limb from posterior anchor through the posterior portal).
- Place remnant inside limbs through lateral row anchors. This will tension the medial seal stitch.

6.4.4 SpeedBridge Preparation

- Abduct arm during preparation of bone for lateral row anchors. Do not exceed more than 60°.

- External and internal rotation of arm to aid in anterior and posterior anchor placement, respectively.
- Tap the punched holes, especially for lateral row anchors, to reduce the chance of fracture and anchor failure, especially in good bone quality.

6.4.5 Dog-Ear

- Can use a free stitch for dog-ear (i.e., FiberLink, Arthrex) in luggage tag fashion to reduce and incorporate into the lateral row anchor.
- If dog-ear is expected, a preloaded sliding suture from the lateral anchor can be used to reduce it.

6.4.6 Patch Augment

- We use a bioinductive implant from the bovine Achilles tendon (Rotation Medical, Plymouth, MN) on top of the repair site. We find this system to be an easy and user-friendly delivery system.[1]
- Can anchor to bone (greater tuberosity) as well as soft tissue (cuff repair).

6.5 Pitfalls/Complications

6.5.1 Medial Seal Failure

- Medial seal stitch can fail in two ways:
  - Do not unload the anchor. One loaded FiberWire (Arthrex) from each anchor is used for the medial seal. It is a sliding suture. Care should be taken to avoid unloading the anchor.
  - Make sure good knot and loop security is achieved prior to sliding inside through the cannula. In our experience, this requires at least five alternating half hitches, but any secure knot will do. Check security by simultaneously tightening both superior limbs then both inferior limbs of knot. Be careful not to unload the anchor or significant length on remnant limbs will be lost. Tie extra knots as needed until completely secure.

6.5.2 Failure of Repair

If too much tension on tissue or significant arm abduction is required to reduce the footprint, tissue will tear through the sutures. Consider separate anterior fixation of the leading edge of the supraspinatus first. This is done prior to SpeedBridge repair to decrease tension on the repair and simplify the remaining repair.

6.6 Rehabilitation

- Conservative.
- Universal abduction sling at all times postoperatively for 4 weeks.
- Gentle passive range of motion in the scapular plane from weeks 4 to 8.
- Active-assisted range of motion from weeks 8 to 12.
- Begin strengthening at 12 weeks.
- Return to normal activities at 6 months.
- Full recovery takes 1 year.

6.7 Rationale and/or Evidence for Approach

- Medial seal stitch reduces soft tissue to bone, blocking fluid interposition and promoting tissue to bone healing.
- Double-row repair has shown a higher load to failure than single-row and keeps lateral tissue down to bone, increasing the contact area to bone and decreasing acromial impingement with abduction.[2,3]
- Augmentation of repair with anterior fixation of the leading edge helps decrease tension on the repair and reduces anterior gap formation with external rotation forces.[4] It also converts the massive retracted tear to a more manageable U-shaped tear, which decreases tension on repair and makes for technically easier repair.
- Patch augmentation has shown good short-term results for augmenting the biology of repair for compromised tissue.

References

[1] Washburn R, III, Anderson TM, Tokish JM. Arthroscopic rotator cuff augmentation: Surgical technique using bovine collagen bioinductive implant. Arthrosc Tech. 2017; 6(2):e297–e301

[2] Duquin TR, Buyea C, Bisson LJ. Which method of rotator cuff repair leads to the highest rate of structural healing? A systematic review. Am J Sports Med. 2010; 38(4):835–841

[3] Henry P, Wasserstein D, Park S, et al. Arthroscopic repair for chronic massive rotator cuff tears: A systematic review. Arthroscopy. 2015; 31(12):2472–2480

[4] Garcia IA, Jain NS, McGarry MH, Tibone JE, Lee TQ. Biomechanical evaluation of augmentation of suture-bridge supraspinatus repair with additional anterior fixation. J Shoulder Elbow Surg. 2013; 22(7):e13–e18

7 Two-Anchor, Double-Row Rotator Cuff Repair with Incorporated Biceps Tenodesis

Michael J. O'Brien and Felix H. Savoie

Summary

The two-anchor, double-row rotator cuff repair is a surgical technique to repair large and massive rotator cuff tears with fewer anchors to limit anchor material in the bone and maximize the contact area between tendon and bone. Recurrent rotator cuff tears are a devastating outcome to patients. One common reason for recurrent tears is failure of the primary repair to heal. The rotator cuff insertion on the greater tuberosity footprint occupies a limited surface area of the bone. Use of multiple anchors may fill this finite space with anchor material, limiting the contact area between tendon and bone, which is necessary for healing to occur. For this reason, we have developed a two-anchor, double-row rotator cuff repair technique for large and massive tears. This technique can be utilized on large and massive tears to facilitate healing by providing excellent footprint coverage with limited anchor material to maximize contact area between the tendon and greater tuberosity bone while also being able to tenodese the biceps tendon at the rotator cuff repair site.

Keywords: double-row, footprint coverage, healing, rotator cuff repair, two-anchor

7.1 Patient Positioning

- Rotator cuff repair surgery may be performed in either the beach chair or lateral decubitus position.
- The patient position is largely surgeon-dependent based on experience and comfort level.

7.2 Portal Placement

- Standard shoulder arthroscopy portals are utilized.
- The procedure begins with a standard posterior viewing portal, placed in the soft spot of the raphe of the infraspinatus.
- An anterior portal is established in the rotator interval, in line with the acromioclavicular joint, using an outside-in technique with a spinal needle.
  - The portal is placed just cephalad to the subscapularis, in a position where a lesser tuberosity anchor may be inserted if necessary.
- A lateral portal is created 3–4 cm off the anterolateral edge of the acromion.
- Accessory anterolateral and posterolateral portals are established in line with the standard lateral portal.
  - These portals are utilized for performing anterior and posterior releases, manipulating the rotator cuff tendons with a grasper, reducing the rotator cuff to the greater tuberosity footprint, and suture passage.

7.3 Surgical Technique (Step-by-Step Approach)

7.3.1 Posterior Viewing Portal

- A posterior portal is established for the arthroscope. The scope is introduced into the glenohumeral joint and diagnostic arthroscopy is performed.
- Using an outside-in technique with a spinal needle, an anterior portal is established in the rotator interval, in line the with acromioclavicular joint.
- All intraarticular pathology is addressed as indicated.
- The rotator cuff tear is identified from inside the joint.
- In the setting of a massive retracted rotator cuff tear, a 360° capsular release is performed to allow the humeral head to drop to a reduced position in the glenohumeral joint and facilitate reduction of the rotator cuff tear.
- Once all intraarticular pathology has been addressed, the blunt trocar is used to advance the arthroscope into the subacromial space.
- Using a spinal needle with an outside-in technique, a lateral portal is established 3–4 cm off the anterolateral corner of the acromion.
- The motorized shaver is introduced through the lateral portal.
  - A limited bursectomy is performed to allow visualization of the rotator cuff tear. A complete bursectomy is not performed as this decreases blood supply to the rotator cuff.
  - If a lateral overhang is present on the acromion, it is resected now with the shaver or bur.
  - The greater tuberosity footprint is lightly decorticated.[1,2]
- Care is taken not to remove the cortical layer of bone on the greater tuberosity, as this may weaken the suture anchor attachment.

7.3.2 Lateral Viewing Portal

- The arthroscope is then moved to a lateral viewing portal.
- It is the authors' observation that the rotator cuff tear is best appreciated viewing from the lateral portal (▶ **Fig. 7.1**).
  - The rotator cuff tear pattern can be identified: crescent-shaped, V-shaped, L-shaped, reverse-L-shaped.
  - Laminations in the tear can be visualized.
  - Sutures can be placed accurately in the tendon for an anatomic repair.
- Accessory anterolateral portals and posterolateral portals can be established with a spinal needle.
- The accessory lateral portals can be used to:
  - Secure the tear edges with a grasper to identify the tear pattern.
  - Assess tear retraction and mobility.
  - Perform anterior and posterior releases.
  - Reduce the tendon to the greater tuberosity footprint.
- The tendon edges are lightly debrided, and the greater tuberosity footprint is lightly decorticated.
- An acromioplasty is performed at the discretion of the surgeon (▶ **Fig. 7.2**).
  - Acromioplasty may be beneficial to improve visualization, increase the working space, remove osteophytes that may cause external impingement, and create a bleeding acromion bed to bathe the rotator cuff repair site.

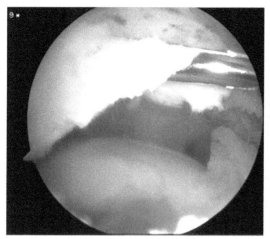

Fig. 7.1 Viewing from the lateral portal in a right shoulder in the beach chair position, a reverse-L-shaped full-thickness supraspinatus tear can be visualized. The tear can be manipulated with a grasper to determine tear pattern, check tendon mobility, and reduce the tendon to the greater tuberosity.

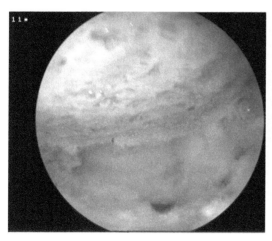

Fig. 7.2 A view from the lateral portal in a right shoulder after completion of acromioplasty. We routinely perform acromioplasty to improve visualization, create more working space, remove any sources of external impingement, and create a bleeding acromion bed to bathe the rotator cuff repair site.

7.3.3 Repair

- A triple-loaded anchor is placed into the greater tuberosity footprint just lateral to the articular cartilage margin (▶ **Fig. 7.3**).
  - We prefer an open architecture anchor, such as the Healicoil (Smith & Nephew, Andover, MA), to allow bone marrow and blood products to flow out of the marrow canal and bathe the repair site to promote healing (▶ **Video 7.1**).
- A small awl or punch is used to microfracture the greater tuberosity footprint.
  - Microfracture allows bone marrow contents to bathe the repair site and facilitate healing.[3,4]
  - Avoid microfracture in osteopenic bone, as this may compromise anchor purchase.
- A grasper can be utilized, if necessary, though an anterior portal to reduce the rotator cuff tendon during suture passage.
- A retrograde suture passer is placed percutaneously to pass and retrieve sutures through the rotator cuff tendons.

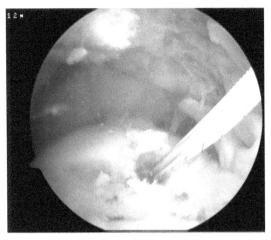

Fig. 7.3 A motorized shaver is used to create a bleeding trough of bone in the medial tuberosity, and a triple-loaded, medial-row anchor is placed just lateral to the articular cartilage margin.

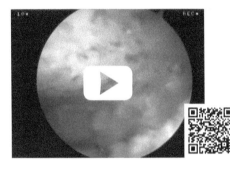

Video 7.1 This video demonstrates an arthroscopic rotator cuff repair and biceps tenodesis in a right shoulder in the beach chair position, utilizing a two-anchor double-row rotator cuff repair with incorporated biceps tenodesis.

- We prefer to pass sutures with the IDEAL Suture Grasper (Mitek Sports Medicine, DePuy Synthes, Raynham, MA).
- Sutures are place in mattress fashion, evenly spaced across the tear (► **Fig. 7.4**).
- Care is taken to place the sutures in the tendon, and not at the muscle–tendon junction.
- Overtensioning of the medial row sutures may lead to a type-II failure.
- If a biceps tenodesis is also to be performed, the anterior suture can also be passed through the long head of the biceps tendon.
    - The suture grasper is passed through the rotator cuff tendon, and then through the biceps tendon, before retrieving the suture.
    - The biceps tenodesis is performed to the greater tuberosity anchor, and the biceps tendon sits between the rotator cuff tendon and greater tuberosity bone.
- The three mattress sutures are tied, leaving all suture tails long.
- For the lateral row anchor, either both limbs from each mattress (six limbs) or one limb from each mattress (three limbs) can be incorporated into the anchor, depending on the anchor type and how many sutures it can accommodate.
- The remaining sutures are then incorporated into one lateral row anchor. The anchor is placed into an anatomic location to decrease tension on the repair.
- The lateral row anchor is impacted, tensioned, and deployed (► **Fig. 7.5**).

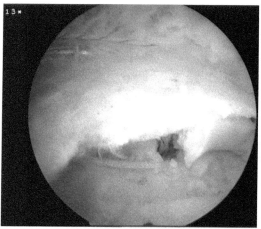

Fig. 7.4 Three mattress sutures are placed evenly across the torn tendon. Take great care not to place sutures too medial at the muscle–tendon junction, as overtensioning of the repair may cause a type-II failure with tearing at the muscle–tendon junction.

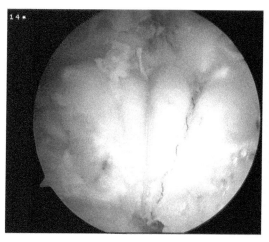

Fig. 7.5 Final view from the lateral portal of a right shoulder two-anchor, double-row rotator cuff repair. One limb of each medial-row suture is left long and incorporated into one lateral-row anchor.

- This technique anatomically repairs the rotator cuff tear, with excellent tension of the tendon to the bone.
- The two-anchor, double-row repair allows for anatomic reduction of the rotator cuff tendon, with excellent footprint coverage and tendon to bone contact area, while decreasing the amount of bone occupied by plastic anchors.

7.4 Surgeon Tips and Tricks (Use of Specific Instrumentation)

- Viewing from the lateral portal allows for complete visualization of the tear, to identify tear pattern and any delamination.
- A triple-loaded, medial-row anchor allows six sutures to be passed through the tendon, in mattress fashion, with only one anchor placed.

- Use of retrograde suture passers allows for quick suture passing and retrieval while viewing from the lateral portal.
  - This allows for very accurate suture placement.
- After the mattress sutures are tied, if a dog-ear is present, re-pass one of the suture limbs through the dog-ear before incorporation into the lateral row anchor, to tension and reduce the dog-ear.
- Choose a lateral row anchor that allows six sutures to be passed through one anchor; thus, suture options will not be limited with lateral row fixation.

7.5 Pitfalls/Complications

- Do not debride the tuberosity bone too much or you will weaken the anchor purchase.
- In elderly patients with osteoporotic bone.
  - Do not perform a microfracture to the tuberosity bone as the bone integrity may be compromised.
  - Do not overtighten lateral row sutures, as the sutures may cut though the osteoporotic bone and compromise the fixation of the lateral row anchor.
- Space the sutures evenly across the tendon to avoid dog-ears.
- Do not place medial-row sutures at the muscle–tendon junction or overtighten the medial row. Overtensioning the repair may lead to a type-II failure with tearing at the muscle–tendon junction.

7.6 Rehabilitation

- Abduction pillow sling for 6–8 weeks depending on tear size, chronicity, tendon quality, and revision surgery.
  - Pillow sling full time. May remove to shower, dress, and perform home exercises.
- First visit at 7–10 days post-op: begin passive range of motion (PROM) exercises with external rotation to neutral, shoulder rolls, and shoulder retraction.
- Ultrasound performed in office at weeks 6 and 12, to progress physical therapy.
- Week 6: begin physical therapy for PROM and active assisted range of motion (AAROM), shoulder retraction, and posture training.
- Week 8: begin AAROM all planes, progress as tolerated.
- Week 12: begin rotator cuff and periscapular strengthening.
- Months 5–6: plyometrics, progress scapular strengthening.

7.7 Rationale and/or Evidence for Approach

- Limited bony area for rotator cuff to heal.
- Multiple anchors may fill bone with plastic anchors, limit contact area between tendon and bone, and limit potential healing.
- The use of too many anchors may be a cause for rotator cuff tendons not healing and re-tearing after surgery.[1,2]

References

[1] Curtis AS, Burbank KM, Tierney JJ, Scheller AD, Curran AR. The insertional footprint of the rotator cuff: An anatomic study. Arthroscopy. 2006; 22(6):609.e1

[2] Mochizuki T, Sugaya H, Uomizu M, et al. Humeral insertion of the supraspinatus and infraspinatus. New anatomical findings regarding the footprint of the rotator cuff. J Bone Joint Surg Am. 2008; 90(5):962–969

[3] Osti L, Del Buono A, Maffulli N. Microfractures at the rotator cuff footprint: A randomised controlled study. Int Orthop. 2013; 37(11):2165–2171

[4] Milano G, Saccomanno MF, Careri S, Taccardo G, De Vitis R, Fabbriciani C. Efficacy of marrow-stimulating technique in arthroscopic rotator cuff repair: A prospective randomized study. Arthroscopy. 2013; 29(5): 802–810

8 Arthroscopic Transosseous Equivalent Rotator Cuff Repair: Key Points of Surgical Technique

Thomas "Quin" Throckmorton

Summary
Various surgical techniques have been described in arthroscopic rotator cuff repair. Traditional single row repairs were initially reported and were then followed by double row repairs in an effort to improve fixation. However, concerns arose with the double row technique. In particular, the placement of medial row sutures led to cases of failure at this fixation point. When medial row failure occurred, the resultant segment of tendon available for revision repair was often very short and nearly at the musculotendinous junction. To address this concern, the double-row transosseous equivalent (TOE) repair was developed. This technique has the advantage of the double-row repair in that the sutures provide compression across the entire rotator cuff footprint. However, it mitigates concerns about medial row failure because two rows of fixation are not employed. This chapter will describe the operative technique employed at our center for this repair.

Keywords: beach chair position, rotator cuff repair, traction, transosseous equivalent

8.1 Operative Technique: Patient positioning (▶ Video 8.1)

- Beachchair position.
  - When sitting the patient up to the beachchair position, we take care to control the chin for proper head positioning.
  - In the coronal plane, check carefully to keep the nose, chin, and sternum in line before securing the head.
  - Avoid neck extension. If any is noted, apply gentle pressure to the chin to bring the neck into neutral flexation.
- 12 lb of traction are placed to distract the joint and to facilitate visualization.
  - We use a pulley kit for traction similar to what is used for the arthroscopy in the lateral decubitus position.

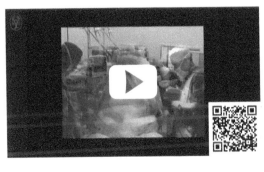

Video 8.1 This video details the surgical technique of arthroscopic single row, transosseous equivalent (tension band) rotator cuff repair.

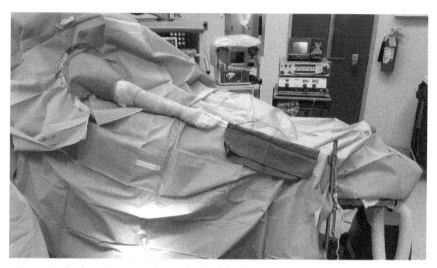

Fig. 8.1 12 lb of traction are applied to the shoulder through a suspension kit to improve arthroscopic visualization.

- The pole and pulley are attached with standard clamps to the operating room table (▶ **Fig. 8.1**).
- We avoid prolonged traction more than 90–120 minutes.

8.2 Portal Placement (▶ Fig. 8.2)

- Our working viewing portal is the posterior portal.
  - A posterolateral viewing portal through the subacromial space may be used and is helpful for small, anterior supraspinatus tears.
- We use an anterior working portal for intraarticular work such as biceps tenodesis and debridement.
- The lateral or anterolateral working portal is used with an 8 mm cannula for most subacromial procedures.
  - Subacromial debridement.
  - Suture placement.
  - Subacromial decompression.
- We use a superior working portal just off the lateral acromial edge as an accessory portal.
  - Suture anchor placement.
  - Suture storage.

8.3 Surgical Technique

- Subacromial debridement.
  - We establish a lateral portal and perform a thorough bursectomy with electrocautery.

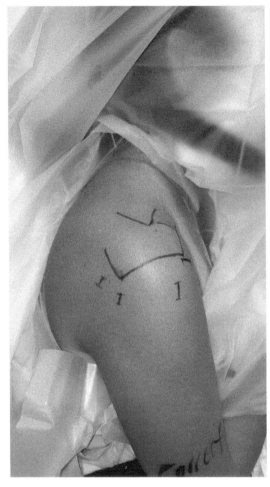

Fig. 8.2 Standard arthroscopic portals are utilized for transosseous equivalent RCR. In particular, the anterosuperior portal functions well for suture storage and allows suture anchor placement at the optimal angle of insertion.

- Once the bursa is cleared, electrocautery is used to outline the anterior and lateral edges of the acromion. It is then examined for any evidence of subacromial spurring or impingement lesion.
  - We do not perform a full release of the coracoacromial ligament.
- After the bony exposure is completed, we then identify the rotator cuff tear margins and establish the tear shape.
- Rotator cuff repair (transosseous equivalent, inverted mattress, lateral row with tape suture).
  - We enlarge the lateral portal and place an 8 mm cannula. Using electrocautery and shaver, the greater tuberosity is debrided to create a bony bed for healing.
  - Superficial and deep releases of any adhesions around the rotator cuff are performed as needed to mobilize it for repair.
  - A suture passer is used to place two inverted mattress stitches using tape suture.
  - The anterosuperior portal is established by needle localization to identify anchor sites. The sutures are retrieved and stored through this portal.

- The middle two limbs are then crossed to create a tension band, transosseous equivalent construct.
- The suture anchors are placed through the anterosuperior portal.
  - We aim for at least a 1 cm bone bridge between anchors.
  - We attempt to place anchors at 45°–60° angle for optimal fixation.
  - Subacromial decompression (optional).

8.4 Surgeon Tips and Tricks

- Thorough bursectomy.
  - We pay special attention to the lateral bursa, which can interfere with suture passage and cannula placement if not thoroughly cleared.
- Suture management.
  - The anterosuperior portal can function as a waiting room portal for previously placed sutures.
- Portal placement.
  - We carefully study the sagittal images on the preoperative magnetic resonance imaging to identify the location of the rotator cuff tear. We use that information to establish our lateral portal to ensure that our suture passer can access the entire width of the tear.
  - We use needle localization to ensure that the superior portal can place both suture anchors with an appropriate bone bridge between them.

8.5 Pitfalls and Complications

- Inadequate bursectomy will interfere with visualization, suture passage, and anchor placement.
- Avoid suture tangles by using the anterosuperior portal for suture storage.
- If the anterosuperior portal is not placed correctly, it can interfere with suture anchor placement. This in turn may result in an inadequate bony bridge between anchors, which place the construct at risk for fracture.
- Repair failure.

8.6 Rehabilitation

- Our program is based on the premise that the repair is at risk for re-tear up to 6 months following surgery.
- First 2 weeks.
  - Sling immobilization and Codman's exercises only.
- Weeks 2–6.
  - The patient continues wearing a sling at all times when not in physical therapy.
  - We begin formal physical therapy with active assisted range of motion (AAROM) and passive range of motion (PROM) up to 90° of forward elevation and external rotation to 30°.
- Weeks 6–12.
  - The patient comes out of the sling for daily activities in front of the body.
  - Light activities such as driving and desk work are permitted.
  - Physical therapy continues with advancement of AAROM and PROM to full forward elevation and external rotation.

- Weeks 12–24.
  - The patient is out of the sling full time with a 10 lb weight limit for daily activities.
  - Physical therapy continues with advancement of active range of motion and PROM in all planes. Isometric strengthening with a 10 lb limit is initiated.
- Week 24.
  - The patient is released to unrestricted activities.

8.7 Literature Review

- Biomechanics of transosseous equivalent (TOE) repair are favorable to single- and double-row repairs.
  - These studies indicate that TOE provides repair "self-reinforcement."[1,2]
- TOE has been reported to have a lower re-tear rate than single- and double-row repairs. However, this difference was not statistically significant.[3]
- Knotless and knotted TOE constructs have both been studied with good outcomes. However, a lower re-tear rate was noted after knotless repair.[4]
- Rotator cuff repairs are at risk for re-tear up to 6 months after surgery. But re-tears are uncommon thereafter.[5]

References

[1] Park MC, Mc Garry MH, Gunzenhauser RC, Benefiel MK, Park CJ, Lee TQ. Does transosseous-equivalent rotator cuff repair biomechanically provide a "self-reinforcement" effect compared with single-row repair? J Shoulder Elbow Surg. 2014; 23(12):1813–1821

[2] Park MC, Peterson AB, Mc Garry MH, Park CJ, Lee TQ. Knotless transosseous-equivalent rotator cuff repair improves biomechanical self-reinforcement without diminishing footprint contact compared with medial knotted repair. Arthroscopy. 2017; 33(8):1473–1481

[3] Mc Cormick F, Gupta A, Bruce B, et al. Single-row, double-row, and transosseous equivalent techniques for isolated supraspinatus tendon tears with minimal atrophy: A retrospective comparative outcome and radiographic analysis at minimum 2-year followup. Int J Shoulder Surg. 2014; 8(1):15–20

[4] Millett PJ, Espinoza C, Horan MP, et al. Predictors of outcomes after arthroscopic transosseous equivalent rotator cuff repair in 155 cases: A propensity score weighted analysis of knotted and knotless self-reinforcing repair techniques at a minimum of 2 years. Arch Orthop Trauma Surg. 2017; 137(10):1399–1408

[5] Iannotti JP, Deutsch A, Green A, et al. Time to failure after rotator cuff repair: A prospective imaging study. J Bone Joint Surg Am. 2013; 95(11):965–971

9 Arthroscopic Double-Row Transosseous Equivalent Repair of Large Rotator Cuff Tears

Ajay S. Padaki, Daniel J. Song, Pinkawas Kongmalai, and William N. Levine

Summary

Operative treatment of rotator cuff tears has increased in the past several decades in response to biomechanical and clinical evidence, supporting repair of symptomatic full-thickness tears in patients who have failed nonoperative management. As our understanding of rotator cuff anatomy, biology, pathophysiology, and biomechanics improves along with the technological advances in orthopedic biologics, implant material, and design, there is constant evolution in the surgical treatment of rotator cuff tears. Although the arthroscopic approach is most commonly used today, the traditional open or mini-open rotator cuff repair remains a viable approach to rotator cuff repairs. Technological advances have provided orthopedic surgeons with a variety of surgical techniques to repair rotator cuff tears. Surgical techniques should be carefully selected and used after evaluating patient factors, tear size, tear pattern, tissue pathology, and surgeon experience to create the optimum repair construct. The arthroscopic, double-row transosseous-equivalent repair of rotator cuff tears is a commonly used technique for rotator cuff tears that allows anatomic repairs with a large tendon to a bone interface that is theoretically and biomechanically superior to other rotator cuff repair techniques. This chapter will provide a concise, easy-to-follow approach, highlighting the pearls and pitfalls of the technique.

Keywords: double row repair, rotator cuff, shoulder surgery, transosseous equivalent

9.1 Patient Positioning

9.1.1 Standard Supine Beach Chair Positioning

- Preparation.
    - Bilateral venodynes for deep vein thrombosisprophylaxis; leg ramp.
    - Ensure neutral neck alignment following intubation.
    - Perform exam under anesthesia.
    - Assemble limb positioner of choice at ipsilateral hip.
    - Hang extremity; soap scrub followed by chlorhexidine scrub.
    - Sterile draping per institutional protocol and limb positioner attachment.
    - Mark the posterolateral and anterolateral acromial border, coracoid, and acromioclavicular joint.

9.2 Portal Placement

9.2.1 Posterior

- Inject wheal into all portal sites with lidocaine with 1% epinephrine.
- Palpate soft spot 1 cm medial and 2 cm posterior to posterolateral acromion.
- 1 cm scalpel incision through skin only.
- Trocar through deltoid with fleck of glenoid before insertion toward coracoid.

9.2.2 Anterior

- Under direct visualization, place an 18G spinal needle 1 cm lateral to lateral coracoid through the rotator interval.
- 1 cm scalpel incision through skin only.
- Switching stick, dilator, and cannula placement.

9.2.3 Lateral

- Mark two to three fingerbreadths lateral to the lateral acromion.
- Insert an 18G spinal needle under direct visualization after transition to subacromial space.

9.3 Surgical Technique (Step-by-Step Approach)

9.3.1 Diagnostic Arthroscopy from the Posterior Portal

- Insert probe into anterior portal.
- Assess integrity of superior labrum with probe.
- Move probe superior to biceps tendon and pull traction with probe to examine biceps tendon for tear, tendinitis, and instability.
- Examine humeral head cartilage laterally and glenoid cartilage medially.
- Visualize middle glenohumeral ligament and subscapularis at humerus.
- Rotate inferiorly and examine inferior glenohumeral ligamentand inferior labrum.
- Assess capsular ligament insertions along the humerus before traversing inferior pouch and ruling out the presence of loose bodies.
- Gently rotate to visualize posteroinferior labrum and posterosuperior labrum.
- Place the arm in slight abduction and external rotation and evaluate rotator cuff for tears.
- Address labral, cartilage, and biceps pathology as indicated.

9.3.2 Subacromial Space

- Remove posterior scope and place trocar directly under acromion.
- Sweep trocar medially and laterally to improve visualization before placing the trocar at the coracoacromial (CA) ligament.
- Establish lateral portal as delineated above, then insert a 7 mm cannula.
- Identify anterolateral acromial edge.
- Debride bursa with combination of shaver and electrocautery to optimize visibility while alternating visualization between the posterior and lateral portals.
- Perform acromioplasty if needed to help visualization of rotator cuff.
- Visualizing from the lateral portal, evaluate the rotator cuff tear including tear pattern, mobility, and reducibility.
- Visualizing from the posterior portal, debride adhesions to rotator cuff as needed to gain sufficient excursion to reapproximate the anatomic footprint.
- Prepare the rotator cuff footprint until cancellous bone is visible to maximize healing potential.
- Insert the spinal needle directly adjacent to the acromion to assess the angle of medial suture anchor placement.

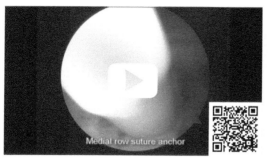

Video 9.1 Surgical demonstration of an arthroscopic double row transosseous equivalent repair of a large rotator cuff tear.

- Create a small incision to place anterior and posterior medial anchors just off the articular margin.
- Pass sutures starting from anterior to posterior utilizing the Scorpion suture passing device.
- Pass one limb each from the anterior and posterior suture anchor out of the lateral portal.
- Load these sutures into a Swive Lock suture anchor.
- Using electrocautery, remove soft tissue off the lateral greater tuberosity to ensure ease of anchor placement.
- Tap into desired lateral row anchor and place suture anchor with appropriate tension using the cannula as a guide.
- Cut suture limbs flush.
- Repeat this process for the remaining two sutures from the medial row anchors.
- Evaluate for additional tears or "dog-ears" anterior or posterior to the repair and utilize sutures from the lateral anchors to further repair or reduce the rotator cuff.
- Perform acromioplasty as indicated.
- Close skin with 4–0 subcutaneous Biosyn (▶ **Video 9.1**).

9.4 Surgeon Tips and Tricks (Use of Specific Instrumentation)

- Place 0 Prolene through suspected or partial rotator cuff tear from the glenohumeral space to ease localization in the subacromial space.
- Perform thorough subacromial bursectomy and possible acromioplasty to ensure adequate visualization of the entire rotator cuff tearthroughout the case.
- Maintain hemostasis throughout the case.
- Ensure optimal suture management at all times with specific protocol.
- Hold cannula directly over the awl so swivel lock placement is not difficult.
- After repair, ensure footprint restored from glenohumeral joint.

9.5 Pitfalls/Complications

- Inadequate visualization of rotator cuff tear secondary to inadequate subacromial bursectomy.
- Poor suture management.
- Inappropriate tension (under- and overtensioning).

9.6 Rehabilitation

- Remain non-weight-bearing on the operative arm for 6 weeks in a pad sling.
- Pendulum exercises with no other shoulder range of motion (ROM) during this 6-week period.
- Active-assisted ROM with physical therapy at weeks 6–12.
- Active ROM and strengthening at weeks 12–20.
- Continued strengthening and home exercise program at weeks 20 and beyond.
- 2-week follow-up for wound inspection, 6-week follow-up to initiate physical therapy, and 3- and 6-month follow-ups to evaluate for rotator cuff integrity and progress with physical therapy.

9.7 Rationale and/or Evidence for Approach

9.7.1 Repair Technique

- The authors prefer double-row repair because double-row rotator cuff repair increases the bone–tendon interface.[1]
- The double-row repair also has been shown to increase fixation strength of the tendon[2] with less gapping.[3]
- Anatomic restoration of the footprint is critical for rotator cuff repair, and double-row repair best reapproximates the footprint.[4,5,6]
- While not clinically significant, double-row repair has demonstrated greater tendon healing on magnetic resonance imaging than the single-row technique.[7]
- Despite these cadaveric studies, however, clinical investigations show marginal, if any, benefit of double-row repair.[8,9]

9.7.2 Postoperative Therapy

- Despite protocols[10] advocating for early ROM, the authors recommend 4–6 weeks of immobilization to minimize gapping following repair.[11]
- While accelerated early movement may increase short-term results, no long-term effects have been demonstrated.[12,13,14]
- Standard immobilization after surgery also may increase early tendinous strength.[15]
- Rate of re-tear has been shown to be equivocal between the two groups with some studies showing a nonsignificant trend in increased re-tears in the early movement cohort.[12,15]

References

[1] Meier SW, Meier JD. Rotator cuff repair: The effect of double-row fixation on three-dimensional repair site. J Shoulder Elbow Surg. 2006; 15(6):691–696

[2] Kim DH, Elattrache NS, Tibone JE, et al. Biomechanical comparison of a single-row versus double-row suture anchor technique for rotator cuff repair. Am J Sports Med. 2006; 34(3):407–414

[3] Ahmad CS, Kleweno C, Jacir AM, et al. Biomechanical performance of rotator cuff repairs with humeral rotation: A new rotator cuff repair failure model. Am J Sports Med. 2008; 36(5):888–892

[4] Dines JS, Bedi A, ElAttrache NS, Dines DM. Single-row versus double-row rotator cuff repair: Techniques and outcomes. J Am Acad Orthop Surg. 2010; 18(2):83–93

[5] Mazzocca AD, Millett PJ, Guanche CA, Santangelo SA, Arciero RA. Arthroscopic single-row versus double-row suture anchor rotator cuff repair. Am J Sports Med. 2005; 33(12):1861–1868

[6] Tuoheti Y, Itoi E, Yamamoto N, et al. Contact area, contact pressure, and pressure patterns of the tendon–bone interface after rotator cuff repair. Am J Sports Med. 2005; 33(12):1869–1874

[7] Sugaya H, Maeda K, Matsuki K, Moriishi J. Repair integrity and functional outcome after arthroscopic double-row rotator cuff repair. A prospective outcome study. J Bone Joint Surg Am. 2007; 89(5):953–960

[8] Burks RT, Crim J, Brown N, Fink B, Greis PE. A prospective randomized clinical trial comparing arthroscopic single- and double-row rotator cuff repair: Magnetic resonance imaging and early clinical evaluation. Am J Sports Med. 2009; 37(4):674–682

[9] Lapner PL, Sabri E, Rakhra K, et al. A multicenter randomized controlled trial comparing single-row with double-row fixation in arthroscopic rotator cuff repair. J Bone Joint Surg Am. 2012; 94(14):1249–1257

[10] Düzgün I, Baltacı G, Atay OA. Comparison of slow and accelerated rehabilitation protocol after arthroscopic rotator cuff repair: Pain and functional activity. Acta Orthop Traumatol Turc. 2011; 45(1):23–33

[11] Millett PJ, Wilcox RB, III, O'Holleran JD, Warner JJ. Rehabilitation of the rotator cuff: An evaluation-based approach. J Am Acad Orthop Surg. 2006; 14(11):599–609

[12] Cuff DJ, Pupello DR. Prospective randomized study of arthroscopic rotator cuff repair using an early versus delayed postoperative physical therapy protocol. J Shoulder Elbow Surg. 2012; 21(11):1450–1455

[13] Kim YS, Chung SW, Kim JY, Ok JH, Park I, Oh JH. Is early passive motion exercise necessary after arthroscopic rotator cuff repair? Am J Sports Med. 2012; 40(4):815–821

[14] Parsons BO, Gruson KI, Chen DD, Harrison AK, Gladstone J, Flatow EL. Does slower rehabilitation after arthroscopic rotator cuff repair lead to long-term stiffness? J Shoulder Elbow Surg. 2010; 19(7):1034–1039

[15] Lee BG, Cho NS, Rhee YG. Effect of two rehabilitation protocols on range of motion and healing rates after arthroscopic rotator cuff repair: Aggressive versus limited early passive exercises. Arthroscopy. 2012; 28(1):34–42

10 Arthroscopic Rotator Cuff Repair Using a Suture-Bridge Technique and Associated Open Subpectoral Biceps Tenodesis

Catherine M. Rapp, Alexander Vara, Brett P. Wiater, and J. Michael Wiater

Summary

Rotator cuff and long head of the biceps brachii (LHB) pathology are frequently concomitant. Successful surgical treatment requires appropriately addressing both issues. While many techniques exist, the authors have found the use of a suture-bridging repair of the rotator cuff tendon in conjunction with an arthroscopically assisted open subpectoral LHB tenodesis to provide a minimally invasive technique that is straightforward to perform and results in excellent patient outcomes. Step-by-step instructions for both procedures, including patient positioning, incision sites, and intraoperative techniques, will be displayed using videography. Tips, pitfalls, and postoperative considerations will also be reviewed.

Keywords: rotator cuff repair, shoulder arthroscopy positioning, subpectoral biceps tenodesis

10.1 Patient Positioning

- Dependent upon preoperative surgical planning, including patient factors and surgeon preference. The patient presented here has a full thickness tear of the supraspinatus tendon (SST), loose bodies within the synovium of the long head of the biceps brachii tendon (LHBT), and painful acromioclavicular joint (ACJ) degeneration and osteolysis (▶ Fig. 10.1, ▶ Fig. 10.2).
- Standard beach chair[1] (▶ Fig. 10.3):
  - Patient is sat fully upright to aid in visualization, not a semi-upright position.

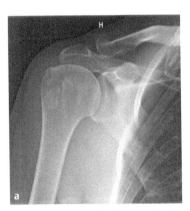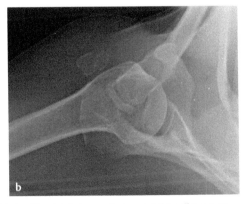

Fig. 10.1 Radiographs of the patient's right shoulder. **(a)** Anteroposterior, and **(b)** axillary views demonstrating multiple, large loose bodies.

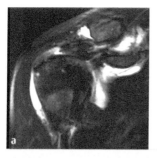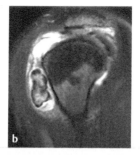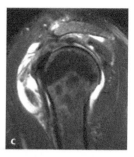

Fig. 10.2 Magnetic resonance imaging of the patient's right shoulder. **(a)** Coronal oblique, and **(b)** sagittal far lateral images demonstrate a full thickness tear of the supraspinatus tendon (SST) with multiple large loose bodies in the subacromial space and biceps synovium. **(c)** Sagittal medial image demonstrates impingement of the anterior acromion on the SST with deformation of the tendon.

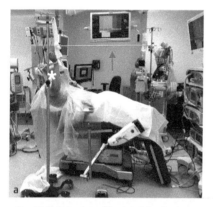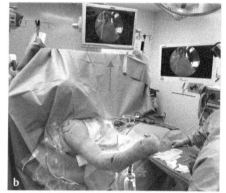

Fig. 10.3 Patient positioning **(a)** prior to preparation, and **(b)** after draping. Beach chair position with bed slightly flexed. Arthroscopy tower and equipment are positioned at the foot of the bed. Note position of arm holder (SPIDER2, Smith & Nephew, Andover, MA) with the proximal portion of the mechanical arm positioned such that it will unobtrusively fit under the bed, out of the way, during the case (*red asterisk*). A horizontal bar placed between two IV poles will allow the patient to be draped and still have easy anesthesia access. One arthroscope monitor can be positioned just above this bar (*red arrow*). To ease preparation, the arm can be hung with a kerlix loop and IV pole (*yellow asterisk*). The hand is prepped at the surgeon's discretion. It need not be prepped if carefully covered with an impervious stockinet, taking care not to contaminate the shoulder/arm.

– Head and neck carefully placed in a neutral and well-padded position.
– Nonoperative arm support. Arm relaxed at side. Shoulder slightly forward flexed. Elbow less than 90°.
– Lower back in contact with the chair. An extra table pad placed under the patient's thighs will help prevent the patient from slipping down the bed as well as contribute to hip/knee flexion. Additional table flexion is also helpful.
– Bilateral lower leg sequential compression devices on and functioning.
• An operative arm holder is useful and unobtrusive. Attach the arm holder to the side bed rail on the section with the patient's feet. Angle the body of the holder with the mechanical arm 45° toward the floor from the bed (▶ **Fig. 10.3**a).

- Draping
  - On anesthesia's side of the bed, a horizontal bar between two IV poles allows the drapes to be out of the operative field, maintain sterility, and give anesthesia easy access to the patient (▶ **Fig. 10.3**b).

10.2 Portal and Incision Placement

- Portal placement is chosen based on preoperative planning (▶ **Fig. 10.4**). For a rotator cuff repair, we routinely use one posterior, one anterior, and one lateral small working portal; one large lateral working portal; and one accessory portal for anchor placement. Care should be taken to keep the skin incision the same size as the cannula. Too large an incision will lead to fluid extravasation around the cannula, increased blood flow, and poor visibility because of the Bernoulli effect.[2] To help maintain pressure in the system, place closed cannulas in portal sites not currently in use.
  - Posterior portal. Midacromial line approximately 3 cm below the posterior acromion. Just below the "soft spot." This is the only portal placed without direct visualization. Keeping this portal low will prevent hinging on the acromion, especially in larger individuals.
  - Anterior portal. Made under direct visualization using a spinal needle for localization staying superior and lateral to the coracoid to protect neurovascular structures. Placement depends on how this portal will be used. For instance, in this case of distal clavicle excision, the portal was placed externally in line with the ACJ and internally just below the LHBT. A small diameter, smooth, rigid cannula was used.

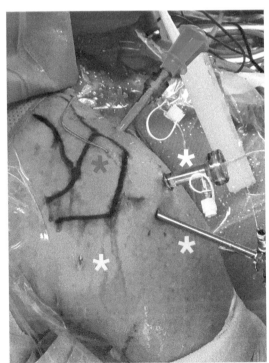

Fig. 10.4 Portal placement from external view. Anterior portal with small diameter, smooth, rigid cannula (*red asterisk*). Anterolateral large working portal with large diameter, rigid, screw-in style cannula (*yellow asterisk*). Posterolateral small viewing portal (*green asterisk*). Posterior viewing portal (*blue asterisk*). Accessory portal for anchor placement (*purple asterisk*).

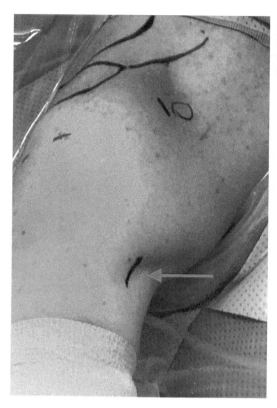

Fig. 10.5 Approach to the long head of the biceps brachii tendon (LHBT) subpectoral tenodesis (*red arrow*).

- Lateral portals. It is important to place these portals low to prevent hinging on the acromion, approximately 2 cm below the lateral acromion.
  - Posterior portal is just anterior to the posterior edge of the acromion and small; it is a viewing portal for the arthroscope.
  - Anterior portal is at the anterior edge of the acromion and larger; it is a working portal. A large-diameter, typically 8 mm, cannula is used. In this case, a rigid, screw-in style cannula was utilized; flexible cannulas are also available.
- Accessory portal. Placed under direct visualization using a spinal needle for percutaneous anchor placement. Typically, they are just off the edge of the lateral acromion. Because of soft tissue swelling during the case, the portal is often medial to surgical markings.
• Approach to the subpectoral LHBT tenodesis is placed with the arm in full external rotation, medial to the long head of the biceps brachii (LHB) muscle belly. The proximal edge is at the inferior border of the pectoralis major tendon (PMT). It is 2–3 cm in length (▶ **Fig. 10.5**).

10.3 Surgical Technique Step-by-Step

• Preincision considerations:
  - Confirm universal protocol for correct site, correct procedure, correct patient.

- Single, weight-appropriate dose of IV antibiotics: cefazolin, clindamycin, or vancomycin. We do not use postoperative antibiotics in the setting of arthroscopic outpatient surgery in an otherwise immunocompetent patient.
- Tranexamic acid 1 g IV prior to incision and again at the end of the case for all patients.
- First, 9 L of saline are dosed with epinephrine at 1:300,000.
  - Fluid pressure set-at 40 mmHg. We will fluctuate between 30–60 mmHg based on intraoperative visualization. Anesthesia will maintain systolic blood pressure < 110 mmHg based on patient characteristics.
  - Exam under anesthesia to document preoperative passive motion, perform manipulation and/or lysis of adhesions if necessary.
- Standard diagnostic arthroscopy is performed, which has been well described.[1]
  - Posterior and anterior portals are placed first as described above.
  - Note LHBT anchor degeneration (▶ **Fig. 10.6**) and SST tear (▶ **Fig. 10.7**).
    - LHBT tenotomy is completed using a radiofrequency ablation (RFA) device that is heat-sensitive with a continuous flow of fluid to prevent overheating of the articular cartilage.[3]
    - The anterolateral working portal is placed at this point. A spinal needle is used to localize the SST tear such that the portal is directly in line with the tear. The footprint is then debrided via this portal using a combination of a motorized arthroscopic 4.5-mm smooth shaver, 4.5-mm shaver with teeth, and 5.5-mm oval bur (▶ **Fig. 10.7**). Note that the structural integrity of the footprint is maintained by removing only the soft tissue down to punctate bleeding cortical bone; it is not carried down to trabecular bone. Also, the rotator interval is left intact as this patient had no pre-op motion limitation.
- Subacromial space is entered via the posterior portal.
  - Impingement lesion on acromion is noted (▶ **Fig. 10.8**). Complete subacromial bursectomy with lateral and anterior acromioplasty[4,5,6] is performed using the RFA device in combination with the motorized arthroscopic shavers and bur.

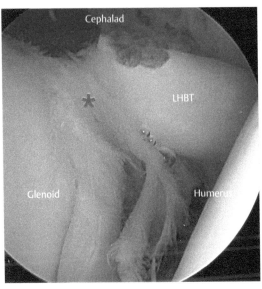

Cephalad

*

LHBT

Glenoid

Humerus

Fig. 10.6 The glenohumeral joint as viewed from the posterior portal with fraying and degeneration of the superior labrum and biceps anchor consistent with a type 1 SLAP (*red asterisk*).

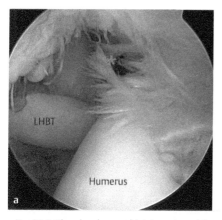
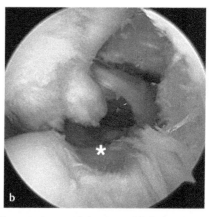

Fig. 10.7 The glenohumeral joint as viewed from the posterior portal showing a full thickness, crescent tear of the supraspinatus tendon (*red asterisk*) before **(a)**, and after **(b)** footprint debridement (*yellow asterisk*).

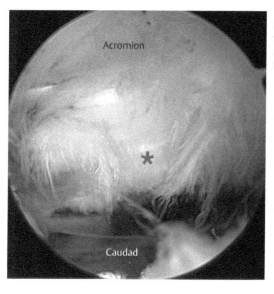

Fig. 10.8 Subacromial space as viewed from the posterior portal showing an anterior acromion impingement lesion (*red asterisk*).

- Multiple loose bodies are removed using an arthroscopic grasper.
- The goal is complete visualization of the SST tear and footprint (▶ **Fig. 10.9**).
- RTC repair—Transosseous equivalent using a suture-bridge technique.[7]
  - The accessory portal is made as described above, under direct visualization to optimize medial anchor placement at the articular margin (▶ **Fig. 10.4**, ▶ **Fig. 10.10**).
    - For the medial row, we utilized 4.75 mm vented, double-loaded, screw-in suture anchors.[8] A simple punch followed by a screw-in tap was used prior to anchor placement. Alternatively, only the screw-in tap can be used.

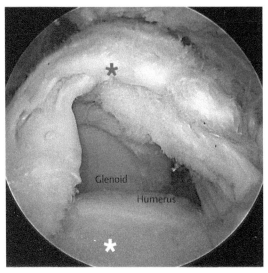

Fig. 10.9 Subacromial space after bursectomy and acromioplasty as viewed from the posterolateral viewing portal, showing the full thickness crescent tear of the supraspinatus tendon (*red asterisk*) and debrided footprint (*yellow asterisk*).

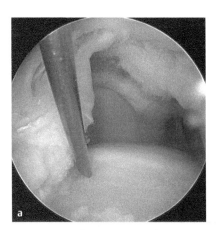
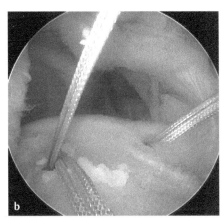

Fig. 10.10 Medial row anchor placement along the greater tuberosity as viewed from the posterolateral viewing portal. **(a)** Localization with a spinal needle. **(b)** After double-loaded anchor placement.

- Suture management is critical. Ensure the sutures are not wrapped around each other or the tendon prior to tying. Using the anterior and posterior portal to hold sutures while they are not in use is helpful.
- A suture passer is used for passing and retrieving the sutures through the rotator cuff. Because of the size of the tear and intrasubstance delamination (▸ **Fig. 10.9**), all eight arms of the two double-loaded anchors were passed.
- The medial row was tied[9,10] using a sliding Tennessee knot followed by half-hitches.
- Each knotless, interference-type, screw-in lateral anchor accepted one arm of each suture, four in each of the two anchors. Anchors were placed approximately 1 cm

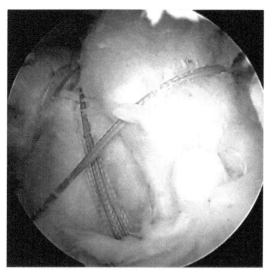

Fig. 10.11 Final construct for transosseous equivalent supraspinatus tendon repair.

distal to the greater tuberosity with adequate separation in line with the pull of the rotator cuff. Sutures were tensioned such that the cuff would be flush to the greater tuberosity but not so tight as to create an avascular state (▶ **Fig. 10.11**).

- Distal clavicle excision is completed with the motorized arthroscopic 5.5 mm bur after clearing the soft tissue from the undersurface of the distal clavicle using the RFA device. Take care to leave the posterior and superior portions of the ACJ ligaments intact. The anterior lateral and direct anterior portals are used alternately for viewing and working. Ensure complete resection of the most superior portion of the clavicle by visualizing with the camera in the anterior portal.
- Skin closure of the portal sites consists of wound closure tape (SteriStrip Reinforced Adhesive Skin Closure, 3 M, St. Paul, MN) for small portal sites. Large working portals are additionally closed with a single deep dermal stitch using a 4–0 monofilament absorbable suture (MONOCRYL Sutures, Ethicon Inc., Johnson & Johnson Medical N.V., Belgium).
- Open subpectoral tenodesis was performed using a cortical button (BicepsButton, Arthrex, Naples, FL) as previously described.[11,12] This method was chosen because of the patient's pathology with loose bodies in the LHBT sheath.
  - The skin is incised in the site described above; subcutaneous tissues are dissected down to the fascia. Fascia is incised overlying the LHB distal to the PMT. At this point, blunt dissection is completed in a blind fashion with a finger, finding the posterior aspect of the PMT and following it laterally to its insertion on the humerus. At this point, the LHBT is found lying directly over the humerus within the bicipital groove. It can be delivered using a Schnidt tonsil or right-angle clamp to dissect between the bone and tendon and subsequently pulling it free.
  - Whipstitch the tendon using a looped #2 nonabsorbable suture on a straight needle (FiberLoop, Arthrex) starting at the musculotendinous junction and progressing proximally ~2 cm; excise the remaining proximal tendon. Divide the suture loop and pass the ends through the cortical button.
  - The site of tenodesis is chosen at the midportion of the PMT using an army–navy retractor under the tendon for visualization; this should place the LHB

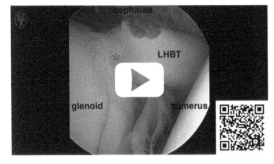

Video 10.1 Surgical demonstration featuring transosseous equivalent arthroscopic repair of the supraspinatus tendon followed by open subpectoral biceps tenodesis.

musculotendinous junction at approximately the inferior border of the PMT. The tenodesis site is prepared using a 3.2 mm guidewire, which is drilled unicortically at first. The tendon is sized, in this case, 5.5 mm in diameter. A reamer is sized the same as the tendon is then passed over the guidewire and through the near cortex only. The guidewire is then passed through the far cortex. By passing the guidewire in two steps, it will prevent plunging through the far cortex. The button is passed through the far cortex and the suture ends are toggled to advance the proximal whipstitched LHBT through the near cortex and into the intramedullary canal. Once appropriate tension has been achieved, the suture ends are tied. One arm of the suture is then passed through the biceps tendon using a free needle and the ends are tied again to reinforce the repair. There is no need for an interference screw in addition to the button.[11,12]

– The site is irrigated and closed using 4–0 monofilament absorbable suture (MONOCRYL) in a deep dermal stitch followed by wound closure tape (SteriStrip Reinforced Adhesive Skin Closure) (▶ **Video 10.1**).

10.4 Surgeon Tips and Tricks

- Arthroscopic instrumentation. Products are available from multiple vendors. While we have listed the vendors utilized at our facility, we recognize that other companies have equally suitable equipment and we do not endorse any one brand.
  - Cannulas (Arthrex):
    - ○ Small working portal: 5.5 mm smooth.
    - ○ Large lateral working portal: 8.25 mm × 9 cm rigid twist-in or 8 mm × 3–5 cm PassPort (Arthrex) flexible.
  - Fluid pump (DualWave Arthroscopy Pump, Arthrex).
  - RFA device (ArthroCare SportsMedicine, Sunnyvale, CA).
  - Motorized arthroscopic shavers (Arthrex).
    - ○ 4.5 mm smooth shaver is used within the glenohumeral joint on the least aggressive jaw opening setting to prevent unwanted debridement. Oscillation is used for soft tissue debridement, and forward spin (1500 rpm) is used to debride the footprint.
    - ○ 4.5 or 5.5 mm shaver with teeth is used with the most aggressive oscillating setting in the subacromial space during bursectomy.
    - ○ 5.5 mm oval bur is used in a forward or reverse spin for acromioplasty and distal clavicle excision.

- Suture passing devices:
  ○ FIRSTPASS (Smith & Nephew, Andover, MA).
  ○ BirdBeak or Penetrator (Arthrex).
  ○ Variably angled SutureLasso device (Arthrex).
- Other arthroscopic instrumentation: probe, knot pusher, small and large graspers, suture retriever, suture cutter, tape cutter both with and without tails, and scissors.
- Anchors:
  ○ Medial row: double-loaded (either two suture or one suture and one tape) screw-in anchor is standard. Used here is a 4.75-mm vented anchor (Healicoil Regenesorb Suture Anchor, Smith & Nephew).
  ○ Lateral row: 4.5-mm screw-in interference anchor (SwiveLock, Arthrex).
- Preferred knots: sliding Tennessee followed by half-hitches. The Tennessee is a simple sliding knot to perform. It is low profile to prevent impingement on the acromion.
- Making anchor placement easier.
  - Arm position.
    ○ Adduct the arm when putting in medial anchors and passing the suture.
    ○ Abduct for the lateral anchors.
    ○ Internally rotate for posterior anchors.
    ○ Externally rotate for anterior anchors.
  - Use percutaneous accessory portals for anchor passage rather than the working or viewing portals.
    ○ Off the lateral acromion for SST/infraspinatus repairs.
    ○ Anterolateral for subscapularis repair.

10.5 Pitfalls/Complications

- Be careful not to incorporate the LHBT with the rotator cuff repair when passing the anterior sutures.
  - If LHBT is left intact, unrecognized incorporation of the tendon into the repair can be a source of postoperative pain and motion limitations.
  - If planning a tenodesis, it will prevent delivery of the tendon to the planned site.

10.6 Rehabilitation

- Weeks 0–4: Brief period of immobilization with passive shoulder external rotation and abduction either patient- or therapist-directed.[13]
  - Extend this period to 6 weeks for large tears.
  - No shoulder extension.
  - Active elbow/wrist/hand range of motion without weight.
- Weeks 4–8.
  - Progress to full passive motion and initiate active and active-assist range of motion.
  - Isometrics at 4 weeks, wall push-ups at 6 weeks.
  - Scapular facilitation.
- Weeks 8–12.
  - Joint mobilization.
  - Start theraband exercise for rotation with arm at side.
  - Proprioceptive neuromuscular facilitation active assist.

- Weeks 12 +.
  - Aggressive strengthening.
  - Theraband in flexion and rotation with arm at 90° abduction.
  - Proprioceptive neuromuscular facilitation active.
  - Sport-specific training.

10.7 Rationale

- Transosseous equivalent with a double-row, suture-bridge technique.[7]
  - Transosseous equivalent repair is supported by biomechanical studies over traditional double-row and single-row repairs, suggesting improved early fixation strength and footprint coverage.[14,15,16,17] However, improved functional outcomes between fixation strategies have not been shown by meta-analysis of clinical studies with short-to-medium-term follow-up of less than 5 years.[18,19,20] These analyses have, however, suggested lower re-tear and improved healing rates, especially in larger tears, when a double-row technique is used. A systematic review[21] and a meta-analysis[22] of arthroscopic cuff repairs have suggested that a healed tendon leads to a superior clinical outcome. Thus, it may be possible that longer-term studies will correlate a lower re-tear rate as the result of a transosseous equivalent technique with improved long-term clinical outcome.
  - For the technique, we prefer to tie the medial row prior to draping the sutures over the cuff and into the lateral anchors. This will limit extravasation of synovial fluid between the tendon and the bone and has been shown to be biomechanically superior in gap formation, mean failure, and contact pressure.[9,10]
  - The use of a vented medial suture anchor has been shown to improve bone in-growth and tendon healing.[8]
- Subacromial decompression. We recognize that this technique is controversial. Meta-analysis of clinical studies with short-term, 2-year follow-up did not find significantly different outcomes between groups undergoing acromioplasty and those that did not.[23] However, acromioplasty may have a long-term protective effect on the cuff, preventing tears.[4] Also, large lateral acromion extension appears to be detrimental to cuff integrity.[5] Because there appears to be little downside and a possible long-term positive effect, we prefer to complete the decompression for those with an impingement lesion and/or bursal-sided tear. Care is taken during the procedure to leave the deltoid origin intact. It is done as a limited anterior and lateral acromioplasty without coracoacromial ligament transection, which should limit contact pressures between the cuff and acromion without potentially causing anterosuperior escape.[6,24]
- Biceps tenodesis.[11,12] Patients undergoing an LHB tenotomy or tenodesis at the time of cuff repair have been shown to have superior clinical outcomes at short-term follow-up.[25] Determination of the type of procedure is based on pathology of the LHBT as well as surgeon and patient preference. No specific procedure is routinely recommended because of equivalent clinical results.[26] In general, when doing a tenodesis, we prefer to do a subpectoral procedure as it is easily reproducible and theoretically eliminates any potential pathology within the groove as a source of continued anterior shoulder pain.

References

[1] Abrams JS, Phillips J. Arthroscopy shoulder surgery: Anatomy, setup, and equipment. In: Miniaci A, Iannotti JP, Williams GR, Zuckerman JD, eds. Disorders of the Shoulder. Diagnosis and Management: Sports Injuries, 3rd ed. Baltimore, MD: Lippincott Williams & Wilkins; 2014:79–90

[2] Burkhart SS, Denard PJ. Rotator cuff repairs: Arthroscopic management. In: Miniaci A, Iannotti JP, Williams GR, Zuckerman JD, eds. Disorders of the Shoulder. Diagnosis and Management: Sports Injuries. 3rd ed. Baltimore, MD: Lippincott Williams & Wilkins; 2014:291–324

[3] Zoric BB, Horn N, Braun S, Millett PJ. Factors influencing intra-articular fluid temperature profiles with radiofrequency ablation. J Bone Joint Surg Am. 2009; 91(10):2448–2454

[4] Björnsson H, Norlin R, Knutsson A, Adolfsson L. Fewer rotator cuff tears fifteen years after arthroscopic subacromial decompression. J Shoulder Elbow Surg. 2010; 19(1):111–115

[5] Nyffeler RW, Werner CML, Sukthankar A, Schmid MR, Gerber C. Association of a large lateral extension of the acromion with rotator cuff tears. J Bone Joint Surg Am. 2006; 88(4):800–805

[6] Katthagen JC, Marchetti DC, Tahal DS, Turnbull TL, Millett PJ. The effects of arthroscopic lateral acromioplasty on the critical shoulder angle and the anterolateral deltoid origin: An anatomic cadaveric study. Arthroscopy. 2016; 32(4):569–575

[7] Park MC, Elattrache NS, Ahmad CS, Tibone JE. "Transosseous-equivalent" rotator cuff repair technique. Arthroscopy. 2006; 22(12):1360.e1–1360.e5

[8] Clark TR, Guerrero EM, Song A, O'Brien MJ, Savoie FH. Do vented suture anchors make a difference in rotator cuff healing. Ann Sport Med Res. 2016; 3(3):1068

[9] Mall NA, Lee AS, Chahal J, et al. Transosseous-equivalent rotator cuff repair: A systematic review on the biomechanical importance of tying the medial row. Arthroscopy. 2013; 29(2):377–386

[10] Nassos JT, ElAttrache NS, Angel MJ, Tibone JE, Limpisvasti O, Lee TQ. A watertight construct in arthroscopic rotator cuff repair. J Shoulder Elbow Surg. 2012; 21(5):589–596

[11] Meadows JR, Diesselhorst MM, Finnoff JT, Swanson BL, Swanson KE. Clinical and sonographic evaluation of bicortical button for proximal biceps tenodesis. Am J Orthop. 2016; 45(5):E283–E289

[12] Snir N, Hamula M, Wolfson T, Laible C, Sherman O. Long head of the biceps tenodesis with cortical button technique. Arthrosc Tech. 2013; 2(2):e95–e97

[13] Osborne JD, Gowda AL, Wiater B, Wiater JM. Rotator cuff rehabilitation: Current theories and practice. Phys Sportsmed. 2016; 44(1):85–92

[14] Park MC, ElAttrache NS, Tibone JE, Ahmad CS, Jun BJ, Lee TQ. Part I: Footprint contact characteristics for a transosseous-equivalent rotator cuff repair technique compared with a double-row repair technique. J Shoulder Elbow Surg. 2007; 16(4):461–468

[15] Park MC, Tibone JE, ElAttrache NS, Ahmad CS, Jun BJ, Lee TQ. Part II: Biomechanical assessment for a footprint-restoring transosseous-equivalent rotator cuff repair technique compared with a double-row repair technique. J Shoulder Elbow Surg. 2007; 16(4):469–476

[16] Quigley RJ, Gupta A, Oh JH, et al. Biomechanical comparison of single-row, double-row, and transosseous-equivalent repair techniques after healing in an animal rotator cuff tear model. J Orthop Res. 2013; 31(8):1254–1260

[17] Park MC, Mc Garry MH, Gunzenhauser RC, Benefiel MK, Park CJ, Lee TQ. Does transosseous-equivalent rotator cuff repair biomechanically provide a "self-reinforcement" effect compared with single-row repair? J Shoulder Elbow Surg. 2014; 23(12):1813–1821

[18] Saridakis P, Jones G. Outcomes of single-row and double-row arthroscopic rotator cuff repair: A systematic review. J Bone Joint Surg Am. 2010; 92(3):732–742

[19] Millett PJ, Warth RJ, Dornan GJ, Lee JT, Spiegl UJ. Clinical and structural outcomes after arthroscopic single-row versus double-row rotator cuff repair: A systematic review and meta-analysis of level I randomized clinical trials. J Shoulder Elbow Surg. 2014; 23(4):586–597

[20] Mascarenhas R, Chalmers PN, Sayegh ET, et al. Is double-row rotator cuff repair clinically superior to single-row rotator cuff repair: A systematic review of overlapping meta-analyses. Arthroscopy. 2014; 30(9):1156–1165

[21] Slabaugh MA, Nho SJ, Grumet RC, et al. Does the literature confirm superior clinical results in radiographically healed rotator cuffs after rotator cuff repair? Arthroscopy. 2010; 26(3):393–403

[22] Yang JJ, Robbins M, Reilly J, Maerz T, Anderson K. The clinical effect of a rotator cuff retear: A meta-analysis of arthroscopic single-row and double-row repairs. Am J Sports Med. 2017; 45(3):733–741

[23] Song L, Miao L, Zhang P, Wang W-L. Does concomitant acromioplasty facilitate arthroscopic repair of full-thickness rotator cuff tears? A meta-analysis with trial sequential analysis of randomized controlled trials. Springerplus. 2016; 5(1):685

[24] Denard PJ, Bahney TJ, Kirby SB, Orfaly RM. Contact pressure and glenohumeral translation following subacromial decompression: How much is enough? Orthopedics. 2010; 33(11):805

[25] Watson ST, Robbins CB, Bedi A, Carpenter JE, Gagnier JJ, Miller BS. Comparison of outcomes 1 year after rotator cuff repair with and without concomitant biceps surgery. J Arthrosc Relat Surg. 2017; 33(11):1928–1936

[26] Leroux T, Chahal J, Wasserstein D, Verma NN, Romeo AA. A systematic review and meta-analysis comparing clinical outcomes after concurrent rotator cuff repair and long head biceps tenodesis or tenotomy. Sports Health. 2015; 7(4):303–307

11 Transosseous Repair

J. Gabriel Horneff and Mark D. Lazarus

Summary

Transosseous rotator cuff repair remains the gold standard of repair. As arthroscopic techniques have evolved, the majority of repairs have been performed through the use of anchor-based techniques. This chapter describes an arthroscopic transosseous tunneling technique used to repair rotator cuff tears with no implant use that best recreates the "gold standard" that was performed in the days of open rotator cuff repair. This technique requires careful suture management and familiarity with the use of a tunneler device but, ultimately, results in stronger, cheaper, and better repairs.

Keywords: arthroscopic cuff repair, posterosuperior cuff repair, rotator cuff repair, transosseous repair, tunneler

11.1 Patient Positioning

- The patient is placed in the beach chair position. This is our preference but a lateral decubitus position with 5 to 10 pounds of distraction on the operative arm is also acceptable depending on surgeon preference.
- The operative extremity is prepped and draped in the typical sterile fashion.
- A mechanical arm holder can be utilized to position the operative extremity in space (this is for our preferred beach chair positioning).

11.2 Portal Placement

- There are five main portals utilized for this approach to rotator cuff repair.
- Standard posterior portal.
  - Created first in the posterior soft spot about 1–2 cm inferior and medial from the posterolateral edge of the acromion.
  - Initial viewing portal for diagnostic scope of the glenohumeral joint and subacromial space.
  - Serves as the retrieval portal for the posterior tunnel sutures.
  - Serves as the portal for tying the medial limbs of the posterior tunnel horizontal mattress "rip-stop" sutures.
- Standard anterior portal.
  - Created second in the rotator interval under spinal needle localization.
  - Serves as the initial working portal for use of the arthroscopic shaver and electrocautery.
  - Serves as the retrieval portal for the anterior tunnel sutures.
  - Serves as the portal for tying the medial limbs of the anterior tunnel horizontal mattress "rip-stop" sutures.
- Lateral portal.
  - Created third with spinal needle localization with the needle parallel to the horizontal of the floor. It is typically located in line with the anterior edge of the acromion.

- Serves as the main working portal for subacromial space.
- Enlarged for placement of the tunneling device for drilling of the lateral tunnels, shuttling of the sutures through the tendon edge, and lateral knot tying.
- Posterolateral portal.
  - Typically created fourth for placement of the arthroscope during tunneling and suture management of the rotator cuff repair.
- Medial (acromial edge) portal.
  - Used for spinal needle localization and drilling of the medial tunnel drill holes.

11.3 Surgical Technique (Step-by-Step Approach)

- Prior to incision, a surgical timeout should always be performed to correctly identify the patient, procedure, and correct operative limb.
- A standard posterior portal is created and the arthroscope is introduced into the glenohumeral joint. An anterior portal is immediately created in the rotator interval. A diagnostic arthroscopy is performed to assess the rotator cuff, labrum, articular surface, and remaining structures.
- If the subscapularis tendon is torn, this should be repaired as best as possible by the surgeon's preferred technique.
- Once all intraarticular work is completed, the arthroscope should be redirected to the subacromial space.
- A lateral portal is created under spinal needle localization in line with the anterior border of the clavicle.
- A combination of arthroscopic shavers, burs, and electrocautery are used via the lateral portal to remove any debris from the undersurface of the acromion. Any large subacromial spurs can be smoothed. The arthroscopic tools can then also be used to remove any soft tissue attached to the exposed greater tuberosity footprint. The arthroscopic bur is used to lightly decorticate the greater tuberosity to encourage healing of the repaired cuff. An arthroscopic grasper can be brought in to ascertain the excursion and quality of the torn tendon tissue.
- The posterolateral portal is created for placement of the arthroscope for visualization during the repair.
- A spinal needle is brought into the shoulder off the lateral edge of the acromion to determine the number and spacing of the medial holes for tunnel placement. Once the proper localization is identified, a small portal is created and the medial row drill guide from the Tornier ArthroTunneler TunnelPro System (Wright Medical Group, Memphis, TN) is used to guide the placement of the medial holes with the drill.
- The medial holes for all the planned tunnels are drilled to the stop on the drill making sure to not violate the articular bone. The holes should be placed just adjacent to the lateral edge of the articular cartilage near the tuberosity.
- The holes are then smoothed with the medial row awl so as to remove any bony debris and prevent sharp edges of bone from cutting the sutures.
- The lateral portal is enlarged enough to allow for placement of the tunneling device. The medial hook on the tunneler is placed into a medial hole and the retractable lateral guide is positioned adjacent to the lateral portion of the greater tuberosity (the white pegs on the handle allow for retraction). Once in the proper position, the white pegs are held in place to ensure that the guide is firmly held to

the lateral portion of the tuberosity and the blue switch is engaged in the forward position on the handle. This switch deploys the metal suture lasso that will capture the shuttling suture.

- The lateral drill bit is placed through the tunneler handle to drill the tunnel. The drill is removed and the metal shuttle suture passer is placed in the handle. The blue switch is then retracted as the suture passer is removed slowly to allow for capture of the shuttling suture. The tunneler is then removed from the lateral portal with the loop of the shuttling suture captured out of the medial tunnel.
- The loop of the shuttling suture is loaded with the appropriate number of repair sutures (three for outer tunnels and four for inner tunnels) and the free limbs of the shuttling suture are pulled through the lateral portal to load the sutures through the tunnel. Each of the sutures placed in the tunnel are of different type/color to allow for organization. The first two sutures are used for simple suture patterns while the third (and fourth sutures depending on number of tunnels) are used for horizontal mattress "rip-stop" stitches that are tied to the same type of suture found in an adjacent tunnel.
- For anterior tunnel sutures, the medial and lateral suture limbs are brought out through the anterior portal and tagged outside of the shoulder with hemostats (one hemostat for medial limbs and two hemostats for lateral limbs). We have designed a color-coded hemostat system to help organize the suture limbs outside of the shoulder, which is described in the Tips and Tricks section.
- Only the most posterior tunnel will have its suture limbs brought out through the posterior portal and tagged with hemostats.
- A large working cannula is placed into the lateral portal.
- Starting posteriorly, each medial suture limb is separately retrieved through the lateral working cannula and passed through the rotator cuff tendon via a suture passing device. Once passed through the tendon, the limbs are retrieved out of their respective anterior or posterior portals and retagged with the appropriate hemostat.
- A small cannula is placed in the posterior portal and the corresponding medial limbs of horizontal mattress "rip-stop" sutures from the most posterior tunnels are retrieved. These matching suture type/color medial limbs are then tied outside of the shoulder with a square knot and the excess suture is trimmed.
- The lateral limbs of these horizontal mattress sutures are then retrieved out of the lateral cannula. A grasper is used to reduce the cuff via the lateral portal as the lateral limbs are pulled taut. The horizontal mattress knot is visualized into placed and the grasper is removed. The lateral limbs are then tied in a nonsliding knot via alternating half hitches with an arthroscopic knot pusher.
- The medial and corresponding lateral limbs of the remaining sutures in the tunnels that just had a horizontal mattress tied are retrieved and tied sequentially from posterior to anterior in a simple suture pattern, with the lateral limbs serving as the post during arthroscopic knot tying.
- The small cannula is placed in the anterior portal and the process is repeated for the remaining tunnels with the horizontal mattress knots between adjacent tunnels tied first followed by the simple sutures.
- Remove all instrumentation from the shoulder and close the portal sites with a nonabsorbable suture and dress with sterile dressings to preference.
- The patient is placed in an abduction sling prior to awakening from anesthesia and then taken to the recovery room (▶ **Video 11.1**).

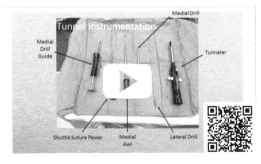

Video 11.1 Surgical demonstration of an arthroscopic transosseous rotator cuff repair technique.

11.4 Surgeon Tips and Tricks

- Larger tears often require more tunnels with most cases requiring anywhere between two and four tunnels. All peripheral tunnels are loaded with three sutures while inner tunnels (one tunnel in a three-tunnel repair and two tunnels in a four-tunnel repair) require four sutures.
- Suture management is the key to success with this technique. We use a color-coded hemostat system to organize suture limbs outside of the shoulder. Depending on how many tunnels are being used determines how many colors are involved. The following is our proposed color-coding scheme.
    - Two tunnels:
        - Tunnel 1 (anterior): three sutures →medial (one red hemostat); lateral (one white hemostat).
        - Tunnel 2 (posterior): three sutures →medial (one black hemostat); lateral (one white hemostat).
    - Three tunnels:
        - Tunnel 1 (anterior): three sutures →medial (one red hemostat); lateral (two red hemostats).
        - Tunnel 2: four sutures →medial (one white hemostat); lateral (two white hemostats).
        - Tunnel 3 (posterior): three sutures →medial (one blue hemostat); lateral (two blue hemostats).
    - Four tunnels:
        - Tunnel 1 (anterior): three sutures →medial (one red hemostat); lateral (two red hemostats).
        - Tunnel 2: four sutures →medial (one white hemostat); lateral (two white hemostats).
        - Tunnel 3: four sutures →medial (one blue hemostat); lateral (two blue hemostats).
        - Tunnel 4 (posterior): three sutures →medial (one green hemostat); lateral (two green hemostats).
- We find that some abduction of the shoulder prior to drilling of the tunnels helps to engage stronger bone laterally.
- Suture placement through the cuff tendon should be carefully performed. For the simple sutures, the medial limbs should be placed into the tendon slightly anterior or posterior to the line of the tunnel and medial to the placement of the horizontal mattress suture limbs. The medial limbs of the horizontal mattress sutures are placed

more in line with the tunnels (between the anterior and posterior simple suture limbs) and slightly more lateral. The purpose of this lateralization of the horizontal mattress sutures is so they serve as a "rip-stop" to prevent cutout of the simple sutures through the tendon.

11.5 Pitfalls/Complications

- Usual possible risks that come along with arthroscopic shoulder surgery (i.e., infection, bleeding, wound healing, etc.).
- One concern with the use of transosseous tunnels is the potential for suture cutout if the bone quality is poor. To combat this, we will employ the use of tape-like sutures, which are less likely to cut through the bone. We also recommend making sure that the tunneler is completely seated before drilling the lateral hole to prevent a shallow tunnel in the weaker proximal bone of the greater tuberosity.
- Conversely, the bone can also cut sutures because of sharp edges near the tunnel holes. We recommend the use of the arthroscopic awl to help smooth the edges of the tunnel and, again, can use tape-like sutures, which are less likely to rupture.
- There have been studies showing that knot strength varies considerably among arthroscopic surgeons.[1] One disadvantage of the transosseous technique is that it is heavily dependent upon the surgeon's ability to tie secure knots. Therefore, one must be comfortable with the knot-tying technique.

11.6 Rehabilitation

- Weeks 0–6: Sling worn at all times. Portal sutures removed at the first postoperative visit. Passive range of motion (PROM) began with supine passive forward elevation to 90° and supine passive external rotation to 30°. This can be started as early as week 2 depending on tear size.
- Weeks 6–12: Discontinuation of the sling. Patient can actively use arm for light waist-level activity not heavier than a coffee cup. Continue PROM with elevation to 140° and external rotation to 40°. May also begin scapular strengthening and phase 1 cuff strengthening. Formal physical therapy (PT) is started with a concurrent home exercise program.
- Weeks 12–18: Add internal rotation stretches. Continue strengthening. No lifting greater than 10 pounds with both hands.
- Weeks 18–24: The PT regimen is advanced to full strengthening (phase 2) with transition to a home-based program. No lifting greater than 20 pounds with both hands.
- Week 24 and beyond: Can return to full activity with no weight restrictions. May begin sports-/work-specific strengthening if necessary.

11.7 Rationale and/or Evidence for Approach

- The use of transosseous tunnel repair significantly reduces the cost of rotator cuff surgery.[2,3] Seidl et al found that the mean cost for rotator cuff repair was nearly $950 less when using a tunneler over arthroscopic anchors.[2] This cost difference was magnified in the instances of larger tears where more anchors would need to be used.

- Transosseous repair has been shown to have a low re-tear rate of about 6% with minimal complications compared to anchor-based repair.[3]
- Patients undergoing transosseous repair have been found to have a faster decrease in their postoperative pain compared to anchor repair, which may be sign of improved repair.[4]
- The use of bone tunnels may improve blood flow to the repaired cuff tendon and contribute to better biological healing of the repair.[5]
- Instances of revision repair may be easier because no anchors have been used to limit the amount of bony purchase left available in the greater tuberosity footprint.

References

[1] Hanypsiak BT, DeLong JM, Simmons L, Lowe W, Burkhart S. Knot strength varies widely among expert arthroscopists. Am J Sports Med. 2014; 42(8):1978–1984

[2] Seidl AJ, Lombardi NJ, Lazarus MD, et al. Arthroscopic transosseous and transosseous-equivalent rotator cuff repair: An analysis of cost, operative time, and clinical outcomes. Am J Orthop. 2016; 45(7):E415–E420

[3] Kuroda S, Ishige N, Mikasa M. Advantages of arthroscopic transosseous suture repair of the rotator cuff without the use of anchors. Clin Orthop Relat Res. 2013; 471(11):3514–3522

[4] Randelli P, Stoppani CA, Zaolino C, Menon A, Randelli F, Cabitza P. Advantages of arthroscopic rotator cuff repair with a transosseous suture technique: A prospective randomized controlled trial. Am J Sports Med. 2017; 45(9):2000–2009

[5] Urita A, Funakoshi T, Horie T, Nishida M, Iwasaki N. Difference in vascular patterns between transosseous-equivalent and transosseous rotator cuff repair. J Shoulder Elbow Surg. 2017; 26(1):149–156

12 True Transosseous Hybrid Rotator Cuff Repair

Brett Sanders

Summary

Transosseous and anchor-based cuff repair methods each have specific technical advantages, which can be used synergistically in rotator cuff repair, like two sides of the same coin. Transosseous fixation offers double-row, 2-point fixation per tunnel, small diameter marrow vents, multiple sutures per tunnel, and unlimited fixation points per case with no cost ceiling. Anchors may have improved biomechanics in some settings and offer knotless fixation, which may be used in conjunction with transosseous approaches. Clinical literature has never demonstrated a fundamental difference in healing rates between the two methods. This chapter discusses a novel hybrid technique to provide double-row, anatomic footprint reconstruction at the healing interface of the rotator cuff with no inert anchor burden to the tuberosity, while capitalizing on biomechanical advantages of a single knotless lateral row anchor, which also serves to independently tighten and backup primary transosseous fixation. This construct allows for a high fixation point per surface area repair, excellent access to biologically active marrow elements, no inert material in the footprint to consider in the revision setting, and redundant high-strength fixation. Moreover, cost reproducibility may be achieved regardless of tear size in the value-based era of surgery. This chapter describes an all-arthroscopic technique for "true" transosseous rotator cuff repair, utilizing a gold standard technique with five fixation points, but only one anchor. This repair combines many desirable qualities namely double-row fixation excellent biological considerations with bone marrow vents accessing repair site, dense fixation point per surface area repair, independent fixation, and cost reduction per fixation point.

Keywords: hybrid rotator cuff repair, rotator cuff repair, transosseous, true transosseous hybrid rotator cuff repair, value-based medicine

12.1 Patient Positioning

The patient may be positioned in either beach chair or lateral decubitus position. We prefer a beach chair with a mechanical arm holder, especially to allow for controlled rotation and forward flexion of the arm during biceps tenodesis.

12.2 Portal Placement

The standard posterior portal and anterior superior portal are utilized. Specific portals for the technique include (see ▶ **Fig. 12.1**):
- Low anterolateral portal for introduction of tunneling device during cuff repair and biceps tenodesis.
- Midlateral portal v. in ▶ **Fig. 12.1**. for viewing during biceps tenodesis.
- Accessor anterior–inferior instrumentation portal iii in ▶ **Fig. 12.1** to aid in suture passage through the biceps portal iv in ▶ **Fig. 12.1**.

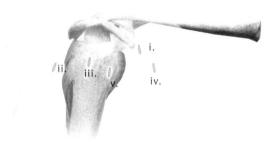

Fig. 12.1 Portals for transosseous cuff repair and biceps tenodesis. i. standard anterosuperior portal; ii. standard posterior portal; iii. midlateral viewing portal; iv. accessory anterior-inferior instrumentation portal; v. low anterolateral working portal.

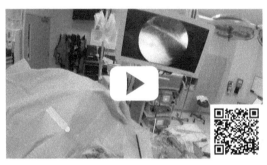

Video 12.1 True transosseous hybrid arthroscopic cuff repair of a right shoulder is shown in the beachair position. This technique offers triple row fixation, no inert material at the healing interface, decreased cost per fixation point, cortical augmentation, and the chance to retension the construct at the final step.

12.3 Surgical Technique (Hybrid Cuff Repair)

- The cuff tear pattern is mobilized and assessed in the standard fashion (▶ **Video 12.1**).
- Footprint preparation: The footprint surface is prepared with a shaver to optimize healing. The geometry of the footprint reconstruction and placement of the fixation points are planned at this phase.
- Medial fixation points: A 2.9 mm awl is placed through an accessory portal just lateral to the acromion to create two medial fixation points just adjacent to the articular surface of the humeral head. These would be in the location of a medial row anchor. While the awl is in the subacromial space, the tuberosity may be microfractured to create more bone marrow vents to aid in ingress of biologically active marrow cells.
- Tunnel creation: The low anterolateral portal is localized by placing a spinal needle just above the tuberosity. The TransOs tunneler is introduced in an inverted fashion, penetrating the subdeltoid fascia low on the tuberosity. The tip is then rotated up into the previously created medial fixation point. Simultaneous tunnel creation and shuttle suture delivery are performed with the reusable tunneling device (TransOs, Tensor Surgical, Chattanooga, TN).
- Suture passage: The doubled suture is pulled through the superior awl portal and used to shuttle three high-strength sutures of different color through the tunnel for this "Xbox" style repair. The inferior tails of the sutures are clipped to the surgical drapes to prevent them from sliding or unloading. The sutures may now be managed intraarticularly, similar to an anchor-based repair.

- The previous two steps are repeated for the second, posterior tunnel. There are now two tunnels with three sutures (referred to as "triplets") in each tunnel.
- Suture passage through the tendon: Simple sutures are passed through the tendon with standard antegrade or retrograde techniques. They are stored in the anterior or superior portals.
- Creation of mattress, or "box" stitch: A different-colored medial suture tail from the anterior and posterior tunnel are retrieved from the lateral cannula and tied together outside the cannula. The inferior tails are used to slide the knot back into the joint and position the knot where it is most advantageous for the repair. This creates the medial mattress limb that compresses the tendon between the two tunnels and excludes synovial fluid from the repair. The lateral limbs of the box are left untied.
- Creation of "X" stitch: A superomedial tail from the posterior tunnel and an inferolateral tail from the anterior tunnel are retrieved through the lateral cannula and tied together. Pulling on the posterior inferolateral tail of the posterior tunnel and the superomedial tail of the anterior tunnel will reduce the knot into the joint at the medial footprint of the cuff wherever it is desired by the surgeon. The tails are left untied.
- Tying the simple sutures: Both tails of the anterior tunnel simple suture are retrieved through the lateral cannula and tied with a locking, sliding knot, using a lateral post based on the inferolateral tuberosity. The posterior simple stitch is then tied in the same manner. This step will reduce the cuff to its anatomic footprint by circumferential transosseous compression.
- Tying the mattress and crossing "X" stitch: The remaining tails of these two sutures are then tied lateral on the tuberosity. At this phase, the medial tails that have been left long can be positioned between the tunnel fixation points, optimizing cuff surface area compression from the lateral anchor. The lateral sutures of these limbs may be tied and cut.
- Anchor placement: The repair is now fully complete as a transosseous repair, which could be used as a stand-alone repair. However, the long medial tails offer an extra opportunity to independently and mechanically back up the construct with a single cost-effective anchor and also provide final tightening of the construct. The medial tails are brought through the lateral cannula and a knotless anchor is used to place them below the mattress stitch on the inferior portion of the tuberosity, creating a self-reinforcing construct based in the harder bone of the lower portion of the tuberosity. If dog-ears in the cuff are present, additional sutures may be incorporated to reduce them with the lateral anchor at this time.

12.4 Surgeon Tips and Tricks (Use of Specific Instrumentation)

- Keep the portal more inferior than an anchor portal by localizing a spinal needle just over the greater tuberosity. This angle makes it easier to achieve a large bone bridge in the hardest bone and works with the force of the deltoid to rotate the device lower on the humerus.
- Techniques may be used with simple sutures alone or knotless lateral row anchors early in the learning curve.
- Snap the inferior limbs of the sutures to the drapes to ease suture management in the suture passing step and prevent inadvertent unloading of the tunnel.

- Use sutures of different colors to ease suture management.
- If a suture unloads, more can be shuttled into the tunnel if there are any sutures left in the tunnel, or it may be retunneled. Unloading of a tunnel does not destroy the anchor point as does an unloaded anchor in the same position. This fact holds true for revision cases as well.
- Any tunnel can be substituted for an anchor if there is concern over soft bone with no repercussions. The 2.9/5.5 diameter mismatch will give the anchor higher torque in soft bone. If the awl can be inserted without the use of a mallet, we consider anchor augmentation; otherwise, transosseous fixation is sufficient for mechanical stability.
- Tapes may be used in the tunnel for the simple stitches to decrease plastic deformation of the bone and provide higher surface area compression.
- The anterior two-thirds of the proximal humerus may be tunneled from the anterior lateral portal; if a posterior tunnel is desired for a three-tunnel massive tear, the posterolateral portal is utilized to place the tunnel.

12.5 Pitfalls/Complications

- Suture cutting through soft bone: In our experience, this rarely happens with modern indications and instrumentation that avoids drilling and removing bone. If a tunnel does cut through intraoperatively, any other feasible fixation paradigm may be used as the diameters of the tunnels are small and bone-conserving. Lateral row anchors, buttons, screws, and tapes are all options for fixation in osteoporotic bone. Unlike loose hardware, fixation loss from suture cut through in the post-op phase would not necessarily result in revision surgery.
- Suture management: Suture management is facilitated by colored sutures, controlling/organizing the sutures on the field, and placing a cannula in the instrumentation portal, which serves to stabilize the inferior sutures.
- Revision concerns: Hybrid techniques are easily revised, as the tuberosity bone is conserved. Anchors may be placed into previous tunnels, or they may be retunneled. Revision of a tunneled repair is usually a type 1 failure, which conserves tendon substance. In severe bone defects, additional support can be achieved with screw fixation distally.
- Rehabilitation: No active motion for 6 weeks. Elbow range of motion and pendulums only. A graduated stretching and strengthen program are then implemented.

12.6 Rationale and/or Evidence for Approach

- Arthroscopic methods to achieve the gold standard transosseous cuff repair have now been described, which have similar biomechanics and clinical results, but decreased implant burden relative to anchor-based techniques.[1,2,3,4,5,6,7,8,9,10,11,12] Anchor-based and transosseous techniques for cuff repair may be used synergistically in the surgeon's armamentarium to treat complicated rotator cuff tears in the value-based era of medicine.[13,14,15,16,17] This hybrid approach is designed to maximize the number of fixation points per repair while minimizing complications and cost.[18,19,20,21,22,23]
- Basic science has supported several principles for rotator cuff repair: high initial fixation strength, adequate resistance to cyclic loading, and anatomic footprint reconstruction with crossing sutures meant to provide compression and decrease

shear forces at the tendon–bone interface.[24,25,26,27,28] Transosseous-equivalent techniques use anchors to mimic the desirable cerclage effect about the footprint created by true transosseous repair[29]. Because one anchor per fixation point is necessary, multiple anchors must be used to achieve this goal, increasing cost in the episode of care and potential hardware problems in the greater tuberosity. Many anchors achieve high strength and stiffness in adequate bone. However, some potential concerns regarding anchor fixation are tissue strangulation,[30] stress concentration,[31,32,33,34] and modulus mismatch at the anchor–suture–tendon interface. As the rotator cuff tissue is typically the weak link in the repair construct, certain very rigid anchor constructs may create an abrupt stress and strain transition that could lead to tendon transection at the medial anchor. Previous authors have described this "type 2" failure mode to be associated with, if not unique to, anchor constructs.[26,27] Transosseous techniques offer the advantage of high-density, double-row fixation points within a repair, excellent access to biologically active marrow elements through small diameter marrow vents, satisfactory biomechanics, and lower implant burden. A true transosseous, single-anchor hybrid technique could offer the clinical advantages of both paradigms to a maximal degree while achieving cost reproducibility in the episode of care. While the exact interplay of tension, vascularity, stiffness, ultimate failure strength, and other variables necessary in a rotator cuff repair remain unknown, it may be inferred that delivering a sufficiently strong biologically active repair in a sustainable manner is a key concern.

References

[1] Garrigues GE, Lazarus MD. Arthroscopic bone tunnel augmentation for rotator cuff repair. Orthopedics. 2012; 35(5):392–397

[2] Cicak N, Klobucar H, Bicanic G, Trsek D. Arthroscopic transosseous suture anchor technique for rotator cuff repairs. Arthroscopy. 2006; 22(5):565.e1–565.e6

[3] Kim KC, Rhee KJ, Shin HD, Kim YM. Arthroscopic transosseous rotator cuff repair. Orthopedics. 2008; 31(4): 327–330

[4] Garofalo R, Castagna A, Borroni M, Krishnan S. Arthroscopic transosseous (anchorless) rotator cuff repair. Knee Surg Sports Traumatol Arthrosc. 201 2; 20(6):1031–1035

[5] Fox MP, Auffarth A, Tauber M, Hartmann A, Resch H. A novel transosseous button technique for rotator cuff repair. Arthroscopy. 2008; 24(9):1074–1077

[6] Burkhart SS, Nassar J, Schenck RC, Jr, Wirth MA. Clinical and anatomic considerations in the use of a new anterior inferior submaxillary nerve portal. Arthrsocopy. 1996; 12(5):634–637

[7] Kuroda S, Ishige N, Mikasa M. Advantages of arthroscopic transosseous suture repair of the rotator cuff without the use of anchors. Clin Orthop Relat Res. 2013; 471(11):3514–3522

[8] Nho SJ, Shindle MK, Sherman SL, Freedman KB, Lyman S, MacGillivray JD. Systematic review of arthroscopic rotator cuff repair and mini-open rotator cuff repair. J Bone Joint Surg Am. 2007; 89 Suppl 3:127–136

[9] Black EM, Lin A, Srikumaran U, Jain N, Freehill MT. Arthroscopic transosseous rotator cuff repair: Technical note, outcomes, and complications. Orthopedics. 2015; 38(5):e352–e358

[10] Sanders B. Novel reusable transosseous tunnel based soft tissue repair techniques about the shoulder: A rational, value-based approach. Ortho Rheumatol. 2016; 5(1):00164

[11] Srikumaran U, et al. Arthroscopic transosseous anchorless vs anchored rotator cuff repair: A comparison of clinical and patient reported outcomes, structural integrity, and costs. Arthroscopy. 2016; 32(6):e22–e23

[12] Flanagin BA, Garofalo R, Lo EY, et al. Midterm clinical outcomes following arthroscopic transosseous rotator cuff repair. Int J Shoulder Surg. 2016; 10(1):3–9

[13] Churchill RS, Ghorai JK. Total cost and operating room time comparison of rotator cuff repair techniques at low, intermediate, and high volume centers: Mini-open versus all-arthroscopic. J Shoulder Elbow Surg. 2010; 19(5):716–721

[14] Genuario JW, Donegan RP, Hamman D, et al. The cost-effectiveness of single-row compared with double-row arthroscopic rotator cuff repair. J Bone Joint Surg Am. 2012; 94(15):1369–1377

[15] Adla DN, Rowsell M, Pandey R. Cost-effectiveness of open versus arthroscopic rotator cuff repair. J Shoulder Elbow Surg. 2010; 19(2):258–261

[16] Vitale MA, Vitale MG, Zivin JG, Braman JP, Bigliani LU, Flatow EL. Rotator cuff repair: An analysis of utility scores and cost-effectiveness. J Shoulder Elbow Surg. 2007; 16(2):181–187

[17] Narvy SJ, Ahluwalia A, Vangsness CT, Jr. Analysis of direct cost of outpatient arthroscopic rotator cuff repair. Am J Orthop. 2016; 45(1):E7–E11

[18] Jost PW, Khair MM, Chen DX, Wright TM, Kelly AM, Rodeo SA. Suture number determines strength of rotator cuff repair. J Bone Joint Surg Am. 2012; 94(14):e100

[19] Kummer FJ, Hahn M, Day M, Muslin RJ, Jazrawi LM. Laboratory comparison of a new arthroscopic transosseous rotator cuff repair technique to a double row transosseous equivalent repair using anchors. Bull Hosp Jt Dis. 2013; 71(2):128–131

[20] Bisson LJ, Manohar LM. A biomechanical comparison of transosseous-suture anchor and suture bridge rotator cuff repairs in cadavers. Am J Sports Med. 2009; 37(10):1991–1995

[21] Srikumaran U, Hannan C, Kilcoyne K, Petersen S, Mcfarland E, Zikria B. Arthroscopic anchored versus transosseous cuff repair: A comparison of clinical outcomes and structural integrity. Arthroscopy. 2016; 32(6):e22

[22] Russell RD, Knight JR, Mulligan E, Khazzam MS. Structural integrity after rotator cuff repair does not correlate with patient function and pain: A meta-analysis. J Bone Joint Surg Am. 2014; 96(4):265–271

[23] Kilcoyne KG, Guillaume SG, Hannan CV, Langdale ER, Belkoff SM, Srikumaran U. Anchored transosseous-equivalent versus anchorless transosseous rotator cuff repair: A biomechanical analysis in a cadaveric model. Am J Sports Med. 2017; 45(10):2364–2371

[24] Jo CH, Shin JS, Park IW, Kim H, Lee SY. Multiple channeling improves the structural integrity of rotator cuff repair. Am J Sports Med. 2013; 41(11):2650–2657

[25] Milano G, Saccomanno MF, Careri S, Taccardo G, De Vitis R, Fabbriciani C. Efficacy of marrow-stimulating technique in arthroscopic rotator cuff repair: a prospective randomized study. Arthroscopy. 2013; 29(5):802–810

[26] Cho NS, Yi JW, Lee BG, Rhee YG. Retear patterns after arthroscopic rotator cuff repair: Single-row versus suture bridge technique. Am J Sports Med. 2010; 38(4):664–671

[27] Trantalis JN, Boorman RS, Pletsch K, Lo IK. Medial rotator cuff failure after arthroscopic double-row rotator cuff repair. Arthroscopy. 2008; 24(6):727–731

[28] Lee TQ. Current biomechanical concepts for rotator cuff repair. Clin Orthop Surg. 2013; 5(2):89–97

[29] Franceschi F, Papalia R, Franceschetti E, et al. Double-row repair lowers the retear risk after accelerated rehabilitation. Am J Sports Med. 2016; 44(4):948–956

[30] Christoforetti JJ, Krupp RJ, Singleton SB, Kissenberth MJ, Cook C, Hawkins RJ. Arthroscopic suture bridge transosseus equivalent fixation of rotator cuff tendon preserves intratendinous blood flow at the time of initial fixation. J Shoulder Elbow Surg. 2012; 21(4):523–530

[31] Panella A, Amati C, Moretti L, Damato P, Notarnicola A, Moretti B. Single-row and transosseous sutures for supraspinatus tendon tears: A retrospective comparative clinical and strength outcome at 2-year follow-up. Arch Orthop Trauma Surg. 2016; 136(11):1507–1511

[32] McCarron JA, Derwin KA, Bey MJ, et al. Failure with continuity in rotator cuff repair "healing." Am J Sports Med. 2013; 41(1):134–141

[33] Sano H, Yamashita T, Wakabayashi I, Itoi E. Stress distribution in the supraspinatus tendon after tendon repair: Suture anchors versus transosseous suture fixation. Am J Sports Med. 2007; 35(4):542–546

[34] Sanders B, Lavery KP, Pennington S, Warner JJP. Clinical success of biceps tenodesis with and without release of the transverse humeral ligament. J Shoulder Elbow Surg. 2012; 21(1):66–71

13 All-Arthroscopic Anchorless Transosseous Rotator Cuff Repair

Aydin Budeyri, Raffaele Garofalo, and Sumant "Butch" Krishnan

Summary

Open transosseous rotator cuff repair was traditionally the gold standard technique for repair of the torn rotator cuff. All-arthroscopic transosseous (anchorless) rotator cuff repair is an exciting breakthrough over the last decade that combines the advantages of open techniques with a minimally invasive approach. It offers simple, biomechanically reliable, and anatomic tendon-to-bone healing. This all-arthroscopic anchorless approach also uniquely preserves bone tuberosity if a revision procedure ever becomes necessary.

Keywords: all-arthroscopic rotator cuff repair, anchorless, rotator cuff tear, transosseous

13.1 Case and Scope

The case and the scope of this chapter demonstrates a step-by-step instructional video guide (▶ **Video 13.1**) featuring the senior author's novel all-arthroscopic anchorless transosseous rotator cuff repair technique. The presented case specifically highlights key elements for a combined supraspinatus and anterior infraspinatus "L"-shaped complete tendon tear.

Chapter sections are the history, physical examination findings, preoperative radiologic findings, operative planning, patient positioning, preoperative work-up and equipments, intraoperative findings, technical steps, tips and pearls, postoperative period, physical therapy and rehabilitation, final functional status of the patient, and scientific evidence.[1]

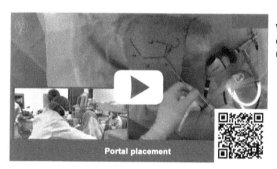

Video 13.1 Surgical demonstration of an all-arthroscopic transosseous rotator cuff repair.

Reference

[1] Flanagin BA, Garofalo R, Lo EY, et al. Midterm clinical outcomes following arthroscopic transosseous rotator cuff repair. Int J Shoulder Surg. 2016; 10(1):3–9

Suggested References

Post M, Silver R, Singh M. Rotator cuff tear: Diagnosis and treatment. Clin OrthopRelat Res. 1983(173):78–91

Ramsey ML, Getz CL, Parsons BO. What's new in shoulder and elbow surgery. J Bone Joint Surg Am. 2010; 92(4): 1047–1061

Garofalo R, Castagna A, Borroni M, Krishnan SG. Arthroscopic transosseous (anchorless) rotator cuff repair. Knee Surg Sports TraumatolArthrosc. 2012; 20(6):1031–1035

14 Fully Arthroscopic Transosseous Rotator Cuff Repair: A Reverse-Guided Technique

Jean Kany

Summary

The transosseous rotator cuff repair has been the gold standard since the very beginning of the open surgery. This chapter describes a fully arthroscopic transosseous procedure for small and medium-sized rotator cuff tears and highlights the above key elements (tips and tricks) as part of the repair. No anchors are implanted; therefore, there is no risk of implant loosening. There is no medial row; therefore, there is less risk of tendon necrosis or re-tear. We also describe the standard portals and rehabilitation process and typical timeline.

Keywords: rotator cuff repair, rotator cuff tear, transosseous suture

14.1 Patient Positioning and Portals (▶ Fig. 14.1)

Under general anesthesia supplemented by local nerve block for better postoperative analgesia in the beach chair position with the arm in a pneumatic arm holder (Spider, Smith & Nephew), a U-drape is placed around the shoulder starting from the neck. A rectangular drape is applied above the shoulder to connect legs of the U-drape, and, finally, arthroscopy drapes are placed. The following portals are used (see ▶ Fig. 14.1, ▶ Fig. 14.2, ▶ Fig. 14.3):

- The posterior (A): palpate the soft spot created by glenoid medially, the humeral head laterally and the rotator cuff superiorly. A general arthroscopic examination is done to assess the GH joint, address the rotator cuff tears and to manage biceps pathology.
- The anterolateral (B): 1 cm lateral to the anterolateral corner of the acromion, frontal to the AC joint. The long head biceps tenotomy (or tenodesis) is done with refreshment of the footprint of the supraspinatus. A bursoscopy, a debridement, and an acromioplasty (with resection of the coracoacromial ligament) are performed.
- Lateral portal (C): 4 cm lateral to the acromion in line with the posterior aspect of the clavicle. This portal shall create a parallel access to the footprint area. Draw an

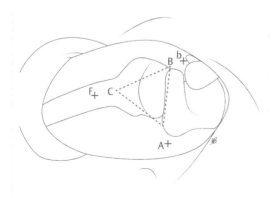

Fig. 14.1 Portals. "A" Soft point. "B" Anterosuperior portal (debridement and acromioplasty). "b" Superior working portal (Taylor Stitcher entry). Frontal to the AC joint. "C" Lateral portal (scope position, frontal to the cuff tear). "F" Shuttle-retrieving portal.

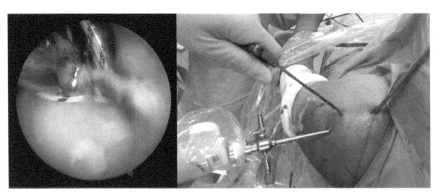

Fig. 14.2 Superior view. The switching stick is inserted through portal "b" and aligned with the humeral shaft while the suture grasper comes from portal "B" and arrives tangent to the footprint.

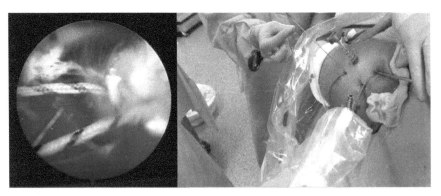

Fig. 14.3 Knots are tightening through the most distal portal "F" to prevent any bone-cutting fracture and to optimize the cuff reduction.

equilateral triangle at the base of the lateral edge of the acromion as from figure. Insert a smooth 8 mm clear cannula with a tapered obturator for an Express view grasper (Smith & Nephew).

- The superior anteromedial portal (b): superior working portal (Taylor Stitcher entry). Frontal to the AC joint.
- The posterolateral (F): in line with B (see ▶ Fig. 14.1), three fingers distally. Use this portal to retrieve sutures.
- Portal P: in line with B (see ▶ Fig. 14.1), two fingers distally. Use this portal to tie knots.

14.2 Surgical Technique

14.2.1 Debride and Prepare the Footprint

- Before inserting, check for the lateral aspect of the tuberosity. A working volume on the side is needed for a clear view and management of the sutures. (Place the shoulder at 20°–30° of abduction and 15°–20° of forward flexion.)

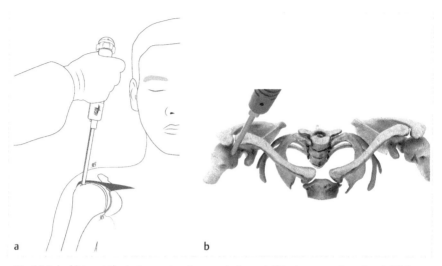

Fig. 14.4 (a, b) Insert the instrument main cannula through this above-mentioned portal "b" (superior anteromedial) and align it with the diaphysis (humeral shaft and long axis of the device must be as parallel as possible).

- Retract the superelastic transosseus needle (STN) needle by turning counterclockwise the gray knob in the tail of the Taylor Stitcher. Check for the correct STN tip exposure once completely within the cannula. Insert a shuttle (e.g., pds size 1) or directly load sutures.
- Use a needle to identify the superior anteromedial portal ("B"), frontal to the AC joint, to ascertain the long axis of the humeral shaft and simultaneously to be as perpendicular as possible to the supraspinatus footprint and close to the cartilage (▶ Fig. 14.4a,b).
- The rotator cuff tissue is evaluated for quality and mobility. How well it can be brought laterally without undue tension is assessed with a grasper. The natural tension of the rotator cuff tissue is respected. Ideally, the rotator cuff is supposed to be anatomically reduced onto its footprint. Gentle releases may be performed, especially release of the coracohumeral ligament from the superior edge of the coracoid process to help mobilize the rotator cuff reduction and decrease its tension after the repair.
- A starter punch is placed in the chosen tunnel position close to the cartilage of the humeral head.
- If needed, a second tunnel is placed depending on the size of the tear.

14.2.2 Deploy the Instrument

- Insert the instrument main cannula through this above-mentioned portal (superior anteromedial) and align it with the diaphysis (humeral shaft and long axis of the device must be as parallel as possible).
- Note: you may or may not use the targeting device. The punch included in the instrument kit can be used to create a pre-hole in the footprint area (optional).
- Check the laser mark on the flat surface of the guide containing the STN needle and orient this in the exit direction.

- Prepare to deploy the needle by gently taping the posterior part of the piston until the STN tip emerges in the lateral aspect of the tuberosity at 15–20 mm distally. Be careful to keep the guide in contact with the bone, avoiding being rejected and displaced during STN deployment.
- Once the STN needle emerges on the lateral side, act on the gray knob to slightly retrieve the STN needle and fold the shuttle. Grab the shuttle with a grasper by entering a distal and lateral portal (F) and completely retract the STN needle in the stainless-steel cannula (by turning the knob clockwise). Tighten knots from this distal and lateral portal (P) to prevent any bone cutting.
- Number of tunnels and sutures adopted depend on the lesion type, tear size, grade of retraction, elasticity and quality of the tissues, and type of repair configuration.

14.3 Surgeon Tips and Tricks

- Proper portal placement is important to optimizing a successful surgery. The lateral portal in the subacromial space placed at the midpoint of the rotator cuff tear ensures good visualization of the rotator cuff repair.
- Knots are tightening through the most distal portal (F) to prevent any bone-cutting fracture and to optimize the cuff reduction.
- Sutures are supposed to be convergent from medial to lateral, in the direction of the tunnel entry, reproducing the natural anatomy of the cuff.
- Before tying a sliding suture knot, take a suture grasper to reduce the cuff and slide both limbs of the sutures fully back.

14.4 Pitfalls/Complications

In case of soft bone with fracture while tightening sutures, we suggest using a double row knotless implant more laterally.

14.4.1 Rehabilitation

- The first goal is to protect the repair during the first 4 weeks to allow the repaired tissue to heal. Immobilization using an abduction sling will help accomplish this goal by allowing tension-free healing. The sling is worn 23–24 hours a day with gentle daily passive and pendular mobilization.
- After 4 weeks, active mobilization may be initiated with strengthening, typically 2–4 months after surgery depending on the patient recovery.

14.4.2 Rationale and/or Evidence for Approach

- Arthroscopic single-row rotator cuff repairs demonstrated a failure to heal of 20% to 30%.[1,2] It can restore only 67% of the anatomic surface of the footprint.[3]
- Arthrocopic double-row repair techniques were described to restore the native anatomy of the footprint[4] and biomechanical studies tend to prove a better and stronger coverage footprint fixation to improve healing rates.[5,6] The rate of cuff healing seems superior to the single-row technique.[7,8]
- However, multiple level I and II studies fail to demonstrate a difference in clinical outcomes and re-tear rates when comparing the two techniques.[9,10]

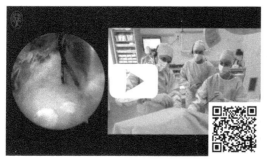

Video 14.1 Surgical demonstration of fully arthroscopic transosseous rotator cuff repair: a reverse- guided technique.

- Moreover, double-row short-term results have shown a high rate of re-tear larger than the primary lesion, probably because contact pressure that is too high with the medial-row mattress sutures induce which may a possible necrosis of the cuff tendon.
- Measurement of bone–tendon contact pressure in a continuous way with piezoelectric pressure gauges have shown that ideal pressure should be homogeneously spread onto the footprint.[11]
- Based on the aforementioned studies, Garofalo et al have strongly encourage a low tension repair performed best with a transosseous suture.[12] They try to (arthroscopically) reproduce the previous (open) gold standard techniques described by Codman, McLaughlin, Neer, De Palma, Rowe, Hawkins, and Graig.
- We describe a modification of the original Garofalo technique with a reverse guided transosseous technique (▸ **Video 14.1**).

14.5 Conclusion

If the cuff is anatomically reducible without any tension onto its footprint, we propose our aforementioned transosseous suture technique instead of a classical double-row technique. If the cuff is not anatomically reducible, we propose a classical single-row technique, as tension that is too high could induce tendon cuff necrosis and a larger re-tear than the primary lesion. If there are only tendons with a fatty muscle belly infiltration, we propose a fully arthroscopic latissimus dorsi tendon transfer.[13]

References

[1] Boileau P, Brassart N, Watkinson DJ, Carles M, Hatzidakis AM, Krishnan SG. Arthroscopic repair of full-thickness tears of the supraspinatus: Does the tendon really heal? J Bone Joint Surg Am. 2005; 87(6): 1229–1240

[2] Flurin PH, Landreau P, Gregory T, et al. Cuff integrity after arthroscopic rotator cuff repair: Correlation with clinical results in 576 cases. Arthroscopy. 2007; 23:340–346

[3] Apreleva M, Özbaydar M, Fitzgibbons PG, Warner JJ. Rotator cuff tears: The effect of the reconstruction method on three-dimensional repair site area. Arthroscopy. 2002; 18(5):519–526

[4] Lo IK, Burkhart SS. Double-row arthroscopic rotator cuff repair: Re-establishing the footprint of the rotator cuff. Arthroscopy. 2003; 19(5):1035–1042

[5] Meier SW, Meier JD. Rotator cuff repair: The effect of double-row fixation on three-dimensional repair site. J Shoulder Elbow Surg. 2006; 15(6):691–696

[6] Brady PC, Arrigoni P, Burkhart SS. Evaluation of residual rotator cuff defects after in vivo single- versus double-row rotator cuff repairs. Arthroscopy. 2006; 22(10):1070–1075

[7] Hantes ME, Ono Y, Raoulis VA, et al. Arthroscopic single-row versus double-row suture bridge technique for rotator cuff tears in patients younger than 55 years: A prospective comparative study. Am J Sports Med. 2018; 46(1):116–121

[8] Wade R, Salgar S. Clinico-radiological evaluation of retear rate in arthroscopic double row versus single row repair technique in full thickness rotator cuff tear. J Orthop. 2017; 14(2):313–318

[9] Spiegl UJ, Euler SA, Millett PJ, Hepp P. Summary of meta-analyses dealing with single-row versus double-row repair techniques for rotator cuff tears. Open Orthop J. 2016; 10:330–338

[10] Nicholas SJ, Lee SJ, Mullaney MJ, et al. Functional outcomes after double-row versus single-row rotator cuff repair: A prospective randomized trial. Orthop J Sports Med. 2016; 4(10):2325967116667398

[11] Grimberg J, Diop A, Kalra K, Charousset C, Duranthon LD, Maurel N. In vitro biomechanical comparison of three different types of single- and double-row arthroscopic rotator cuff repairs: Analysis of continuous bone-tendon contact pressure and surface during different simulated joint positions. J Shoulder Elbow Surg. 2010; 19(2):236–243

[12] Garofalo R, Castagna A, Borroni M, Krishnan SG. Arthroscopic transosseous (anchorless) rotator cuff repair. Knee Surg Sports Traumatol Arthrosc. 2012; 20(6):1031–1035

[13] Kany J, Anis H, Werthel JD. Massive irreparable rotator cuff tears: Treatment options, indications, and role of fully arthroscopic latissimus dorsi transfer. Obere Extremität. 2018; 13(89)

15 Double-Row Subscapularis Repair for Full-Thickness Subscapularis Tears

Grant Garcia, Hailey Casebolt, and Anthony Romeo

Summary

The subscapularis is the strongest rotator cuff muscle in the shoulder and, until this recent decade, most surgical repairs were performed through an open approach. In contrast, the reporting of arthroscopic repair techniques and outcomes is relatively limited. This is likely a result of the difficulty in all-arthroscopic repairs and the relative rarity of this injury in comparison to the supraspinatus and infraspinatus tendon. Even when arthroscopic repair is attempted, it can be challenging for an expert surgeon, and attempting a double-row repair adds further levels of complexity. Given these issues, we will provide our technique to improve potential complications that allow for a successful arthroscopic double-row supscapularis repair. This video chapter outlines background on double-row repair, portal placement, surgical technique, and tricks to avoid potential pitfalls.

Keywords: arthroscopy subscapularis, double-row, rotator cuff

15.1 Patient Positioning

- Beach chair position is our preferred technique (▶ **Fig. 15.1**).
  - Lateral decubitus position can be used based on surgeon preference.
- The patient is placed on the edge of the table and secured.
  - Two folded towels are placed behind the scapula.
  - The head is secured with a towel and tape. Care is taken to avoid excess flexion or extension of the neck.
- The shoulder is positioned in an orientation familiar to the surgeon.
  - We ensure the shoulder can move freely without blockage by the table. This is paramount, as maneuverability during the procedure facilitates easier surgical repair.
- Note: If unable to achieve adequate arthroscopic fixation, the beach chair position facilitates simple conversion to an open procedure.

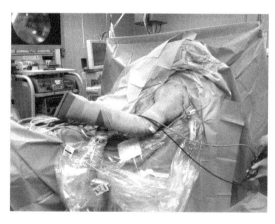

Fig. 15.1 This demonstrates our standard beach chair set-up. In addition, a mobile arm holder is used throughout the case as seen in this image.

15.2 Portal Placement (▶ Video 15.1, Part 1)

- Bony landmarks are drawn on the skin.
  - The acromion-clavicular articulation, clavicle, acromion, spine of the scapula, and coracoid process are identified and marked.
- The posterior portal is placed in the soft spot.
  - 2 cm inferior and 1 to 2 cm medial to the posterior lateral corner of the acromion.
- The anterior portal is just lateral to the coracoid.
  - Directly below the coracoacromial ligament.
- The lateral portal is placed 3 cm inferior to the lateral edge of the acromion.
  - In line with the midpoint of the anteroposterior distance on the acromion.
- An anterosuperior-lateral working portal is placed last.
  - This is two fingerbreadths off the edge of the anterolateral corner of the acromion.
  - In reference to the anterior portal, it is 1–2 cm superior and 2 cm lateral. This portal greatly improves the speed and ease of repair.
- The anterior and anterosuperior-lateral portals are the main working portals.
- The posterior portal is used for viewing.

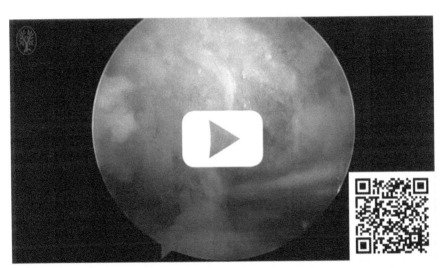

Video 15.1 The patient was placed in the beach chair position. A standard posterior portal was established followed by anterior, direct lateral, and anterosuperior under direct visualization. If significant adhesions are present, dissection of the axillary nerve may be necessary. To improve visualization, the biceps tendon was amputated and coracoplasty is performed with a 4.0-mm arthroscopic burr. The subscapularis was mobilized and the tendon approximated with an arthroscopic grasper. The footprint was prepared with an electrothermal device and 4.0-mm arthroscopic burr. The inferior medial-row anchor was placed. The suture was passed with a suture-passing device through the subscapularis in a medial to lateral angle. The superior medial anchor was placed next. Superior sutures were passed in a similar fashion. A superior mattress stitch may be placed. The bicipital groove was prepared with an electrothermal device and arthroscopic burr. A superior and inferior lateral row anchor was placed in the bicipital groove approximately 1 cm apart. Final fixation was performed through arthroscopic knot tying.

15.2.1 Portal Placement Technique

- All portal sites are injected with 0.25% bupivacaine and epinephrine.
- The posterior portal is placed with a blunt trocar.
- The anterior portal is established with an inside-out technique.
- The anterosuperior lateral portal localized with a spinal needle to allow optimization for repair.
  - Care is taken to avoid its convergence with the anterior portal.

15.3 Surgical Technique (Step-by-Step Approach)

- Basic principles of rotator cuff repair should be followed.
  - This pertains to both a primary and revision setting. This includes tendon mobilization, tear pattern recognition, footprint preparation, and a tension-free repair.
- We prefer a 30° scope throughout the procedure.
  - If there is difficulty with visualization a 70° scope can be used.
- Note: The subscapularis repair is performed first when involved with supraspinatus tear.
  - This is done because swelling can limit visualization and decrease appropriate working space in the anterior shoulder.

15.3.1 Steps

1. A systematic evaluation of the entire glenohumeral joint is performed (▶ **Video 15.1, Part 2**).
   - Any additional pathology requiring surgical repair is noted and will be added to the operative plan at this time.
2. A dynamic exam is performed of all rotator cuff tendons while viewing from the posterior portal.
3. Advancing the posterior scope to the anterior humeral margin improves visualization of the subscapularis.
   - A thorough evaluation of the anterior shoulder is performed.
     - Subscapularis retraction, subluxation of long head of the biceps and conjoint tendon involvement are often present.
   - An arthroscopic evaluation of the axillary nerve may be performed when there is significant retraction of the subscapularis tendon (▶ **Video 15.1, Part 3**).
4. Long head of the biceps tendon removal (▶ **Video 15.1, Part 4**).
   - The long head of the biceps tendon is frequently involved with supscapularis tears.
   - Generally, the medial sling is disrupted and there is subluxation (▶ **Fig. 15.2**).
     - Often there is preexisting pathology in the tendon as well. This is represented by either tendon fraying or edema.
   - Before the subscapularis mobilization, the tendon is amputated with arthroscopic scissors (▶ **Fig. 15.3**).
     - The intra-articular portion is debrided to the superior labrum.
     - The distal portion will later be tenodesed. The type of tenodesis is determined by the age and pathology of the patient. This will be discussed later in the chapter.
   - Removal of the biceps tendon from the groove improves visualization and mobilization of the subscapularis.
     - The proximal bicipital groove is the insertion point for our lateral row.

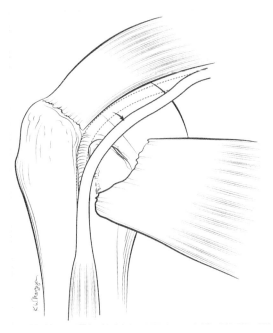

Fig. 15.2 This is a representative drawing of the subscapularis tear allowing for instability of the biceps tendon.

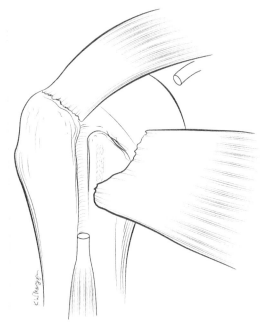

Fig. 15.3 This is a representative drawing of the removal of long head of the biceps tendon that allows for the mobilization of the subscapularis tendon.

5. The rotator interval is resected.
   - This allows better visualization of the coracoid.
     – Additional capsular tissue is also removed.
6. A coracoidplasty is performed from the anterior portal (▶ **Video 15.1, Part 5**).
   - Staying lateral—all fatty tissues are removed until the coracoid is reached.
   - An electrothermal device is used to clear the periosteum on the posterior coracoid (▶ **Video 15.1, Part 6**).
   - A 4.0-mm bur is then used to remove bone from the posterolateral aspect of the coracoid
     – This allows for more space anterior to the subscapularis. This is analogous to the subacromial decompression for the supraspinatus.
       Note: After debridement, there should be 5–10 mm of space between the coracoid and subscapularis.
7. Subscapularis tendon mobilization (▶ **Video 15.1, Part 7**).
   - A 360° release is performed.
     – Superior margin from coracoid.
     – Posterior from anterior capsule and scapular neck.
     – Inferior from axillary nerves and vessels.
     – Anterior from conjoined tendon.
       Note: Care should be taken not to debride the tendon.
   - This can be difficult in chronic retracted tears where the tendon morphology is distorted.
     – Additional release of the coracohumeral ligament structures is often needed for mobilization.
   - Attention is turned to the medial edge of the tendon to allow for further mobilization.
   - A 5.0 shaver is introduced, and all loose tissue is debrided.
   - The tendon edges are also freshened up at this time.
   - The middle glenohumeral ligament is identified and separated from the tendon.
     – This is done with our electrothermal cutting device.
8. Tendon approximation (▶ **Video 15.1, Part 8**).
   - The anterosuperior lateral portal is introduced.
     – An arthroscopic grasper is used from the anterolateral portal to identify maximal excursion of the tendon (▶ **Fig. 15.4**). This can help define the previously distorted anatomy of the tendon.
   - Also, this "excursion test" best defines the repair footprint.
     – A traction stitch can be used if needed.
       Note: If there is good quality tendon tissue without significant retraction, we prefer a double-row repair.
     – If there is significant retraction and tendon tissue loss, we proceed with a tension-free, single-row repair or augment the tendon,
9. Preparation of the footprint (▶ **Video 15.1, Part 9**).
   - This can be performed from an anterosuperior lateral or anterior portal.
     – The arm is internally rotated and abducted to deliver the tuberosity to the bur.
     – A 4.0 bur is used to clear the appropriate footprint.
     – This is performed down to bleeding bone.
     – Bone marrow stimulation is also performed prior to the placement of anchors.
10. Medial row anchor placement.

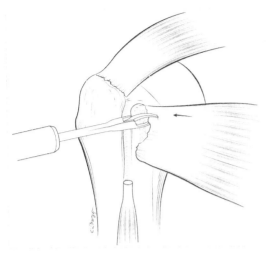

Fig. 15.4 This drawing demonstrates an arthroscopic grasper mobilizing the subscapularis tendon to reapproximate the footprint of the subscapularis.

15.3.2 Tips

- Suture anchors designed for cancellous bone are ideal for repair.
- The anterior portal is used for inserting the suture anchors.
  - Anchors are inserted 5 mm away from the articular surface.
- 4.75 mm SwiveLock anchors (Arthrex, Naples, FL) loaded with FiberTape (Arthrex) are used.
- The first anchor is placed at the inferior portion of the tear.
- All subsequent medial row anchors are placed further superiorly.
  - The number of medial row anchors varies with the size of tear. Generally, two are used.
  - We place one anchor per 1 cm of exposed footprint.

15.3.3 Inferior Medial Anchor Placement (▶ Video 15.1, Part 10)

- The anchor is placed after using a punch to facilitate insertion.
  - All sutures are then pulled through the anterior cannula.
- Using a switching stick, the cannula is removed and the sutures are pulled outside of the cannula through the same portal.
- The cannula is reinserted with the sutures on the outside.
- Suture passage is performed with a 30°SutureLasso (Arthrex) or a Penetrator (Arthrex) (▶ **Video 15.1, Part 11**).
  - A FastPass Scorpion (Arthrex) can greatly improve ease of passage and may be used in more difficult cases.
  - The suture should be passed at an angle medial to lateral through the entire tendon thickness. The articular side is more medial then the bursal side.
- This is usually 1 cm from the medial edge and 1 cm from the inferior portion of the tendon.

- A crochet hook is used to retrieve the shuttle suture from the lasso and the associated anchor sutures.
  - These are passed outside the shoulder through the anterosuperior lateral portal.
- The anchor suture is secured with a loop by the shuttle suture and passed back into the joint through the tendon and outside the cannula of the anterior portal (by a similar technique as previously described).
- All inferior sutures are passed outside of the anterior cannula to prevent tangling and to prepare for passage of the superior medial row.

15.3.4 Superior Medial Suture Placement (▶ Video 15.1, Parts 12 and 13)

- Once all inferior sutures are passed, the same process is repeated for the superior sutures.
- This is done using a second 4.75 SwiveLock anchor (Arthrex) loaded with Fiber Tape (Arthrex).
- The superior suture once passed is taken out though the anterosuperior lateral portal (▶ Fig. 15.5).
  - This separates the medial row sutures and prevents tangling.
1. Superior mattress stitch (▶ Video 15.1, Part 14).
   - Added fixation for the superior limb of the supscapularis is often needed.
     - Using a suture passage device, an inverted mattress suture is passed at the most superior portion of the tendon.
- This stitch reapproximates the rotator interval.
- The mattress stitch is retrieved through the lateral portal (▶ Fig. 15.6).
  - Once passage is completed, this stitch can be secured with a 4.75 SwiveLock (Arthrex) separately. This is placed in the superior lateral row just medial to the bicipital groove (▶ Fig. 15.7).
  - In most cases, this stitch is secured with the superior lateral row fixation along with one limb from each medial row of FiberTape (Arthrex) (▶ Video 15.1, Part 15).

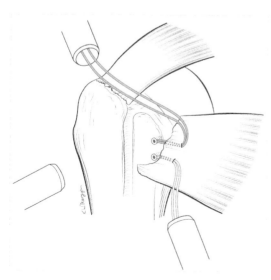

Fig. 15.5 Demonstrates placement of two medial row anchors and then passing these sutures from posterior to anterior through the subscapularis tendon. We typically used FiberTape that is wedged together, making it easier for single passage of both suture limbs.

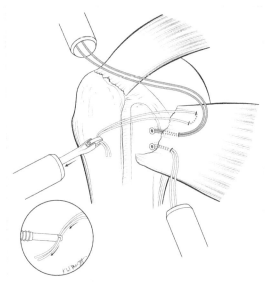

Fig. 15.6 Demonstrates an inverted mattress repair for the upper border of the subscapularis in which the FiberTape suture has been passed anterior to posterior and retrieved through the lateral cannula.

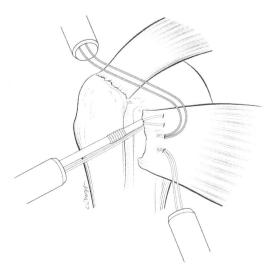

Fig. 15.7 This demonstrates an alternative use of the mattress suture in which the anchor is placed medial to the bicipital groove. Routinely, we place this suture with the superior lateral row anchor.

1. Lateral row fixation (▶ **Video 15.1, Parts 15 and 16**).
   - Once the all medial row sutures have been passed and separated, final fixation is performed.
   - One suture limb from each medial row anchor is retrieved from the lateral portal (▶ **Fig. 15.8**).
     - These are then loaded onto a 4.75-mm SwiveLock (Arthrex).
     - The bicipital groove is prepared with a bur and electrothermal device.
   - The loaded SwiveLock is then placed into the empty bicipital groove for the superior lateral row (▶ **Video 15.1, Part 15**).

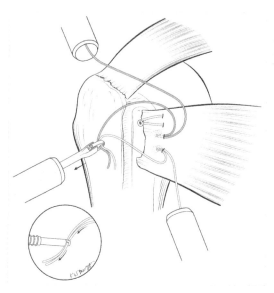

Fig. 15.8 This figure shows the grasping of one limb of each suture and the separation of each to form the superior lateral row.

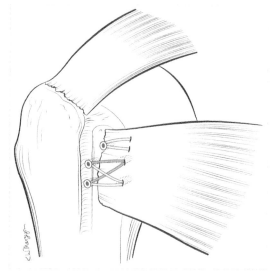

Fig. 15.9 This demonstrates placement of all lateral row anchors and the final repair. The inferior lateral anchor can be used for a biceps tenodesis if needed.

- The remaining medial suture limbs from each anchor are loaded on a second 4.75-mm SwiveLock (Arthrex), and this is placed in the bicipital groove to form the inferior lateral row (▶ **Video 15.1, Part 16**) (▶ **Fig. 15.9**).
2. Final testing (▶ **Video 15.1, Part 17**).
   - Once the original tendon has been secured, the shoulder is put through range-of-motion testing. This is done under arthroscopic visualization to assess the repair.
3. Biceps and supraspinatus repair.
   - Once the supscapularis is repaired, any remaining pathology is addressed. Generally, a double-row repair is also performed for the supraspinatus.

- This is often easier to perform once that the inferior rotator interval has been repaired.
- With most subscapularis tears, the medial sling of the biceps is disrupted. We perform a biceps tenodesis after most subscapularis repairs.
- Our preferred techniques are an arthroscopic tenodesis low in the groove or an open subpectoral tenodesis.

15.4 Surgeon Tips and Tricks

15.4.1 Tips

1. Visualization is key in this procedure.
   - Make sure adequate debridement is performed.
   - Clear the subcoracoid space.
   - A coracoidplasty is essential for adequate visualization and appropriate working room.
   - Make sure to extend full dissection to medial border of subscapularis to assess complete removal of adhesions.
   - Utilization of a 70° scope if necessary.
2. Suture management is very important.
3. Perform a posterior level push for additional space if needed.

15.4.2 Instruments (▶ Fig. 15.10)

- Basic shoulder arthroscopy set (probe, scissors, grasper, switching sticks, tissue punch, suture retriever, crochet hook, knot pusher, knot cutter).
- 30° and 70° arthroscope (4 mm).
- Articulated arm-holding device.
- Arthroscopic shaver and bur.
- Arthroscopic cannulas.
- Arthroscopic radiofrequency ablation device.
- Suture shuttling/passing devices.
- Suture anchors.
  – Medial row sutures: 4.75 mm SwiveLocks loaded with FiberTape (Arthrex).
  – Lateral row sutures: 4.75 mm SwiveLocks (Arthrex) unloaded.

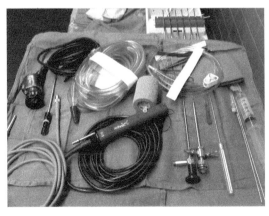

Fig. 15.10 This is an image of our standard arthroscopic set, including all tools necessary to perform all rotator cuff repairs and a biceps tenodesis.

- Sutures (FiberWire, Fibertape, polydioxanonesuture).
- Beach chair or lateral decubitus positioning devices.
- Biceps tenodesis implants (interference screw, anchor, or ENDOBUTTON devices).

15.4.3 Knots

Preferred technique is alternating half hitches. Two initial half hitches are placed, followed by three alternating half hitches.

15.5 Pitfalls/Complications

1. Full thickness tears are easier. Beware of partial tears as it may make it difficult to assess the lower edge of the subscapularis.
2. Poor visualization may occur, especially during a surgeon learning period.
   - A 70° arthroscope may be necessary.
   - Perform all releases and do not skip steps as visualization is very important.
3. Inappropriate tensioning.
   - All soft tissues need to be released.
   - The tendon may have more scarring then standard superior cuff pathology.
4. Overmobilization and neurovascular injury. If the tendon is overmobilized, injury may occur to the neurovascular structures.
5. Increased swelling may occur. Overdebridement of the rotator interval can cause increased swelling. In this case, prompt fixation is needed.
6. Rerupture.
   - Failure to reapproximate the appropriate tendon tension or anatomic footprint may cause failure.
   - Increased tension may increase pull-out risk of anchors.

15.6 Rehabilitation

1. Immediately post-op protocol.
   - Patient is initially placed in a sling. An abduction pillow is slid anteriorly to increase internal rotation. This decreases the strain on the repair.
   - Codman's and pendulums are started to facilitate gentle motion.
     Note: Specific rehabilitation determined based on including the size of the tear, quality of repair, tension on the repair, and variables related to the patient, such as chronic medical conditions.
2. The first 6 weeks, we restrict external rotation to 20° and forward elevation to 140°.
3. After 6 to 12 weeks, passive stretching is performed followed by active-assisted exercises.
4. After 12 weeks, strengthening begins. Specific sport training begins once adequate range-of-motion and strength returns.
5. After 6 to 9 months, full activity and return to sports is allowed.

15.7 Rationale and/or Evidence for Approach

An all-arthroscopic repair of the subscapularis is technically challenging. Appropriate steps to improve visualization and tendon mobilization are mandatory. While more difficult, a double-row repair offers the best success for improved functional outcomes and decreased rerupture rates.[1,2] Additionally, it has been found to biomechanical advantage over a single-row repair.[3] Both our clinical experience and this recent evidence demonstrate why we prefer an all-arthroscopic double-row subscapularis repair.

While double-row repair may have superior outcomes in a handful of studies, it is sometime not possible given certain tendon pathologies. As such, a brief discussion of single-row outcomes is warranted. One of the earliest series by Fox et al[4] reported their results on 14 patients with a single-row repair and greater than 1-year follow-up. Their average age was 56 years and all had good-to-excellent results. They had one failure after a traumatic fall with no other complications. American Shoulder and Elbow Surgeons scores improved from 46 to 82 postoperatively and 79% of patients had excellent Rowe functional scores. Another study by Burkhart and Tehrany[5] with 25 patients reported good results. Their UCLA scores improved from 11 to 31 and their forward flexion increased from 96° to 146°. This cohort was expanded 6 years later with 80% of patients reporting good-to-excellent results at 6 years with over 80% return to work and sport.[6] Bartl et al[7] reported their single-row results on 21 patients with a mean age of 44 years. They had a mean follow-up of 27 months and their lift-off strength (as measured by 100% of normal) improved from 65% to 87% while their belly press improved from 44% to 68%. Additionally, they reported Constant score improvements from 50 to 82. They had one patient with significant postoperative stiffness and one patient with a rerupture. A final study by Heikenfeld et al[8] demonstrated good results on 20 patients treated with a single row performed in the lateral position. Their mean age was 42 years with 90% male patients and an average follow-up of 24 months. Their UCLA scores improved from 16 to 33 and their Constant scores improved from 41 to 81. They had three complications including two reruptures and one reoperation.

The technical difficulties in double-row repair may be a reason for the dearth of literature on the topic. Only a few studies have reported results of double-row repair, with many of them combining single-row repair patients in their cohorts. Grueninger et al[9] performed a double-row repair on 11 patients with a mean age of 45 years. They had a mean follow-up of 12 months and 81% of patients were male. Constant scores improved from 43 to 89 postoperatively and lift-off strength and belly press improved from 2.9 to 4.8 (out of 5). They reported no complications. Lafosse et al[10] demonstrated good results in 17 patients with a mean age of 47 years. Their mean follow-up was 29 months with 76% male patients. They had a mixed cohort with 64.7% of these patients (11/17) receiving a double-row repair. Constant scores improved from 52 to 85 and UCLA scores changed from 16 to 32. Lift-off strength improved from 2.4 to 4.1 and belly press improved from 2.5 to 4.4. They reported two reruptures and two patients with complex regional pain syndrome, but all of these patients were in the single-row group. Lanz et al[11] reported on six patients with a mix of double- (two) and single-row (four) repairs. They had a mean follow-up of 29 months. Their Constant scores improved from 46 to 77 and UCLA scores improved from 14 to 30. No strength scores were reported, and they had no complications. A systematic review by Saltzman et al[2] evaluated all-arthroscopic subscapularis studies. They had eight studies that met their criteria and of these only three used a double-row repair in a portion of their patients. Overall, they found a lower rerupture rate with a double-row repair (0%) compared to a single-row technique (5%–10%). In addition, they reported better Constant strength score improvements with a double row (a change of 14) compared to a single row (a change of 9). Finally, they also found patients with the double-row technique often had higher grade preoperative tears, demonstrating a preference for a more robust repair with difficult cases.

15.8 Conclusion

As evident from these studies, there is limited literature on arthroscopic repair of the subscapularis tendon, especially in comparison to the infraspinatus and supraspinatus. One explanation may be difficult in an all-arthroscopic approach. While the evidence demonstrates superior pain and function outcomes after arthroscopic repair compared to open approaches,[5,12] it continues to be a topic with limited investigation. Additionally, when reported arthroscopically, a majority of repairs are performed with a single row.[2] More recent studies have found data suggesting better outcomes with a double row but further investigation is still needed.[1,2,13,14] In this chapter, we have outlined our technique to perform an all-arthroscopic, double-row subscapularis repair. Our goal is to improve the feasibility of this procedure to maximize both anatomic repair and integrity, with the potential of improved outcomes.

References

[1] Denard PJ, Burkhart SS. Arthroscopic recognition and repair of the torn subscapularis tendon. Arthrosc Tech. 2013; 2(4):e373–e379

[2] Saltzman BM, Collins MJ, Leroux T, et al. Arthroscopic repair of isolated subscapularis tears: A systematic review of technique-specific outcomes. Arthroscopy. 2017; 33(4):849–860

[3] Wellmann M, Wiebringhaus P, Lodde I, et al. Biomechanical evaluation of a single-row versus double-row repair for complete subscapularis tears. Knee Surg Sports Traumatol Arthrosc. 2009; 17(12):1477–1484

[4] Fox JA, Noerdlinger MA, Romeo AA. Arthroscopic subscapularis repair. Tech Shoulder Elbow Surg. 2003; 4(4):154–168

[5] Burkhart SS, Tehrany AM. Arthroscopic subscapularis tendon repair: Technique and preliminary results. Arthroscopy. 2002; 18(5):454–463

[6] Adams CR, Schoolfield JD, Burkhart SS. The results of arthroscopic subscapularis tendon repairs. Arthroscopy. 2008; 24(12):1381–1389

[7] Bartl C, Salzmann GM, Seppel G, et al. Subscapularis function and structural integrity after arthroscopic repair of isolated subscapularis tears. Am J Sports Med. 2011; 39(6):1255–1262

[8] Heikenfeld R, Gigis I, Chytas A, Listringhaus R, Godolias G. Arthroscopic reconstruction of isolated subscapularis tears: Clinical results and structural integrity after 24 months. Arthroscopy. 2012; 28(12):1805–1811

[9] Grueninger P, Nikolic N, Schneider J, et al. Arthroscopic repair of traumatic isolated subscapularis tendon lesions (Lafosse type III or IV): A prospective magnetic resonance imaging-controlled case series with 1 year of follow-up. Arthroscopy. 2014; 30(6):665–672

[10] Lafosse L, Jost B, Reiland Y, Audebert S, Toussaint B, Gobezie R. Structural integrity and clinical outcomes after arthroscopic repair of isolated subscapularis tears. J Bone Joint Surg Am. 2007; 89(6):1184–1193

[11] Lanz U, Fullick R, Bongiorno V, Saintmard B, Campens C, Lafosse L. Arthroscopic repair of large subscapularis tendon tears: 2- to 4-year clinical and radiographic outcomes. Arthroscopy. 2013; 29(9):1471–1478

[12] Mall NA, Chahal J, Heard WM, et al. Outcomes of arthroscopic and open surgical repair of isolated subscapularis tendon tears. Arthroscopy. 2012; 28(9):1306–1314

[13] Koh KH, Kang KC, Lim TK, Shon MS, Yoo JC. Prospective randomized clinical trial of single- versus double-row suture anchor repair in 2- to 4-cm rotator cuff tears: Clinical and magnetic resonance imaging results. Arthroscopy. 2011; 27(4):453–462

[14] Lapner PL, Sabri E, Rakhra K, et al. A multicenter randomized controlled trial comparing single-row with double-row fixation in arthroscopic rotator cuff repair. J Bone Joint Surg Am. 2012; 94(14):1249–1257

16 Arthroscopic Single-Row Subscapularis Tendon Repair

Howard D. Routman and Jack E. Kazanjian

Summary

Arthroscopic rotator cuff repair of the posterosuperior cuff has become the gold standard for soft tissue repairs in the shoulder during the past decade. This has been borne out in the literature with outcomes and healing rates equivalent to open rotator cuff repair. With the technical advances that have been made arthroscopically, the authors believe that these benefits have improved our ability to treat disorders of the subscapularis as well. All-arthroscopic, single-row repair of the subscapularis is achievable for most tears of the subscapularis. This chapter will take a step-by-step approach through the authors preferred approach to this problem from positioning through postsurgical rehabilitation including surgical tips and tricks.

Keywords: arthroscopically, single row, subscapularis repair

16.1 Patient Positioning

- General anesthesia with interscalene block is utilized routinely.
- The patient is positioned in a beach chair position with a pillow under the knees.
- All bony prominences are padded to avoid contact pressure during the procedure.
- A head-holder is used to support and protect the head and spine.
- A commercial beach chair positioner can be used; otherwise, the patient will need to be placed on the lateral edge of the table ensuring adequate access to the shoulder for portal placement.
- Sequential compression devices are applied to the lower extremities.
- The nonoperative arm is positioned in a well-arm holder or secured to the body in a neutral position.
- After positioning is finalized, the bony landmarks of the shoulder are marked and final confirmation that the positioning allows for camera/drill/instrumentation access.
- Examination under anesthesia is performed and the findings documented.
- Clear U-drapes are placed at the medial most aspects of the field, defining the extent of surgical prep.
- The arm, scapula, and chest are prepped in the usual sterile fashion.
- Surgical U-drapes are used proximally to drape the shoulder.
- A waterproof stockinette is used on the arm above the elbow and then the arm is wrapped in Coban, avoiding tightly wrapping this around the ulnar nerve area.
- A pneumatic arm holder is attached to the patient's arm for positioning during the case.
- Systolic blood pressure is maintained at 90–110 mmHg to maximize intraoperative hemostasis and cerebral oxygenation.

16.2 Surgical Technique

- The anterior and posterior clavicle, coracoid, acromioclavicular joint, and acromion, as well as the anterior and posterior borders of the scapular spine, should be drawn on the skin to assist with portal placement. The location of the conjoined tendon off the tip of the coracoid is noted.

- The shoulder joint is entered with a standard 30° scope via a posterior soft-spot portal. This portal is typically 2 cm inferior and 2 cm medial to the posterolateral corner of the acromion.
- The anterior portal is done via an outside-in technique with an 18-gauge spinal needle. The portal is typically inferior to the palpated coracoid and is just above and lateral to the subscapularis intraoperatively.
- A diagnostic glenohumeral arthroscopy is performed identifying all relevant pathology. The biceps tendon is very frequently subluxed and/or torn. Critical evaluation of preoperative imaging of the biceps with regard to subluxation is important. Only in situations in which the biceps demonstrates that it is in nearly perfect condition should it be spared. For most cases of a known subscapularis tear, a biceps tenotomy is performed initially; later, subpectoral tenodesis can be performed at the end of the procedure if tenotomy is not desired.
- Frequently, a superior rotator cuff tear is encountered during the diagnostic arthroscopy; this makes the subscapularis repair easier as the surgeon can gain access to the joint through the superior defect if needed.
- The subscapularis tear and/or "comma" tissue can readily be identified with a 30° arthroscope.
- In cases of partial tears, a 70° arthroscope is utilized to determine the size of the tear and whether repair is needed.
- The rotator interval tissue is removed using a shaver, specifically avoiding injury to the "comma." The conjoined tendon and coracoid are then identified. At this point, the soft tissue on the posterior coracoid can be released with an electrocautery device to evaluate the bony structure of the undersurface of the coracoid, assess the retro-coracoid space, and determine whether a coracoplasty will be required.
- The undersurface coracoid is subsequently skeletonized being knowledgeable of the relevant adjacent anatomy.
- Even if a coracoplasty is not being performed, this step helps to open up the surgical field for eventual passage and visualization of sutures and makes a difference in suture management.
- If subcoracoid impingement is noted, a gentle posterior coracoplasty can be performed with a bur. Using a 4.2 acromionizer bur working from the anterior portal, a 6- to 8-mm template is created anteriorly and then completed using a cutting block technique posteriorly along the coracoid. A flat surface is created with this technique.
- After adequate retro-coracoid space is confirmed, cannula placement for subscapularis repair is planned.
- A clear cannula can be placed through the portal anteriorly; a second cannula can be placed through the superior rotator cuff tear(if present).
- All secondary portals are performed via an outside-in technique with an 18-gauge spinal needle.
- If the tear is isolated to the subscapularis, a second rotator interval portal can be made adjacent to the superior cuff, just adjacent to the anterolateral corner of the acromion.
- We then switch to a 70° scope for the remainder of the subscapularis procedure.
- A 360° release of the subscapularis is performed utilizing shavers, rasps, liberators, and electrocautery.

- Grasping instruments are then used to assess the tension, mobility, and reparability of the subscapularis.
- Traction sutures can be utilized at this point if needed. The "comma" tissue is usually robust and is a good traction suture location.
- The lesser tuberosity is then prepared; all soft tissue is removed with a shaver and electrocautery. The tuberosity is then prepared with a rasp, shaver, and bursimilar to standard footprint preparation for posterosuperior repairs. Aggressive bone removal is discouraged, only freshening of the bone bed is needed.
- In cases of complete tears, two double-/triple-loaded anchors are utilized for a total of four to six sutures. For partial repairs, one double-/triple-loaded anchor is utilized.
- Anchor placement is performed through the anterior rotator interval cannula starting inferiorly.
- A 90° lasso device is used to penetrate the subscapularis tissue from the anterior cannula. The passing suture is initially brought out through the anterosuperior cannula. Care should be taken to make sure that the subscapularis is not retracted medial to the joint line when using the lasso device, as inadvertent vascular injury can occur. For retracted tears that have been mobilized, penetration of the tendon should be done with the tendon pulled into the field of view to avoid a blind passage of the penetrating device medially.
- The inferior anchor suture placement is typically in a horizontal mattress pattern.
- Once all sutures are passed, the sutures are then tied from inferior to superior using an arthroscopic knot-tying technique.
- We prefer a sliding-locking knot; however, this is not a critical component of the operation. Any arthroscopic knot that the surgeon is comfortable with would be adequate for repair.
- Traction sutures can be helpful to position the tendon precisely during the tying down of the repair.
- If a full tear is present, a second anchor will frequently be required.
- If a second anchor is placed, sutures are passed as a horizontal mattress pattern with the exception of the superior suture on the upper anchor; this is a simple suture pass that loops over the top of the subscapularis tendon, locking it into place.
- If only one anchor is used (for a partial repair), the pattern of suture placement is horizontal inferiorly with a simple suture superiorly.
- The sutures are tied and the repair is completed.
- The scope is switched backed to a 30° scope to visualize and document the repair.
- All remaining procedures are then completed as needed. See accompanying
  - ▶ **Video 16.1** demonstrating this surgical technique.

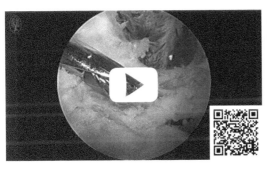

Video 16.1 Surgical demonstration of an arthroscopic single-row subscalpularis tendon repair technique.

16.3 Surgeon Tips and Tricks

- Portals and cannulas should be placed while using the 30° scope.
- The "comma" tissue is the superolateral border of the subscapularis, including the coracohumeral ligament and superior glenohumeral ligament and can be used as a traction suture location.
- Be liberal in removing rotator interval tissue for visualization. If there is the need for more than one anchor and more than four limbs of suture to manage the subcoracoid space, this dissection and clearing of this space helps with suture management.
- Preparation and mobilization of the subscapularis tear should be performed with the 70° scope; be aware of relevant anatomy! The axillary artery/nerve and musculocutaneous nerve are all 25 mm from the coracoid.
- 360° release of the subscapularis involves anterior release from the coracoid, posterior release off the glenoid, and a superior release off of the lateral arch/neck of coracoid. Rasps and liberators work well anteriorly and posteriorly; cautery superiorly.
- Avoid dissection medial to the midportion of the coracoid.
- Traction sutures may not be needed. A grasping instrument from one of the portals can be used to assist in mobilization and suture placement.
- One anchor per square centimeter of the tuberosity is needed—two for full tears, one for partial is a good guideline.
- If difficulty is encountered with anchor or pilot-hole creation because of the patient's head getting in the way, change the rotation of the arm. Consider shoulder flexion, extension, and internal and external rotation changes with a posterior translation on the humerus to achieve an easier passage into the lesser tuberosity.
- Suture management is critical, as the anterior space can be easily congested. Marking the suture pairs and separating the sutures from each individual anchor immediately upon insertion can save a lot of time and frustration.
- Tie each anchor one at a time; it helps reduce the tear and simplifies the procedure.
- If tension is noted on the repair, forward flex and internally rotate the arm.

16.4 Post-Op Rehabilitation

- Initial protection of the repair in an abduction sling for 6 weeks.
- Start formal physical therapy at an average of 4 weeks, being mindful of the tissue quality and tear size.
- Passive range of motion for the first 6 weeks.
- Limit forward flexion to 90°; limit external rotation (ER) to 0°–20° for good quality tissue; however, if tissue quality is poor, more aggressive restrictions can be applied.
- No biceps resistance if tenodesis has been performed for at least 6 weeks.
- At 6 weeks, remove sling and start full active range of motion if tissue quality is good, longer in the sling if the tissue quality is poor.
- At 12 weeks, start resistance.
- At 6 months, unrestricted overhead activities.

16.5 Rationale and Evidence

- The subscapularis is the largest and strongest rotator cuff muscle and plays a very important role for the stability and function of the shoulder joint.[1]

- Open rotator cuff repair frequently missed the presence of subscapularis tearing, and with the introduction of arthroscopic techniques, the normal and abnormal states of the subscapularis were more easily seen.[2]
- With advanced imaging, critical physical examination, and arthroscopic visualization, subscapularis tears are no longer the "forgotten" rotator cuff tear of the shoulder and are more readily recognizable.
- Anatomic repair of the subscapularis should be achievable arthroscopically in the hands of a facile arthroscopist; however, a well-done open subscapularis repair is far better than a poorly done arthroscopic attempt.[3] This technique should be approached as any other arthroscopic technique, learning it incrementally and confirming satisfactory execution with open incisions as needed.
- Arthroscopic single-anchor, single-row repair for upper third subscapularis tears has been shown to have good integrity rates on post-repair imaging.[4]
- Positive clinical subscapularis-specific physical examination findings that are present preoperatively in patients that have a successful repair and rate their results highly may never normalize in some patients.[5,6]
- Arthroscopic repair of isolated subscapularis repairs has been shown to achieve good results,[7] with better outcomes with small full-thickness tears as compared to high-grade partial thickness tears.[8]
- In a systematic review of arthroscopic subscapularis tear repair surgery, Saltzman, et al[9] showed that concomitant treatment of the biceps with tenodesis contributes to better overall results. Surgeons should bear in mind that in the case of a well-repaired subscapularis tear, unaddressed biceps pathology can negatively impact outcomes. Therefore, the threshold for biceps treatment should be considered low in these cases.

References

[1] Keating JF, Waterworth P, Shaw-Dunn J, Crossan J. The relative strengths of the rotator cuff muscles. A cadaver study. J Bone Joint Surg Br. 1993; 75(1):137–140

[2] Bennett WF. Arthroscopic subscapularis repair: a look at primacy from a historical perspective. Arthroscopy. 2014; 30(6):661–664

[3] Mall NA, Chahal J, Heard WM, et al. Outcomes of arthroscopic and open surgical repair of isolated subscapularis tendon tears. Arthroscopy. 2012; 28(9):1306–1314

[4] Rhee YG, Lee YS, Park YB, Kim JY, Han KJ, Yoo JC. The outcomes and affecting factors after arthroscopic isolated subscapularis tendon repair. J Shoulder Elbow Surg. 2017; 26(12):2143–2151

[5] Gerber, Christian, Otmar Hersche, and Alain Farron. "Isolated rupture of the subscapularis tendon. Results of operative repair." JBJS 78.7 (1996): 1015–23

[6] Edwards, T. Bradley, et al. "Repair of tears of the subscapularis." JBJS 87.4 (2005): 725–730

[7] Lafosse L, Jost B, Reiland Y, Audebert S, Toussaint B, Gobezie R. Structural integrity and clinical outcomes after arthroscopic repair of isolated subscapularis tears. J Bone Joint Surg Am. 2007; 89(6):1184–1193

[8] Katthagen JC, Vap AR, Tahal DS, Horan MP, Millett PJ. Arthroscopic repair of isolated partial- and full-thickness upper third subscapularis tendon tears: Minimum 2-year outcomes after single-anchor repair and biceps tenodesis. Arthroscopy. 2017; 33(7):1286–1293, and Millett PJ

[9] Saltzman BA. Collins MJ, Leroux T, et al. Arthroscopic repair of isolated subscapularis tears: A systematic review of technique-specific outcomes. Arthroscopy. 2017;33:849–860

Suggested Readings

Burkhart SS, Tehrany AM. Arthroscopic subscapularis tendon repair: Technique and preliminary results. Arthroscopy. 2002; 18(5):454–463

Fox JA, Noerdlinger MA, Romeo AA. Arthroscopic subscapularis repair. Tech Shoulder Elbow Surg. 2003; 4:154–168

17 Arthroscopic Single Row Subscapularis Repair

Michael Bender and Hussein Elkousy

Summary

This chapter demonstrates an arthroscopic single-row repair technique for tears of the subscapularis tendon. Tears of the subscapularis tendon are often underrecognized and their importance underappreciated. They have been historically treated through open techniques because of the difficulty with visualization, exposure, mobilization, and instrumentation. However, improvements in arthroscopic techniques and instrumentation have allowed us to better diagnose and adequately treat them with an arthroscope. Our technique demonstrates helpful steps for adequate visualization, including arm positioning, camera placement, and portal placement. Mobilization of the tendon and appropriate releases are crucial to restore it to the footprint without excessive tension. Repair techniques vary by numbers of rows, suture patterns, management of the long head of the biceps, type of camera used, and intra- versus extraarticular approaches. We generally prefer to use a single-row, extraarticular technique, using a 30° angle camera for the majority of tears. The corresponding biceps pathology is typically managed with an arthroscopic suprapectoral tenodesis or tenotomy. We demonstrate that subscapularis tears can be successfully repaired via arthroscopic techniques as effectively as open techniques.

Keywords: arthroscopic, biceps tenodesis, extraarticular, rotator cuff repair, rotator interval, single row, subscapularis

17.1 Patient Positioning

- A general anesthetic combined with an interscalene block is typically used.
- The goal of the interscalene block is to allow hypotensive anesthesia to minimize bleeding and improve visualization (▶ **Fig. 17.1**).
- We use a beach chair position with the assistance of an adjustable arm holder (▶ **Fig. 17.2**).
- A specialized bed is used to support the cervical spine, while keeping the shoulder girdle exposed (▶ **Fig. 17.3**, ▶ **Fig. 17.4**, ▶ **Fig. 17.5**).

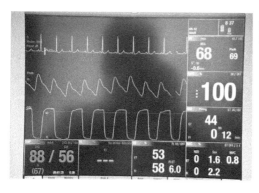

Fig. 17.1 Anesthesia monitor showing hypotensive anesthesia.

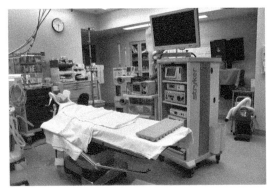

Fig. 17.2 Operating room setup with special bed and arm holder attached.

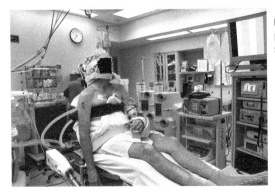

Fig. 17.3 Frontal view of patient positioning and operating room setup.

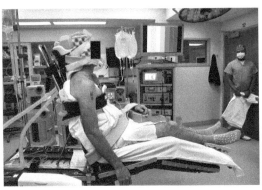

Fig. 17.4 Side view of patient positioning.

17.2 Portal Placement

- Four separate portals are used in the majority of our subscapularis repairs, although this can vary based on additional pathology being addressed at the time of surgery (▶ Fig. 17.6).
- With the exception of the posterior portal, all portals are established with an outside-in technique.

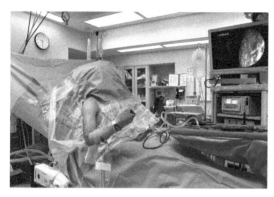

Fig. 17.5 Patient positioning after preparing and draping the operative field.

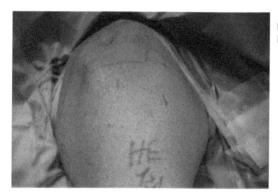

Fig. 17.6 View of proposed portals in a right shoulder.

- Bony landmarks and potential portal sites are marked at the beginning of the case for reference only.
- The posterior viewing portal is established approximately 1 cm inferior and in line with the posterolateral corner of the acromion. This is the initial viewing portal in the glenohumeral joint and on entry into the subacromial space. During subscapularis repair and biceps management, it is used for suture management and for soft tissue traction (rotator cuff or long head of biceps).
- The anterior portal is established second while in the glenohumeral joint. A spinal needle is used to mark the entry point through the lateral aspect of the rotator interval. This portal is used for initial palpation of the subscapularis, mobilization, and release of anterior capsule and adhesions of the subscapularis fossa, excision of the middle glenohumeral ligament (MGHL) when necessary, tenotomy of the proximal biceps, anchor placement in the lesser tuberosity, suture management, and occasionally for suture passage through the subscapularis (▶ **Fig. 17.7**, ▶ **Fig. 17.8**). At the conclusion of glenohumeral arthroscopy, the camera is also placed here for more thorough evaluation of the subscapularis and posterior structures of the glenohumeral joint (▶ **Fig. 17.9**).
- A lateral portal is established after the subacromial space is entered, 2 cm lateral to and at the midline of the lateral border of the acromion. This portal is used for the initial bursectomy but becomes the primary viewing portal for a majority of the bursectomy, biceps management, and subscapularis repair.
- Last, an anterolateral portal is established, typically 3–5 cm inferior to the anterolateral corner of the acromion and in line with the bicipital groove. It is placed

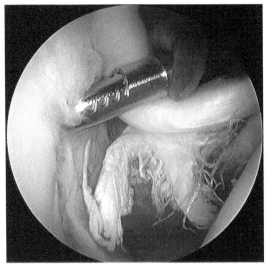

Fig. 17.7 Anterior portal used to assess and address the long head of biceps pathology.

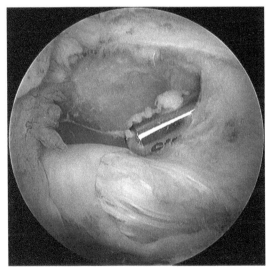

Fig. 17.8 Anterior portal used to debride capsule and expose the subscapularis.

with the arm forward flexed to 70°–90° and in neutral-to-mild external rotation. It is the primary working portal for biceps management, lesser tuberosity footprint preparation, assessment of subscapularis reduction, interval release, and suture passage for the repair (▶ **Fig. 17.10**).

17.3 Surgical Technique

17.3.1 Diagnostic Arthroscopy

- Our posterior viewing portal is first established as described above and the 30° arthroscope is inserted.

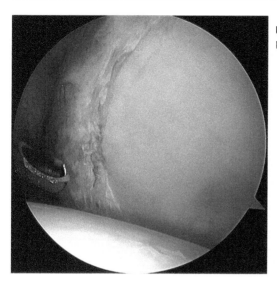

Fig. 17.9 Anterior portal view of the posterior joint compartment.

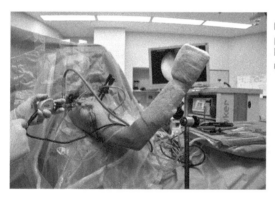

Fig. 17.10 Arthroscope in the lateral portal with all other portals established and the arm in final position for repair.

- The pump pressure is set at 60 mmHg and allowed to distend the capsule.
- A spinal needle is then used to localize and establish the anterior portal through the rotator interval, and a 5.5 mm translucent cannula is inserted.
- A probe is inserted, and a full diagnostic arthroscopy is performed.
- The subscapularis is examined thoroughly from the posterior viewing portal by positioning the arm in flexion and internal rotation. Appreciating the full extent of a subscapularis tear is crucial and can be challenging. Longitudinal splits in the subscapularis tendon are common, easily seen, and may not need to be addressed surgically. But superior third tears of the articular surface or hidden pulley lesions that may impact management can be missed if a thorough assessment is not performed[1,2] (see Surgeon Tips and Tricks).
- A probe is used through the anterior portal to feel the tension on the subscapularis and attempt to lift the lateral tendon off its footprint. A "comma" sign formed by the fibers of the superior glenohumeral ligament and the coracohumeral ligament complex is a common finding to help identify the superior and lateral margin of subscapularis tears, as described by Lo and Burkhart.[3] For larger or more complex

tears, an arthroscopic tissue grasper is helpful in lifting the tendon to see the footprint or pulling more medially retracted fibers laterally to better define the tear. Complete tears are often retracted medially and scarred to the overlying fascia (▶ Fig. 17.11, ▶ Fig. 17.12, ▶ Fig. 17.13, ▶ Fig. 17.14, ▶ Fig. 17.15, ▶ Fig. 17.16, ▶ Fig. 17.17, ▶ Fig. 17.18, ▶ Fig. 17.19, ▶ Fig. 17.20, ▶ Fig. 17.21, ▶ Fig. 17.22).

- The long head of the biceps tendon and its pulley are carefully inspected by pulling the biceps into the joint. If there is significant subscapularis pathology, we will cut the biceps at this point with arthroscopic scissors just above its labral attachment and lightly debride the remaining stump with a shaver. Further biceps management is addressed later (▶ Fig. 17.23, ▶ Fig. 17.24, ▶ Fig. 17.25).

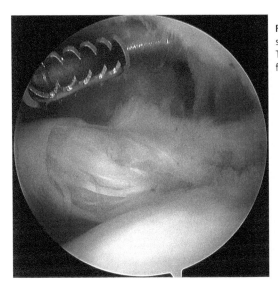

Fig. 17.11 Superior third tear of the subscapularis in a right shoulder. The detachment will be viewed from the subacromial space.

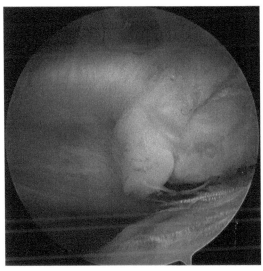

Fig. 17.12 Superior third tear of the subscapularis in a right shoulder with the arm in mild internal rotation.

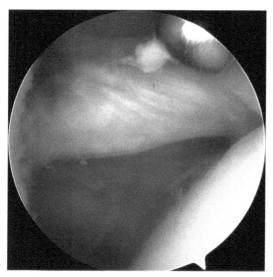

Fig. 17.13 Superior half detachment of the deep surface of the subscapularis in a right shoulder with the arm in external rotation. The inferior one half is attached with a void above it extending to the superior rolled border.

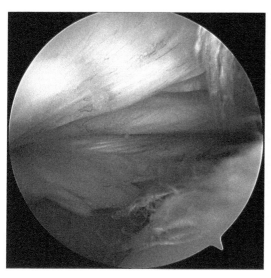

Fig. 17.14 The same shoulder as in ▶ **Fig. 17.13** with the arm internally rotated showing a void and inability to see the attachment suggesting a deep surface tear.

- A shaver and cautery are used to debride adhesions of the subscapularis fossa, excise anterior capsule, excise the MGHL if deemed necessary, expose the conjoint tendon, and partially expose the undersurface of the coracoid.
- The arthroscope is placed through the anterior cannula to complete visualization of the tear prior to entering the subacromial space (▶ **Video 17.1**).

17.3.2 Subacromial Assessment and Decompression

- A blunt trocar is used to redirect the posterior viewing portal into the subacromial space.

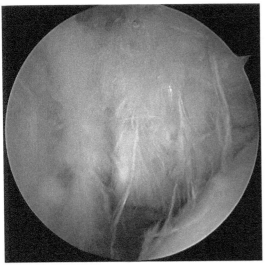

Fig. 17.15 Posterior portal view of a right shoulder showing a macerated long head of biceps stump from the prior spontaneous rupture.

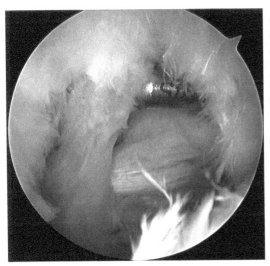

Fig. 17.16 Same shoulder as in ▶ Fig. 17.15 with the biceps stump partially debrided. The middle glenohumeral ligament, subscapularis, and the interval attachment (beneath the shaver) to the superior subscapularis are noted.

- The lateral portal is established, and a 4.5 shaver is used to begin the initial bursectomy. Once subacromial visualization is improved, a switching stick is used to move the arthroscope to the lateral portal.
- 5.5 mm cannulas are then directed into the subacromial space from the previously established anterior and posterior portals.
- A shaver and electrocautery are then used to complete the remainder of the bursectomy and decompression up to the anterior border of the acromion. Any additional rotator cuff pathology is not addressed until after the subscapularis repair.

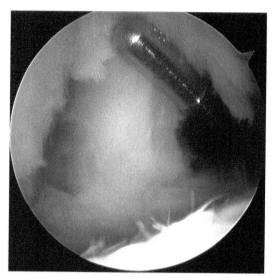

Fig. 17.17 Same shoulder as in
▶ Fig. 17.15 showing the "comma sign."

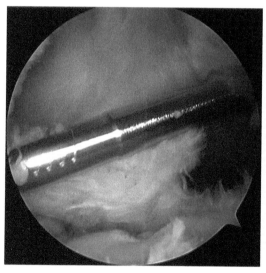

Fig. 17.18 Same shoulder as in
▶ Fig. 17.15 after debridement of the interval showing the conjoined tendon and coracoacromial ligament attachments to the coracoid.

17.3.3 Biceps Management

- We reposition the arm into forward elevation and mild external rotation to bring the bicipital groove into view from the lateral portal.
- Our anterolateral accessory portal is now established by localizing it with a spinal needle over the bicipital groove.
- We place an 8 mm cannula in this portal to accommodate suture-passing devices and instruments (▶ Fig. 17.26).
- The bicipital sheath is first released along the lateral margin with electrocautery. Once exposed, the end of the tendon is grabbed with a tissue grasper from the

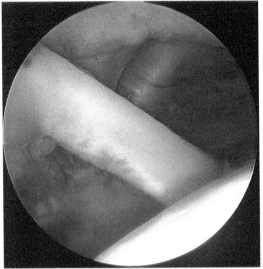

Fig. 17.19 A chronic, retracted subscapularis tear in the right shoulder of a young laborer. The long head of the biceps is subluxated anteriorly. The structure behind it at the 12 to 1 o'clock position is the coracoacromial ligament. The structure at the 11 to 12 o'clock position is the retracted "comma." The subscapularis superior half retracted medially and superiorly and the posterior face is in the left lower quadrant of the image.

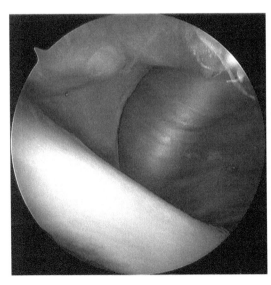

Fig. 17.20 Close-up view of the comma sign, coracoacromial ligament, and long head of the biceps from ► **Fig. 17.19**.

posterior portal to provide tension while we release the sheath more inferiorly (► **Fig. 17.27,** ► **Fig. 17.28,** ► **Fig. 17.29,** ► **Fig. 17.30**).
- The tendon is thoroughly examined. If it is deemed that the tissue quality is poor, a tenotomy is done. If the tissue quality is acceptable, a tenodesis is done. Regardless of the choice, a complete synovectomy is done of the biceps sheath.
- If a tenodesis is chosen, the groove is prepared by debridement with a shaver and rasp to create a healing surface. A metal punch is inserted through the anterolateral portal and impacted low in the groove. A 4.5-mm Healix PEEK

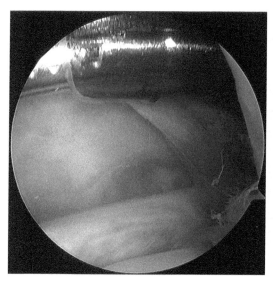

Fig. 17.21 Same shoulder as in ▶ **Fig. 17.19** showing the attached inferior and deep portion of the subscapularis. The tissue on the left and superior to the attached portion is the posterior surface of the torn and retracted subscapularis/interval complex.

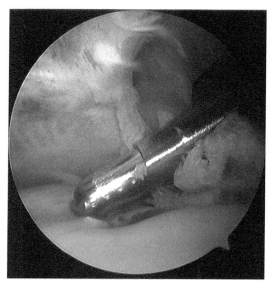

Fig. 17.22 Same shoulder as in ▶ **Fig. 17.19** showing the inferior attached subscapularis distal to the tip of the shaver. The detached subscapularis is between 8:30 and 10:30. The comma sign is superior to that.

double-loaded suture anchor (DePuy Mitek, Raynham, MA) is then inserted, and the suture tails are removed out of the posterior cannula (▶ **Fig. 17.31,** ▶ **Fig. 17.32,** ▶ **Fig. 17.33**).

- An EXPRESSEW III (DePuy Mitek) suture passer is used through the anterolateral portal to pass one limb of one suture through the biceps tendon while it is held under mild tension. This passed suture is then cerclaged around the tendon one time and then tied to the other limb. This is then repeated for the second suture. The excess proximal tendon is then cut and removed (▶ **Fig. 17.34,** ▶ **Fig. 17.35,** ▶ **Fig. 17.36**).

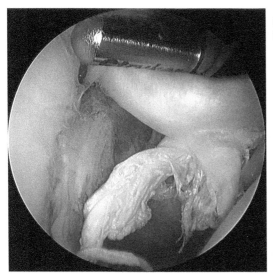

Fig. 17.23 Tear of the long head of the biceps in a right shoulder.

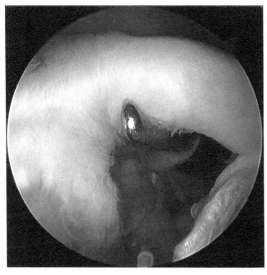

Fig. 17.24 The biceps is cut proximally. It will be assessed more distally for tenodesis versus tenotomy.

17.3.4 Anterior Bursectomy and Tear Mobilization

- The arm is kept in the same forward flexed position. Internal and external rotation can be adjusted as needed (▶ **Fig. 17.37**).
- The cautery is used from the anterolateral portal to follow the groove proximally to enter the glenohumeral and release the interval if it is intact. This is done superior to the superior rolled edge of the subscapularis (▶ **Fig. 17.38**, ▶ **Fig. 17.39**, ▶ **Fig. 17.40**, ▶ **Fig. 17.41**, ▶ **Fig. 17.42**, ▶ **Fig. 17.43**, ▶ **Fig. 17.44**).

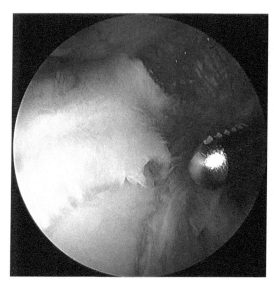

Fig. 17.25 Stump of the biceps after it is cut.

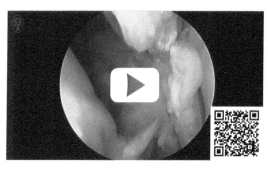

Video 17.1 Surgical demonstration of an arthroscopic single row subscapularis tendon repair technique.

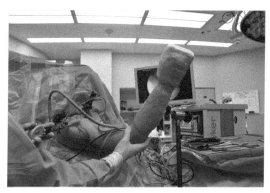

Fig. 17.26 Red 8 mm cannula is in the anterolateral position of a right shoulder.

- Cautery and shaver are then alternated for intraarticular and extraarticular debridement, exposing the undersurface of the acromion, the conjoint tendon, and the lateral and superior borders of the subscapularis.

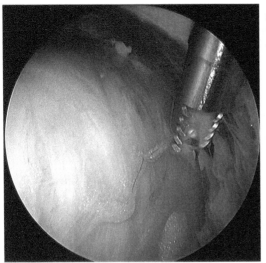

Fig. 17.27 Shaver from the antero-lateral portal palpating the lateral aspect of the biceps groove in a right shoulder.

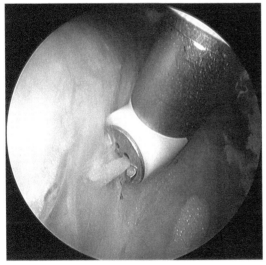

Fig. 17.28 Cautery form the ante-rolateral portal initiating exposure of the biceps sheath in a right shoulder.

- If the tear is retracted, the interval is released to the base of the coracoid. Traction can be placed on the anterior supraspinatus or the subscapularis using graspers in the anterior or posterior portals (▶ Fig. 17.45, ▶ Fig. 17.46, ▶ Fig. 17.47, ▶ Fig. 17.48, ▶ Fig. 17.49).

17.3.5 Tuberosity Preparation and Anchor Placement

- A standard shaver is then inserted through the anterolateral portal to debride any residual interval tissue off the upper border of the tendon and then lightly decorticate the lesser tuberosity footprint. We do not typically find that an aggressive bur is necessary for footprint preparation (▶ Fig. 17.50, ▶ Fig. 17.51).

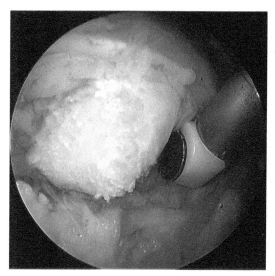

Fig. 17.29 Cut proximal end of the long head of the biceps in a right shoulder.

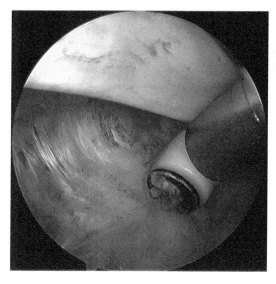

Fig. 17.30 Long head of the biceps pulled proximally and medially to expose the groove in a right shoulder.

- A tissue grasper used through a separate portal can aid in footprint preparation by elevating the subscapularis to improve visibility while using the shaver.
- Depending on the size of the tear, we are usually able to repair the tendon with one or two 4.5-mm Healix PEEK double-loaded suture anchors spaced 1 cm apart.
- The punch for the anchors is inserted through the anterior cannula because this provides the best angle to insert the anchors perpendicular to the bony surface.
- The most inferior anchor is placed first.
- All anchors are generally placed first and they are placed in the lateral third of the prepared footprint. The sutures are then moved to the posterior cannula for suture management purposes (▶ **Fig. 17.52**).

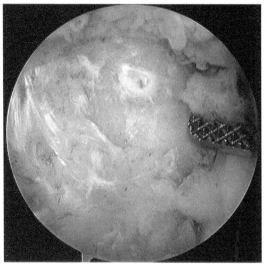

Fig. 17.31 Rasp used to prepare the groove.

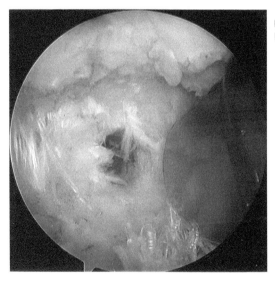

Fig. 17.32 Pilot hole prepared for a PEEK anchor.

17.3.6 Suture Passage and Tendon Repair (▶ Fig. 17.53, ▶ Fig. 17.54, ▶ Fig. 17.55, ▶ Fig. 17.56, ▶ Fig. 17.57, ▶ Fig. 17.58, ▶ Fig. 17.59, ▶ Fig. 17.60, ▶ Fig. 17.61)

- We typically use an EXPRESSEW III (DePuy Mitek) needle-passing device to pass sutures through the torn subscapularis. There are several brands available.
- Occasionally, the needle-passing device does not allow access to attain the angle or depth of passage needed; therefore, a tissue penetrator ("bird beak") is used at times.

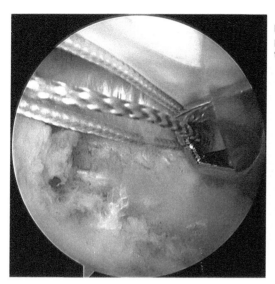

Fig. 17.33 The anchor has been placed and one suture passed for tenodesis.

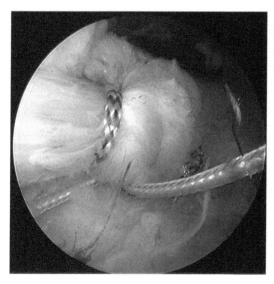

Fig. 17.34 One suture of the tenodesis has been tied in a right shoulder.

- All four limbs of the two sutures from each anchor are passed, starting from the distal or inferior aspect first. A cruciate pattern is created. So, in a right shoulder, the order of suture passage, if facing the shoulder from anteriorly, is at the 6 o'clock, 3 o'clock, 12 o'clock, and 9 o'clock positions.
- Sutures are retrieved through the anterior portal once passed and all four limbs of sutures from one anchor are clamped together.
- All sutures from all anchors are generally passed before they are tied.
- Within each anchor, the sutures are tied first at the 6 o'clock and 12 o'clock positions. This prevents the sutures in line with the subscapularis fibers from pulling through the tendon.

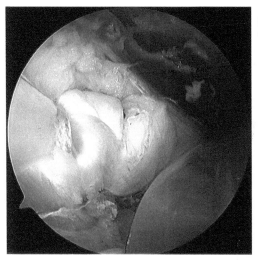

Fig. 17.35 Both sutures of the tenodesis have been tied in a right shoulder.

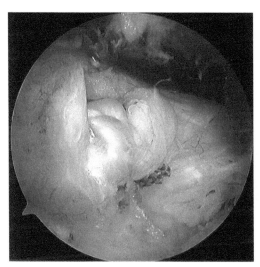

Fig. 17.36 Completed tenodesis in a right shoulder.

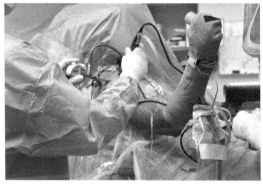

Fig. 17.37 Right arm kept in the forward flexed position for the subscapularis repair.

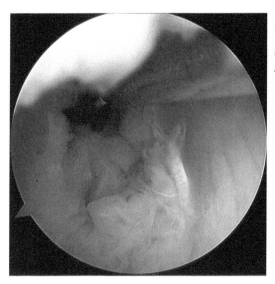

Fig. 17.38 Same shoulder as ▶ Fig. 17.11 finding the interval defect to enter the glenohumeral joint.

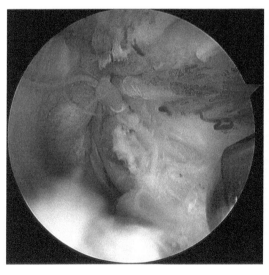

Fig. 17.39 Same shoulder as ▶ Fig. 17.11 with the camera in the joint through the lateral portal and the posterior surface of the subscapularis tear on the right.

- If more than one anchor is placed, the order of tying sutures from each anchor varies based on visualization and ease of reduction. It is often best to tie the superior anchor sutures first to set the reduction.

17.4 Surgeon Tips and Tricks

- The ability to manipulate arm position in the beach chair position is very helpful as opposed to a lateral decubitus position.[4]

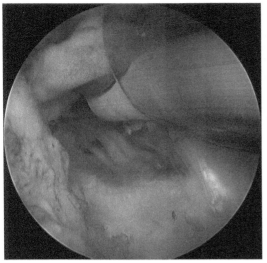

Fig. 17.40 Same shoulder as ▶ **Fig. 17.12** with a more obvious tear and viewing the defect from the subacromial side. The cautery is holding the subscapularis up away from the lesser tuberosity below.

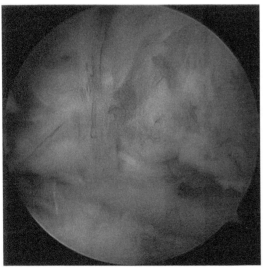

Fig. 17.41 Same shoulder as ▶ **Fig. 17.12** with the camera now in the joint with the subscapularis on the right.

- Despite using an outside-in technique for marking the portals, always outline bony landmarks and potential portal sites at the beginning of the case for reference. Once the soft tissue is swollen from arthroscopy, these markings can be helpful.
- A fluid pump is used generally with the pressure set at 60 mm Hg to allow for good visualization. This can be intermittently and briefly raised if needed.
- The anterior portal is placed in the lateral aspect of the rotator interval so that it allows for a perpendicular approach to the subscapularis insertion for anchor placement and for initiation of release of adhesions and interval tissue in the subscapularis fossa.

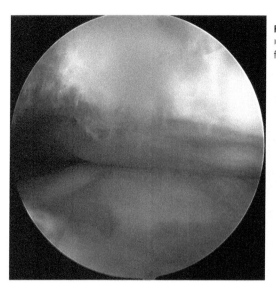

Fig. 17.42 Same shoulder as ▶ **Fig. 17.13** viewing the defect from the subacromial space.

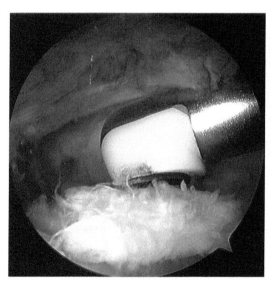

Fig. 17.43 A right shoulder with an associated anterior supraspinatus tear showing the cautery removing the medial attachment of the interval to the biceps groove.

- Much has been written on the difficulty of viewing the subscapularis insertion from a posterior portal using a 30°arthroscope.[5] We have several maneuvers that allow us to assess this insertion relatively thoroughly. First, positioning the arm in mild flexion and internal rotation allows for improved visualization of the attachment site. Having an assistant push the proximal humerus posteriorly and simultaneously pulling the distal humerus anteriorly can further enhance visualization.[5] Moving the arm in internal and external rotation allows us to evaluate whether the subscapularis is moving with humeral motion. This is a functional test and may overlook smaller

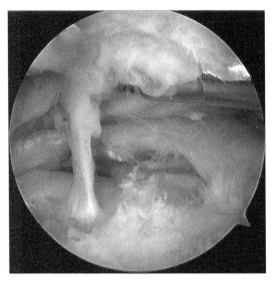

Fig. 17.44 Exposed lesser tuberosity of the same shoulder as ▶ Fig. 17.43.

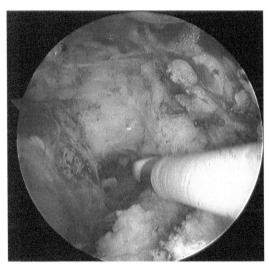

Fig. 17.45 Right shoulder viewed exposing the undersurface of the coracoid to release a scarred subscapularis.

tears. We then place the arthroscope anterior to directly view the subscapular insertion. Finally, we enter the joint via the biceps groove from the subacromial space and examine the subscapularis from this extraarticular position.

- An interval release is key for full mobilization of large retracted tears. This begins in the glenohumeral space using a combination of electrocautery and a 4.5 shaver through the anterior portal to release the rotator interval tissue directly superior to the rolled border of the subscapularis from the coracoid toward the biceps groove laterally. The MGHL is released in these retracted cases. This interval release is completed from the subacromial side by exposing the lateral base of the coracoid using a cautery from the anterolateral portal.

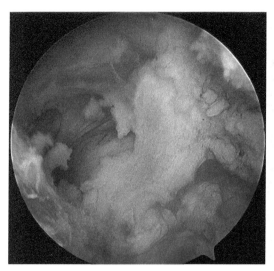

Fig. 17.46 Same shoulder as ▶ **Fig. 17.45** showing the superior border of the subscapularis beneath the exposed coracoid with moderate adhesions still present laterally.

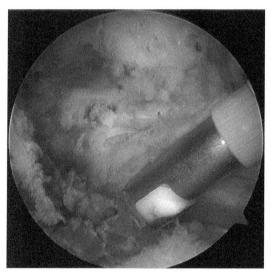

Fig. 17.47 Same shoulder as ▶ **Fig. 17.45** showing better exposure of the subscapularis after partial release is complete.

- We never repair the subscapularis without addressing the long head of the biceps, although the opposite may occur in which the biceps is addressed without repairing the subscapularis.
- Placement of anchors is facilitated by externally rotating the arm and passage of sutures using a needle-passing device is facilitated by internally rotating the arm.
- Using an 8 mm cannula in the anterolateral portal is important to allow the needle-passing device to easily fit through.
- Always visualize the suture pass from both the articular and bursal side of the tendon. This is an advantage afforded by the extraarticular approach taking down the interval.

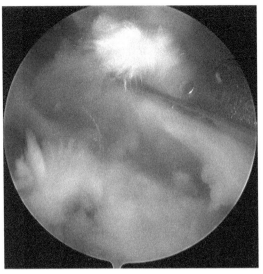

Fig. 17.48 Same shoulder as ▶ **Fig. 17.16**, showing the superior corner of the subscapularis tear being grasped after extensive releases to pull it laterally.

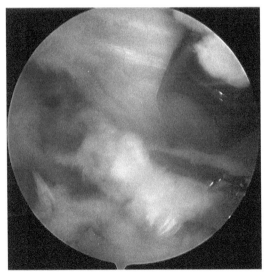

Fig. 17.49 Trial reduction of the subscapularis from the prior figure.

- When a tissue penetrator is used, the suture to be retrieved can be delivered to this instrument using a knot pusher.
- We recommend completing the subscapularis repair before moving on to repair of the supraspinatus or infraspinatus if needed. Because this is typically the most difficult part of the case to visualize and repair, it makes sense to do it first before fluid extravasation and excessive bursal tissue can obstruct one's view. An unrepaired full thickness supraspinatus or infraspinatus tear gives the added benefit of improved articular visualization of the subscapularis tendon from the lateral viewing portal.

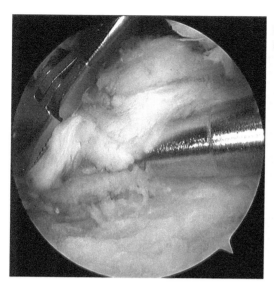

Fig. 17.50 Lesser tuberosity prepared in a right shoulder.

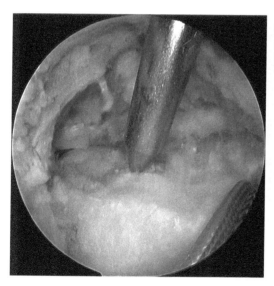

Fig. 17.51 One anchor has been placed inferior and lateral and the pilot hole for the second anchor is being prepared.

- Our preference is to use 4.5 mm PEEK double-loaded suture anchors for the repair. In our experience, this size of anchor is large enough to provide adequate pull-out strength for repairing this large musculotendinous unit, but not too large to limit spacing for multiple anchors if necessary. The PEEK material is preferred over metal anchors to ease any revision procedure and to allow for future magnetic resonance imaging (MRI) assessment if needed.

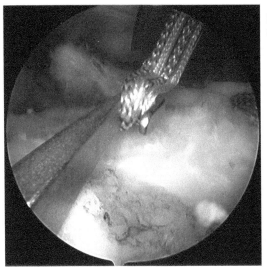

Fig. 17.52 Sutures from the superior anchor moved to the posterior portal.

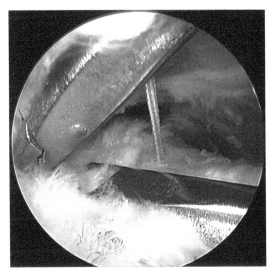

Fig. 17.53 Needle-passing device in a right shoulder with a small tear.

17.5 Pitfalls and Complications

17.5.1 Missed Tears

- MRIs can be less sensitive for subscapularis tears,[6,7] so a thorough physical exam and arthroscopic diagnostic exam should still be performed on the shoulders to uncover many of these hidden lesions and prevent persistent disability.

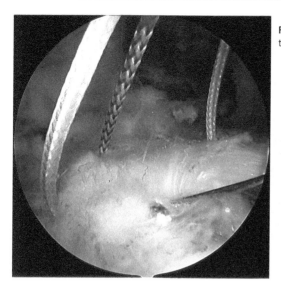

Fig. 17.54 Final suture being passed to create cruciate pattern.

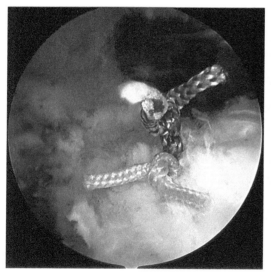

Fig. 17.55 Sutures tied in a right shoulder.

17.5.2 Complete and Retracted Tears

- Often associated with trauma or shoulder dislocation in older patients, complete and retracted tears can be very challenging with delayed treatment.
- Emphasis should be placed on expedited diagnosis with MRI in this clinical scenario and earlier surgical treatment while an arthroscopic repair is still possible. As muscle atrophy and fatty infiltration progress, the results for arthroscopic repairs and healing rates decline.

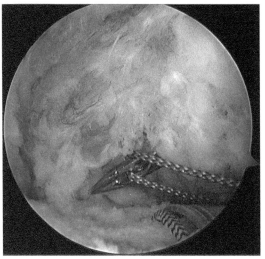

Fig. 17.56 A larger tear with alternative suture-passing technique using a tissue penetrator in a right shoulder.

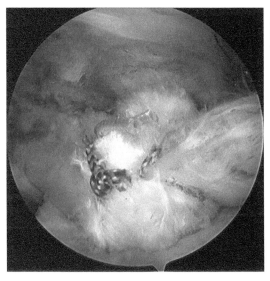

Fig. 17.57 All four suture limbs ties in the completed repair of the tear from ► Fig. 17.16.

- While addressing complete and retracted tears is more difficult, most of these tears can still be repaired arthroscopically with careful and patient tear mobilization.[8] The comma sign as mentioned before can be a guide to find the superior and lateral margin when the tissue planes are difficult to distinguish.[3] Tissue graspers holding tension on the tendon while doing releases can also be helpful.
- Open repair of these tendons is always still an option as a backup plan, but they do come with reported higher infection rates.[9]

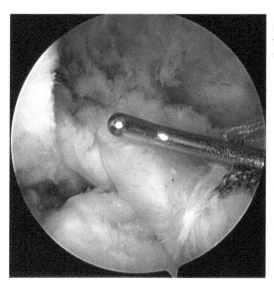

Fig. 17.58 The completed repair from ▶ **Fig. 17.16** showing the tension restored to the subscapularis.

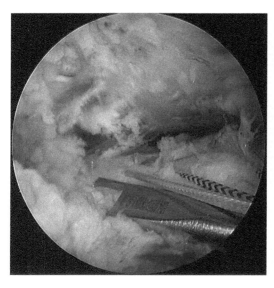

Fig. 17.59 A superior suture being passed in the retracted tear from ▶ **Fig. 17.19** using the more inferior passed sutures for lateral traction.

17.5.3 Re-Tear

- Re-tear rates of isolated subscapularis tears are estimated at 4.8%–11.8% in previously reported studies.[10] Potential factors involved can include tear size, poor tissue quality and biologic factors, fatty infiltration, age, reinjury, or failure to comply with protective rehabilitation protocols.

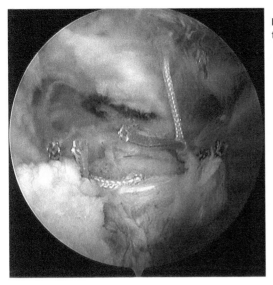

Fig. 17.60 Suture tied down for the tear from ▶ **Fig. 17.19**.

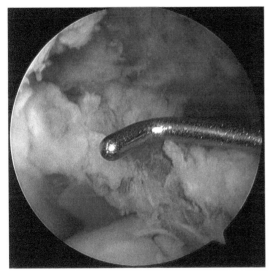

Fig. 17.61 The superior border of the repaired subscapularis from ▶ **Fig. 17.19**.

17.5.4 Infection

- While this can be a devastating complication, it is fortunately a rare occurrence with an estimated incidence of 0.0016%–0.44% in arthroscopic repairs compared with 0.27%–2.45% in open rotator cuff repairs.[9]

17.6 Rehabilitation

- Sling with an abduction pillow for 4 weeks.
- No active elbow flexion for 6 weeks if a biceps tenodesis was done.
- No active internal rotation or passive external rotation beyond 20° for 4 weeks but varies depending on size of tear and tension on repair.
- Passive and active assist range of motion only for the first 8 weeks.
- Active range of motion starts at 8 weeks.
- Gentle strengthening may start at 12 weeks.
- Release to activity at 6 months.
- Rehabilitation protocol adjusted based on other pathology treated, size of the tears, and tissue quality.

17.7 Rationale and Evidence for Approach

- The biceps is always addressed with subscapularis repair because it is either damaged, has caused the subscapularis pathology, or may compromise the repair.
- We can visualize and mobilize the subscapularis as well arthroscopically as we open.[8,10,11]
- We have had success with single-row open subscapularis repairs and find no need for double-row repair.[10,12]
- For a single-row repair, we have found the cruciate pattern to be a very robust repair, with the added benefit of the rip-stop it creates to resist pullout of the tissue in line with the fiber orientation. Five throws of arthroscopic square knots are tied, which we have found to have good knot and loop security.[13]
- The tear is much easier to identify, visualize, and mobilize through the subacromial space than in the glenohumeral joint.
- More cannulae can be used for suture management in the subacromial space than if done all intraarticularly so it is a less complex procedure.
- A criticism is that the disrupted interval may have protected the repair. Our alternative view is that the interval is retracted as evidenced by the comma sign and may actually put tension on the repair if it is not disrupted.
- A suprapectoral biceps tenodesis is done for ease of approach. We are able to identify pathology distal to the pectoralis insertion and have a low threshold for tenotomy if there is any question that tenodesis would incorporate pathologic tissue.[10]

References

[1] Neyton L, Daggett M, Kruse K, Walch G. The hidden lesion of the subscapularis: Arthroscopically revisited. Arthrosc Tech. 2016; 5(4):e877–e881

[2] Walch G, Nove-Josserand L, Levigne C, Renaud E. Tears of the supraspinatus tendon associated with "hidden" lesions of the rotator interval. J Shoulder Elbow Surg. 1994; 3(6):353–360

[3] Lo IK, Burkhart SS. The comma sign: An arthroscopic guide to the torn subscapularis tendon. Arthroscopy. 2003; 19(3):334–337

[4] Nove-Josserand L, Levigne C, Noël E, Walch G. [Isolated lesions of the subscapularis muscle. Apropos of 21 cases]. Rev Chir Orthop Repar Appar Mot. 1994; 80(7):595–601

[5] Denard PJ, Burkhart SS. Arthroscopic recognition and repair of the torn subscapularis tendon. Arthrosc Tech. 2013; 2(4):e373–e379

[6] Malavolta EA, Assunção JH, Guglielmetti CL, et al. Accuracy of preoperative MRI in the diagnosis of subscapularis tears. Arch Orthop Trauma Surg. 2016; 136(10):1425–1430

[7] Foad A, Wijdicks CA. The accuracy of magnetic resonance imaging and magnetic resonance arthrogram versus arthroscopy in the diagnosis of subscapularis tendon injury. Arthroscopy. 2012; 28(5):636–641

[8] Lanz U, Fullick R, Bongiorno V, Saintmard B, Campens C, Lafosse L. Arthroscopic repair of large subscapularis tendon tears: 2- to 4-year clinical and radiographic outcomes. Arthroscopy. 2013; 29(9):1471–1478

[9] Hughes JD, Hughes JL, Bartley JH, Hamilton WP, Brennan KL. Infection rates in arthroscopic versus open rotator cuff repair. Orthop J Sports Med. 2017; 5(7):2325967117715416

[10] Saltzman BM, Collins MJ, Leroux T, et al. Arthroscopic repair of isolated subscapularis tears: A systematic review of technique-specific outcomes. Arthroscopy. 2017; 33(4):849–860

[11] Mall NA, Chahal J, Heard WM, et al. Outcomes of arthroscopic and open surgical repair of isolated subscapularis tendon tears. Arthroscopy. 2012; 28(9):1306–1314

[12] Rhee YG, Lee YS, Park YB, Kim JY, Han KJ, Yoo JC. The outcomes and affecting factors after arthroscopic isolated subscapularis tendon repair. J Shoulder Elbow Surg. 2017; 26(12):2143–2151

[13] Elkousy H, Hammerman SM, Edwards TB, et al. The arthroscopic square knot: a biomechanical comparison with open and arthroscopic knots. Arthroscopy. 2006; 22(7):736–741

18 Arthroscopic Repair of Subscapularis Tear Based on the Tear Types

Chris Hyunchul Jo and Jeong Yong Yoon

Summary

With the advancement of magnetic resonance imaging (MRI) and arthroscopy, the diagnosis of subscapularis tears has become more and more common for arthroscopic surgeons. Nonetheless, arthroscopic technique for subscapularis tendon still remains challenging especially for under-experienced arthroscopists. In this chapter, the authors provide step-by-step approach for arthroscopic repair of subscapularis tear based on the tear types. In addition, we described biological augmentation with platelet-rich plasma and multiple channeling for the enhancement of healing.

Keywords: subscapularis repair, isolated subscapularis tear, platelet-rich plasma, multiple channeling

18.1 Patient Positioning

- The patient is positioned in a beach chair or lateral decubitus position based on surgeon preference.
- The authors prefer to position the patient in the lateral decubitus position.
- Evaluation under anesthesia: the amount of passive shoulder range of motion (ROM) in all directions.
- Gentle manipulation is performed if needed.
- Proper placement of stabilizing devices on the operating table and setup of lateral traction device.
- Rolling patient into a lateral decubitus position.
- Inflation of beanbag device and securing patient with table strap and tape.
- Placement of operative arm in lateral traction device with Spider (Smith & Nephew, Andover, MA).
- Standard sterile prepping and draping.

18.2 Portal Placement

- Anticipated portal sites are drawn out using bony landmarks, including the acromion, clavicle, acromioclavicular joint, and coracoid process.
- Posterior viewing portal: palpated in the "soft spot" of the glenohumeral joint.
- Anterior portal: lateral to the tip of the coracoid process (inside-out and outside-in techniques).
- Lateral subacromial portal: anterior to the usual 50-yard line.
- Posterolateral portal (which provides the Grand Canyon view): 1 cm lateral and anterior to the posterolateral corner of the acromion.

18.3 Surgical Technique (Step-by-Step Approach)

18.3.1 Partial Tear in the Leading Edge

- The arthroscope is introduced through a standard posterior portal.
- Anterior portal: just lateral to the coracoid process under arthroscopic visualization.
- The partial-thickness articular-sided tear is debrided with a mechanical shaver through the anterior portal.
- To visualize the subscapularis footprint better, the assistant can hold the arm in internal rotation and perform a posterior lever push.[1]

18.3.2 Articular-Sided Tear

- The intraarticular approach is appropriate for upper one-third tears.[2]
- The glenohumeral joint was entered and explored through a primary posterior portal.
- If the subscapularis lesion is isolated, without bicipital involvement, repair is performed only if biceps stability is not threatened.
- Frayed partial thickness articular-sided tears were debrided carefully.
- Tendon insertion is reassessed.
- Lesser tuberosity (LT) preparation: the most medial side of the footprint.
- Tissue penetrator is used to pass suture through the upper one-third of the intact tendon.
- The anchor is placed in the previously prepared hole on the LT.
- The sutures are gently tensioned and then impacted, and the anchor–suture construct is screwed into place.

18.3.3 Concealed Bursal-Sided Tear

- Examination of glenohumeral joint and subscapularis tendon insertion: posterior portal as entry portal.
- Debridement: articular side of the subscapularis tendon.
- Reassessment of the tendon.
- Move to bursal side of rotator cuff.
- Removing the biceps tendon away from the groove.
- Arthroscopic exploration: bursal side of the subscapularis tendon.
- If the subscapularis tendon is torn: repair of the tendon.
- In case of associated supraspinatus tendon tear: subscapularis tendon repairs are performed before supraspinatus tendon repair.

18.3.4 Subscapularis Tendon Tear with Supraspinatus Tendon Tear

- Standard posterior portal: status of the rotator cuff (including the subscapularis) and the presence of other intraarticular lesions.
- The retracted subscapularis tendon: comma sign.[3]
- The biceps should be examined along its intraarticular length.
- Biceps instability: tenotomy or tenodesis.

- Detachment of the biceps from its origin enables improved visualization of the subscapularis insertion on the LT.
- The coracoid tip is identified and exposed, the conjoint tendon is identified, and the undersurface of the coracoid is skeletonized with a shaver and electrocautery.
- Coracoplasty: subcoracoid stenosis (coracohumeral distance is < 6 mm).[4]
- The medial sling of the biceps and the superior glenohumeral ligament should be preserved laterally.
- Coracohumeral ligament release around the coracoid.
- Retracted subscapularis tendon tear: anterior, superior, and posterior surfaces are released(three-sided release).[1]
- Three-sided release, using a combination of shaver and electrocautery to release the tendon from the coracoid neck and coracoid base.
- As work proceeds inferiorly in this location, care must be taken to protect the axillary nerve.
- Prepare the LT and greater tuberosity bone bed to a bleeding base.
- For complete tears, two medial anchors were used, and for tears of the upper half of the tendon, one anchor was used.
- The anchors are placed along the medial aspect of the footprint starting inferiorly.
- Sutures are then tied with a slippage-proof(SP) knot, reducing the medial aspect of the subscapularis tendon insertion to bone.[5]
- After the subscapularis tendon is repaired, repair of concomitant rotator cuff tears is performed.
- Depending on the size of the tear, either two or three anchors were applied for the medial row.
- In all tears that have a full-thickness component, we used double-row fixation with a suture bridge technique.

18.3.5 Isolated Subscapularis Tendon Tear

- Standard posterior portal: examination of glenohumeral joint.
- Either tenotomy or tenodesis of the biceps tendon could be performed, depending on the age, gender, and functional requirements of the patient.
- Move to the bursal side of the rotator cuff.
- Subscapularis tendon tear: measure the dimensions and check the excursion.
- Lesion of the retracted subscapularis tendon: releasing the adhesions (three-sided release).
- Traction suture (medial to the comma tissue): facilitates tendon exposure.
- In tears that are still under significant tension after release: a medialization of the bone bed of approximately 5 mm.[6]
- When medialization is necessary, a bur is used to abrade 5 mm of the articular surface to create the new site of tendon attachment.
- Prepare the bone bed of the LT.
- A double-row suture bridge technique was routinely performed for a complete restoration of the footprint (▶ **Video 18.1**).

18.3.6 Biological Augmentation with Platelet-Rich Plasma (PRP)[7,8,9] and Multiple Channeling[10,11]

PRPGel Application
- One day before surgery using a platelet pheresis system.

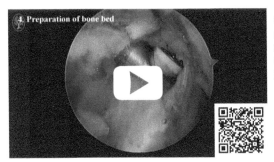

Video 18.1 Arthroscopic repair of subscapularis tear based on the tear types and biological augmentation of rotator cuff repair with platelet rich plasma and multiple channeling.

- Three PRP gels in place, medial row sutures are tied using SP knot if necessary.
- Lateral row was then secured using suture anchors.

Multiple Channeling
- Perform after LT bone bed preparation.
- Thin and long tip bone punch: holes were 4–5 mm apart and 10 mm deep.
- After multiple channeling, suture anchors are placed in the usual manner.

18.4 Surgeon Tips and Tricks (Use of Specific Instrumentation)

- An adequate three-sided soft-tissue release may improve tendon excursion and allow fixation without excessive tension in most repairs.
- The use of an additional 70° arthroscope may also improve the joint view.
- "Hand-on-face" position: achieve an appropriate angle to insert suture anchors
- into the LT.
- We recommend starting with the subscapularis tendon if there are several rotator cuff tendons.
- To produce a gel form of PRP: 0.3 mL of 10% calcium gluconate + 3 mL of PRP.
- The multiple channeling procedure: a kind of the bone marrow stimulation technique.
- Bone punch: thin and long tip is preferred to create channels.

18.5 Pitfalls/Complications

- Well-tolerated procedure with minimal number of complications.
- Small upper border subscapularis tears are often missed on magnetic resonance imaging and definitive diagnosis can be made upon arthroscopy.
- Extreme care should be taken not to pass instruments medial to the coracoid base.

18.6 Rehabilitation

- Immobilized for 4–6 weeks using an abduction brace.
- Immediate post-op: shrugging, protraction, retraction of shoulder girdles, and intermittent exercise of the elbow, wrist, and hand.

- After 4–6 weeks: passive ROM exercise.
- After 3 months: begin strengthening exercise, light sports.
- After 6 months: full return to sports.

References

[1] Denard PJ, Burkhart SS. Arthroscopic recognition and repair of the torn subscapularis tendon. Arthrosc Tech. 2013; 2(4):e373–e379

[2] Denard PJ, Burkhart SS. A new method for knotless fixation of an upper subscapularis tear. Arthroscopy. 2011; 27(6):861–866

[3] Lo IK, Burkhart SS. The comma sign: An arthroscopic guide to the torn subscapularis tendon. Arthroscopy. 2003; 19(3):334–337

[4] Lo IK, Burkhart SS. The etiology and assessment of subscapularis tendon tears: a case for subcoracoid impingement, the roller-wringer effect, and TUFF lesions of the subscapularis. Arthroscopy. 2003; 19(10):1142–1150

[5] Jo CH, Yoon KS, Lee JH, Kang SB, Lee MC. The slippage-proof knot: a new, nonstacking, arthroscopic, sliding locking knot with a lag bight. Orthopedics. 2007; 30(5):349–350

[6] Denard PJ, Burkhart SS. Medialization of the subscapularis footprint does not affect functional outcome of arthroscopic repair. Arthroscopy. 2012; 28(11):1608–1614

[7] Jo CH, Shin JS, Lee SY, Shin S. Allogeneic platelet-rich plasma for rotator cuff repair. Acta Ortop Bras. 2017; 25 (1):38–43

[8] Jo CH, Shin JS, Shin WH, Lee SY, Yoon KS, Shin S. Platelet-rich plasma for arthroscopic repair of medium to large rotator cuff tears: a randomized controlled trial. Am J Sports Med. 2015; 43(9):2102–2110

[9] Jo CH, Shin JS, Lee YG, et al. Platelet-rich plasma for arthroscopic repair of large to massive rotator cuff tears: a randomized, single-blind, parallel-group trial. Am J Sports Med. 2013; 41(10):2240–2248

[10] Jo CH, Shin JS, Park IW, Kim H, Lee SY. Multiple channeling improves the structural integrity of rotator cuff repair. Am J Sports Med. 2013; 41(11):2650–2657

[11] Jo CH, Yoon KS, Lee JH, et al. The effect of multiple channeling on the structural integrity of repaired rotator cuff. Knee Surg Sports Traumatol Arthrosc. 2011; 19(12):2098–2107

19 Arthroscopic Transtendon Double-Row Subscapularis Repair with all Suture Medial Row Anchors

Robert A. Duerr, Tyler J. Hunt, and Laurence D. Higgins

Summary

Arthroscopic transtendon double-row subscapularis repair with use of all suture medial row anchors achieves a biomechanically stable anatomic repair. This repair construct provides compression across a large contact area to recreate the subscapularis footprint and optimize tendon-to-bone healing.

Keywords: all-suture anchor, arthroscopic, subscapularis tear, transtendon repair

19.1 Patient Positioning

Our preferred patient position is in beach chair with a hydraulic powered limb positioner (Spider2, Smith & Nephew, Andover, MA).

19.2 Portal Placement

- Initial posterior viewing portal is placed typically 2 cm inferior and 1–2 cm medial to the posterolateral tip of the acromion in the "soft spot."
- An anterior working portal is established just lateral to the tip of the coracoid through the rotator interval.
- Accessory percutaneous anterior portals will be used for anchor placement directly over the lesser tuberosity.
- From the subacromial space, the anterolateral portal is established for placement of a traction suture to pull in-line with the subscapularis to enable anatomic reduction to the footprint.
- A lateral portal is also established for viewing the entire subcoracoid space to allow thorough debridement and mobilization of the subscapularis.

19.3 Surgical Technique (Step-by-Step Approach)

- Please see accompanying video for detailed description of the surgical technique. Patient is placed in the beach chair position with an adjustable arm holder.
- Diagnostic arthroscopy is performed through a posterior viewing portal.
- An anterior working portal is established to allow thorough diagnostic evaluation.
- Once a subscapularis tear is confirmed, if the long head of the biceps (LHB) tendon remains, this will be cut to remove it from the bicipital groove and later tenodesed.
- The subacromial space is then entered for placement of anterolateral and lateral portals.
- A traction suture is placed in the subscapularis tendon to facilitate mobilization.

- Mobilization of the subscapularis is achieved using combination of electrocautery and a shaver to debride any fibrous adhesions along the anterior capsule and subcoracoid space.
- This is achieved from both subacromial space while viewing from lateral portal and working through anterior and anterolateral portals and from the intraarticular space while viewing from the posterior portal.
- A 70° lens is often used for improved visualization.
- Care must be taken to stay lateral to the coracoid to avoid neurovascular structures.
- Once the subscapularis has been adequately mobilized to allow anatomic reduction to the footprint, the footprint will be prepared using a bur to remove any remaining soft tissues and create a healthy bleeding bone bed for tendon healing.
- The traction suture is then used to reduce the subscapularis to the footprint and is held in place with a clamp from outside the portal.
- Two spinal needles are used to localize placement of the medial row anchors at the articular margin of the humeral head into the lesser tuberosity.
- A small stab incision is made just inferior to the spinal needle, and a FiberTak (Arthrex, Naples, FL) double-loaded soft anchor is placed percutaneously.
- This anchor is preferred for the transtendon technique because of the small diameter (1.6 mm) drill that is needed. These anchors are loaded with a LabralTape and #2 FiberWire (Arthrex).
- Give a gentle pull on the sutures to ensure the anchor is firmly seated.
- These steps are repeated for placement of the second medial row anchor.
- The sutures from the medial row are then tied in a "double-pulley" technique.
- One limb of the free suture from each anchor is brought through the anterior portal and a knot is tied extracorporeal.
- The other two suture limbs are then pulled to shuttle this knot into the medial row.
- These limbs are then brought out through the anterior portal, and a static knot is tied to complete the "double pulley."
- Attention is then turned to the lateral row of the repair construct.
- One limb of the LabralTape from each medial anchor is then retrieved through the anterior portal.
- A 4.75-mm SwiveLock anchor (Arthrex) is loaded with these two LabralTape sutures.
- The lateral row is placed at the lateral aspect of the lesser tuberosity.
- These steps are repeated for placement of a second lateral row anchor, completing the repair construct.
- The repair can be assessed by taking the arm through a range of motion (ROM) to confirm anatomic reduction of the subscapularis.

19.4 Surgeon Tips and Tricks (Use of Specific Instrumentation)

- This technique can be used for both partial and complete tears of the subscapularis.
- In partial tears involving the superior portion of the subscapularis, it is important to identify and anatomically reduce the stump of the remaining tendon.
- We prefer the beach chair position to allow easy access to the anterior shoulder.
- The adjustable arm positioner (Spider2) is an important tool when planning for subscapularis repair as the arm is internally and externally rotated at different points throughout the procedure.

- Tenotomy or tenodesis of the LHB should be performed with all subscapularis repairs.
- Adequate mobilization of the subscapularis is achieved while viewing from both subacromial and intraarticular spaces.
- Placing the subscapularis on tension during mobilization is important to address adhesions long the anterior glenoid and subcoracoid space.
- Accurate placement of the anterolateral portal inline with the subscapularis to allow for a traction stitch to anatomically reduce the tendon to the footprint is imperative for this transtendon repair technique.
- The FiberTak Soft Anchors are easily placed percutaneously and cause minimal damage to the tendon with a 1.6-mm drill hole.

19.5 Pitfalls and Complications

- Neurovascular structures lie just medial and inferior to the coracoid and are at risk during mobilization of the subscapularis.
- Ensure accurate placement of the medial row anchors to avoid penetration of the humeral head.
- Assess the strength and stability of the repair by taking the arm through a full ROM at the conclusion of the repair.

19.6 Rehabilitation

- See www.bostonshoulderinstitute.com for full details.
- Phase 1: immediate postsurgical phase (weeks 1–4).
  - Maintain arm in a sling with abduction pillow at all times and remove only for exercise.
  - Cryotherapy to reduce initial inflammation.
  - At day 21, may begin pendulum exercises and start passive ROM as tolerated under the direction of the physical therapist.
- Phase 2: Protection phase (weeks 4–10).
  - Weeks 4–5: gradually restore full passive ROM.
  - May discontinue sling at end of week 6.
  - Week 6: begin assisted active ROM (AROM).
  - Begin rotator cuff isometrics.
  - Initiate AROM exercises.
- Phase 3: Intermediate phase (weeks 10–14).
  - Weeks 10–12: full AROM.
  - Initiate strengthening program.
  - Week 12: begin light functional activities.
  - Week 14: progress to fundamental shoulder exercises.
- Phase 4: advanced strengthening phase (weeks 16–22).
  - Continue progression of strengthening.
  - Advance proprioceptive, neuromuscular activities.
- Phase 5: return to activity phase.
  - Gradual return to strenuous work activities.
  - Week 26: may initiate interval sport program if appropriate.

19.7 Rationale and Evidence for Approach

- As the anterior force couple of the rotator cuff, the subscapularis plays an important role in shoulder stability and motion, and in isolation was found to produce up to 50% of the rotator cuff force.[1]
- The subscapularis is unique, in that the upper two-thirds of the insertion consists of a tendinous portion at the lesser tuberosity, and a muscular insertion more distal along the humeral metaphysis.[2]
- It is this superior tendinous portion that blends with anterior fibers of the supraspinatus tendon and contributes to the rotator interval and biceps pulley.[3]
- While this superior portion was found to be the strongest of the subscapularis, it is also the most susceptible to injury.[4,5]
- These tears can be missed or overlooked, as they are most often partial tears, and associated with anterior supraspinatus tears that may mimic the symptoms.[6]
- As tears of the subscapularis are more commonly recognized, with incidences up to 43% in one series,[7] it is important to have a knowledge of techniques that can produce a biomechanically stable repair of this important structure.
- The goals of any rotator cuff repair should be to anatomically reduce the tendon to the footprint, maximize tendon–bone contact area, and utilize a biomechanically stable construct that will prevent gapping and allow tendon-to-bone healing.
- Given the biomechanical importance of the subscapularis, we feel that repair techniques should employ these same strategies that have proven effective in supraspinatus and infraspinatus tendon repair.
- Biomechanical studies have demonstrated the advantages of double-row repair versus single-row repair with regard to restoration of the footprint contact area, ultimate load to failure, and resistance to gap formation.[8,9,10,11]
- We feel that a double-row construct is appropriate for subscapularis tears to achieve the above-listed goals.
- This technique in particular has several advantages:
  - Using a traction stitch allows for anatomic reduction of the tendon prior to placement of the transtendon medial row anchors.
  - The double-row construct combined with the medial row "double pulley" provides a large contact area with compression over the entire footprint.
  - The use of a small caliber (1.6 mm) soft anchor causes minimal tendon damage for this transtendon approach.
  - Also, the small soft anchor minimizes the loss of the footprint area that may be associated with larger anchors.
- While further biomechanical and clinical studies are needed to confirm the effectiveness of this technique, we feel that in appropriately selected patients, this technique provides a biomechanically stable construct that is advantageous for tendon-to-bone healing with minimal risk of complications (▶ **Video 19.1**).

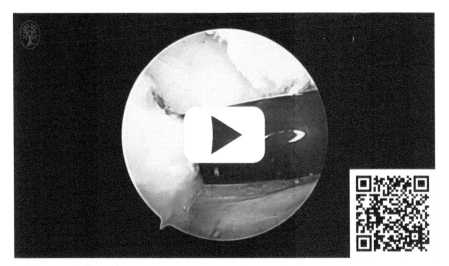

Video 19.1 This video demonstrates our preferred technique for arthroscopic transtendon double-row subscapularis repair. The procedure is on the patient's right shoulder in a beach chair position. The initial view is with a 30 degree lens from a posterior viewing portal. The subscapularis tear is identified and mobilized. Once adequately mobilized the insertion site is prepared and the tendon is held in a reduced position while medial row anchors are placed transtendon. The repair construct is completed using a medial double pulley to compress the tendon and a lateral row in a speed-bridge configuration.

References

[1] Keating JF, Waterworth P, Shaw-Dunn J, Crossan J. The relative strengths of the rotator cuff muscles. A cadaver study. J Bone Joint Surg Br. 1993; 75(1):137–140

[2] Hinton MA, Parker AW, Drez D, Jr, Altcheck D. An anatomic study of the subscapularis tendon and myotendinous junction. J Shoulder Elbow Surg. 1994; 3(4):224–229

[3] Burkhart SS, Esch JC, Jolson RS. The rotator crescent and rotator cable: an anatomic description of the shoulder's "suspension bridge". Arthroscopy. 1993; 9(6):611–616

[4] Arai R, Sugaya H, Mochizuki T, Nimura A, Moriishi J, Akita K. Subscapularis tendon tear: an anatomic and clinical investigation. Arthroscopy. 2008; 24(9):997–1004

[5] Halder A, Zobitz ME, Schultz E, An KN. Structural properties of the subscapularis tendon. J Orthop Res. 2000; 18(5):829–834

[6] Sakurai G, Ozaki J, Tomita Y, Kondo T, Tamai S. Incomplete tears of the subscapularis tendon associated with tears of the supraspinatus tendon: cadaveric and clinical studies. J Shoulder Elbow Surg. 1998; 7(5):510–515

[7] Adams CR, Schoolfield JD, Burkhart SS. The results of arthroscopic subscapularis tendon repairs. Arthroscopy. 2008; 24(12):1381–1389

[8] Tuoheti Y, Itoi E, Yamamoto N, et al. Contact area, contact pressure, and pressure patterns of the tendon-bone interface after rotator cuff repair. Am J Sports Med. 2005; 33(12):1869–1874

[9] Mazzocca AD, Millett PJ, Guanche CA, Santangelo SA, Arciero RA. Arthroscopic single-row versus double-row suture anchor rotator cuff repair. Am J Sports Med. 2005; 33(12):1861–1868

[10] Kim DH, Elattrache NS, Tibone JE, et al. Biomechanical comparison of a single-row versus double-row suture anchor technique for rotator cuff repair. Am J Sports Med. 2006; 34(3):407–414

[11] Smith CD, Alexander S, Hill AM, et al. A biomechanical comparison of single and double-row fixation in arthroscopic rotator cuff repair. J Bone Joint Surg Am. 2006; 88(11):2425–2431

20 Four-Anchor Repair of Massive Subscapularis Tear with Subcoracoid Decompression

Colin P. Murphy, Colin M. Robbins, Connor G. Ziegler, Anthony Sanchez, and Matthew T. Provencher

Summary

Tears involving the muscles of the rotator cuff demonstrate significant variation in severity. Depending on the type of tear, location, muscle quality, and extent of retraction, management of the rotator cuff tear can also differ considerably from patient to patient. In cases where surgical management is indicated, the surgeon has many options, including debridement, arthroscopic repair, mini-open repair, and open repair. At times, surgery may be performed in combination with other procedures, such as a total shoulder arthroplasty. In this chapter, we will describe the surgical management of a massive subscapularis tendon tear, including a subcoracoid decompression. The preparation, technique, and rehabilitation for this unique surgical case will be described in detail and demonstrated through a video presentation.

Keywords: coracoid, rotator cuff, shoulder, subcoracoid decompression, subscapularis

20.1 Patient Positioning[1]

- Beach chair position.
- All bony prominences well padded.
- Operative extremity prepped and draped in usual sterile orthopedic fashion.
- Pneumatic arm positioner to assist with manipulating and holding extremity during the procedure.

20.2 Portal Placement

- Posterior portal.
- Midglenoid anterior portal.
- Midlateral portal placed near midpoint of lateral acromion 1 cm inferior to the acromial edge.
- Accessory anterior portal as needed.

20.3 Surgical Technique[2,3,4]

- Diagnostic arthroscopy.
- Synovectomy and debridement.
  - Performed through anterior portal in the rotator interval.
  - Assess labrum for any degeneration or tears.
  - Take note of any frayed ligaments, tendons, or sheaths.
  - Debride any significant synovitis using a mechanical shaver and radiofrequency (RF) device.

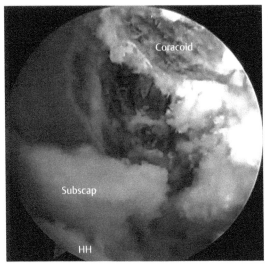

Fig. 20.1 Arthroscopic view of the completed subcoracoid decompression. The arm can be put through full range of motion to ensure that the coracoid will no longer impinge on the subscapularis tendon. Subscap, subscapularis; HH, humeral head.

- Subcoracoid decompression (▶ **Fig. 20.1**).
  - Arthroscope positioned in the posterior portal and the midlateral portal as needed to perform a complete and thorough decompression.
  - Debride any scar tissue, synovitis, and/or inflammation using the combination of an arthroscopic shaver and RF device.
  - Make an indentation in the capsule under the coracoid base medial to the middle glenohumeral ligament (MGHL) with an RF device.
  - Skeletonize coracoid base using an RF or shaver, removing any inflamed bursa.
  - Gently elevate coracoacromial (CA) ligament using an RF device; this preserves the CA ligament.
  - Using an arthroscopic shaver/bur, perform decompression of the coracoid base overlying the subscapularis tendon.
  - A high-speed bone-cutting bur is generally used to remove osteophytes from the coracoid.
- Subscapularis tendon repair.
  - 8 mm cannula inserted into an anterior portal.
  - Debride scar tissue and adhesions along the tendon to maximize tendon excursion.
    - Extend releases medially to the musculotendinous junction as needed but take care superiorly where the subscapular nerve innervates the muscle.
  - Lesser tuberosity bone bed is prepared with a combination of high-speed bone-cutting bur and motorized rasp, which creates a bleeding bed optimal for healing.
  - If a longitudinal tear is present, No. 2 FiberTape suture (Arthrex, Naples, FL) is passed through the tear in a horizontal mattress technique using a Scorpion suture-passing device (Arthrex) to reduce the tear prior to double-row repair (▶ **Fig. 20.2**).
  - Double-row repair using 4.75-mm SwiveLock (Arthrex) anchors.
    1. Suture-loaded anchor placed at the inferomedial aspect of the lesser tuberosity footprint.
    2. Suture-loaded anchor placed at the superomedial aspect of the lesser tuberosity footprint.

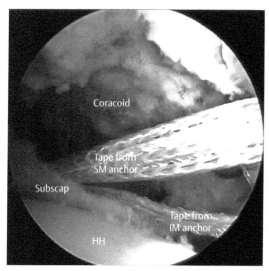

Fig. 20.2 Arthroscopic view showing the FiberTapes from the superomedial (SM) and inferomedial (IM) SwiveLock anchors passed through the subscapularis tendon. The tapes were passed by using a Scorpion suture-passing device. Subscap, subscapularis; HH, humeral head.

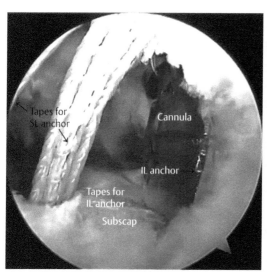

Fig. 20.3 Arthroscopic view showing the placement of the inferolateral (IL) anchor. One end of FiberTape from both the inferomedial and superomedial anchors are placed in the eyelet of the IL anchor. This anchor is placed at the IL aspect of the lesser tuberosity footprint. The FiberTapes for the superolateral (SL) anchor can be seen superior to the IL tapes and anchor. Subscap, subscapularis.

3. One suture strand from each medial row anchor is passed through the eyelet of an unloaded SwiveLock, which is then placed at the inferolateral aspect of the lesser tuberosity footprint. (▶ **Fig. 20.3**).
4. Each remaining suture strand from the medial row anchors is passed through the eyelet of another unloaded SwiveLock, which is then placed at the superolateral aspect of the lesser tuberosity footprint (▶ **Fig. 20.4**).
   – Sutures are cut flush to anchor with an arthroscopic suture cutter.
   – Assess final repair with probe.

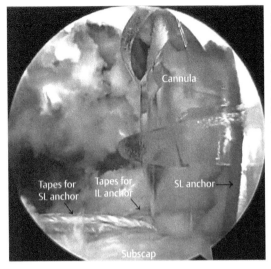

Fig. 20.4 Arthroscopic view showing the placement of the superolateral(SL) anchor. One end of FiberTape from both the inferomedial, and superomedial anchors are placed in the eyelet of the SL anchor. This anchor is placed at the SL aspect of the lesser tuberosity footprint. The FiberTapes for the inferolateral (IL) anchor can be seen inferior to the IL tapes and anchor.- Subscap, subscapularis.

- Wound closure.
  - Copiously irrigate all wounds.
  - Close portal sites with 3–0 Monocryl.
  - Apply sterile gauze and Tegaderm dressings.
  - Place patient in padded abduction sling.

20.4 Surgeon Tips and Tricks

- Proper position of cannulas and use of soft cannulas, such as the PassPort(Arthrex).
- Adequate visualization from the lateral portal.
- Completely release all adhesions from the subscapularis tendon to ensure proper excursion.
  - Inferiorly, superiorly, and laterally.
- Be careful with release of tendon medially as innervation enters subscapularis muscle from superior aspect.
  - Consider turning down RF intensity when working medially.
- Careful and thorough subcoracoid decompression is recommended.
  - First skeletonize coracoid prior to using shaver/bur.
  - A 70° scope can sometimes be helpful.
- The coracoid base is located medial to the glenoid and at the level of the superior aspect of the glenoid.
  - Capsular window to access coracoid base for decompression should be made medial to the MGHL.
- Double-row repair using SwiveLock anchors.
- FiberTape to load anchors and/or may use anchors preloaded with FiberTape.
  - The author prefers knotless and tape construct.
  - May tie two knots with medial row with tape if preferred.
- Place lateral row of SwiveLock anchors at the lateral aspect of the anatomic insertion of the subscapularis tendon.

- Use of suture-passing device.
- Understand the equipment and devices you are using prior to using them on your patient, as there are nuances to every device.
- Creating an accessory anterior portal may be necessary and aid in ease of anchor placement.

20.5 Pitfalls/Complications

- Inadequate soft-tissue release of scarred and retracted subscapularis.
- Incomplete capsular/bony releases off the glenoid.
  - It is essential to perform a complete inferior release.
- Incomplete or inadequate subcoracoid decompression.
- Inadequate exposure/debridement of subscapularis footprint and subsequent suboptimal, nonanatomic repair.
- Inadequate tensioning of lateral row.
  - Ensure the arm is in 20°–30° abduction when tensioning lateral row.
- Poor suture management.
  - Use tape graspers to avoid tangles.
- Leaving proud "dog ears," especially anteriorly.

20.6 Rehabilitation[5]

- Phase I (weeks 1–6): maximal protection, passive range of motion (ROM).
  - Sling (weeks 1–6).
  - No resisted elbow flexion (weeks 1–6).
  - Exercises.
    - Cervical ROM exercises.
    - Elbow/hand/wrist ROM.
    - Ball squeeze.
    - Pendulums.
    - Ankle pumps.
    - Scapular retraction/depression.
    - Aquatherapy for active assist ROM (beginning week 3).
  - Passive ROM (full ROM beginning week 5).
    - External rotation (ER): 30° (weeks 1–2), 60° (weeks 3–4).
    - Forward elevation and scaption: 90° (weeks 1–2), 150° (weeks 3–4).
    - Abduction: 60° (weeks 1–2), 120° (weeks 3–4).
    - Internal rotation: 30° (weeks 1–2), 45° (weeks 3–4).
  - Activities of daily living.
    - Eating/drinking (use uninvolved arm only weeks 7–13).
    - Dressing (use uninvolved arm only weeks 7–13).
    - Washing/showering (use uninvolved arm only weeks 7–13).
    - Computer with supported arm (weeks 1–8).
    - Driving (weeks 3–13).
- Phase II (beginning weeks 6–7): minimal protection, active ROM.
  - Active assist ROM.
    - Internal/ER (weeks 6–8).
    - Flexion/abduction (weeks 6–8).

- Isometrics.
  - Internal/ER (weeks 6–8).
  - Flexion/abduction (weeks 6–8).
- Active ROM.
  - Bench press series (weeks 7–13).
  - Modified military press (weeks 8–13).
  - Side-lying ER (weeks 7–13).
  - Salutes (weeks 7–13).
  - Full can (weeks 8–13).
  - Prone row progression (weeks 7–13).
  - Prone ER90° (weeks 8–13).
  - Prone Ys (weeks 8–13).
  - Prone lift off (weeks 8–13).
  - Open-chain proprioception (weeks 7–13).
- Low load prolonged stretches.
  - Door jamb series (weeks 7–13).
  - Towel internal rotation (weeks 7–13).
  - Cross arm stretch (weeks 7–13).
  - Sleeper stretch(weeks 7–13).
  - TV watching stretch (weeks 7–13).
  - 90°/90°ERstretch (weeks 7–13).
- Activities of daily living.
  - Eating/drinking (weeks 7–8).
  - Dressing (weeks 7–8).
  - Washing/showering (weeks 7–8).
  - Lifting up to 5 lb (weeks 7–13).
• Phase III (beginning week 9): initial resistance, strengthening, and proprioception.
  - Exercises.
    - ER (weeks 9–25).
    - Internal rotation (weeks 9–25).
    - Double arm ER (weeks 9–25).
    - Full can (weeks 9–25).
    - Forward punch w/plus (weeks 9–25).
    - Rows (weeks 9–25).
    - Bicep curl (weeks 9–25).
    - Triceps extension (weeks 9–25).
    - Lat pulldown (weeks 9–25).
    - Initial closed-chain stability (weeks 10–25).
  - Activities of daily living.
    - Overhead activity (weeks 9–13).
• Phase IV (beginning week 10): advanced resistance, strengthening, and proprioception.
  - Exercises.
    - Bear hugs (weeks 10–25).
    - ER at 45° (weeks 10–25).
    - ER at 90° (weeks 10–25).
    - Rhythmic stabilization/neuromuscular control (weeks 10–25).

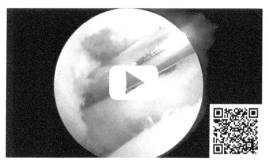

Video 20.1 Preparation, technique, and rehabilitation for the management of a massive subscapularis tendon tear, including a subcoracoid decompression.

- o Advanced closed-chain stability (weeks 17–25).
- o Plyometrics (weeks 21–25).
- o Decelerations (weeks 21–25).
- – Activities of daily living.
- o Lifting > 5 lb (weeks 10–13).
- • Phase V (beginning week 17): return to sports.
- – Criteria.
- o Functional, pain-free active ROM.
- o Maximized strength.
- o Proper scapulothoracic mechanics.
- – Skiing (week 17).
- – Swimming (week 17).
- – Throwing progression (week 25).
- – Overhead and serving sports (week 25).
- – Contact sports (week 25).

20.7 Rationale and/or Evidence for Approach[6]

- • Excellent bony purchase achieved with SwiveLock anchors.
- • Double-row repair provides excellent compression and anatomic restoration of the subscapularis tendon . Please see ▶ **Video 20.1** for demonstration.

References

[1] Provencher MT, Mcintire ES, Gaston TM, Frank RM, Solomon DJ. Avoiding complications in shoulder arthroscopy: Pearls for lateral decubitus and beach chair positioning. Tech Shoulder Elbow Surg. 2018; 11(1):1–3

[2] Kennedy NI, Sanchez G, Mannava S, Ferrari MB, Frangiamore SJ, Provencher MT. Arthroscopic rotator cuff repair with mini-open subpectoral biceps tenodesis. Arthrosc Tech. 2017; 6(5):e1667–e1674

[3] Sanchez G, Chahla J, Moatshe G, Ferrari MB, Kennedy NI, Provencher MT. Superior capsular reconstruction with superimposition of rotator cuff repair for massive rotator cuff tear. Arthrosc Tech. 2017; 6(5):e1775–e1779

[4] Sanchez G, Rossy WH, Lavery KP, et al. Arthroscopic superior capsule reconstruction technique in the setting of a massive, irreparable rotator cuff tear. Arthrosc Tech. 2017; 6(4):e1399–e1404

[5] Ghodadra NS, Provencher MT, Verma NN, Wilk KE, Romeo AA. Open, mini-open, and all-arthroscopic rotator cuff repair surgery: indications and implications for rehabilitation. J Orthop Sports Phys Ther. 2009; 39(2): 81–89

[6] Arce G, Bak K, Bain G, et al. Management of disorders of the rotator cuff: proceedings of the ISAKOS upper extremity committee consensus meeting. Arthroscopy. 2013; 29(11):1840–1850

21 Superior Capsular Reconstruction with Fascia Lata Autograft

Teruhisa Mihata

Summary

In 2007, we developed a new surgical treatment, "superior capsule reconstruction (SCR)," to restore superior stability and muscle balance in the shoulder joint without repairing supraspinatus and infraspinatus tendon tears, consequently improving shoulder function—particularly deltoid muscle function—and relieving pain. The presence of indications for SCR is determined by preoperative magnetic resonance imaging. Goutallier grades 3 and 4 (fatty infiltration equal to, or more than, the muscle volume) are absolute indications. Moreover, in Goutallier grade 2, if the torn tendon is severely atrophied, degenerated, and thin, we recommend SCR. Irreparable rotator cuff tears of Hamada grades 1 to 3 are an absolute indication for "fascia lata "SCR. Factors prognostic of clinical outcome are the degree of graft healing and the level of deltoid function. To decrease the rate of graft tear, a "thick" and "stiff" graft (6 to 8 mm thick) should be made by carefully determining the correct graft size. Concomitant cervical spinal (C5) palsy or axillary nerve palsy worsens clinical outcomes after surgery, resulting in poor shoulder function despite graft healing.

Keywords: autograft, fascia lata, irreparable, reconstruction, rotator cuff, shoulder, superior capsule, tear

21.1 Patient Positioning

Preoperative preparation for superior capsular reconstruction (SCR) is the same as for rotator cuff repair. The surgery can be performed either arthroscopically or by an open approach, and both the lateral decubitus position and the beach chair position are suitable. In my surgery, all procedures are performed under general anesthesia in the lateral decubitus position.

21.2 Portal Placement

Three portals are typically required for arthroscopic SCR. An arthroscope (viewing portal) is placed in a posterior portal from beginning to end. An anterior portal and lateral portal are used as the working portal. For each suture anchor placement, its own small portal (4–5 mm) is created to make the best direction for anchor insertion, which decreases risk of anchor pullout. The graft is inserted though the lateral portal.

21.3 Surgical Technique

21.3.1 Measurement of Defect Size (▶ Fig. 21.1)

Subacromial bursal tissue around the torn tendons is completely removed before measurement of the defect size. The defect is then measured in the mediolateral (5 to 6 cm in most cases: from "the superior glenoid," not the edge of the torn tendon, to the lateral edge of the greater tuberosity) and anteroposterior (from the anterior edge to the posterior edge of the torn tendon) directions. Partial repair of the torn tendons makes the defect size

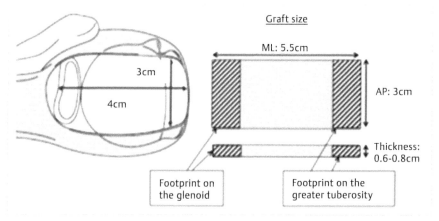

Fig. 21.1 Measurement of defect size and deciding on graft size. The size of the defect is measured in the mediolateral (from the superior glenoid to the lateral edge of the greater tuberosity) and anteroposterior (from the anterior edge to the posterior edge of the torn tendon) directions. The graft length in the anteroposterior direction is determined to be exactly the same as the length of the defect without partial repair of the torn tendon. In the mediolateral direction, the graft should be 15 mm longer than the distance from the superior glenoid to the lateral edge of the greater tuberosity to make a 10 mm footprint on the superior glenoid and allow for 5 mm of latitude in graft size.

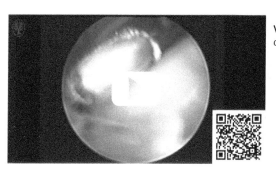

Video 21.1 Surgical demonstration of measurement of defect size.

decrease. However, the partial repair may cause inconsistent clinical results because of overtightening or possible re-tear of the repaired tendon.[1] Therefore, the defect size should be measured without partial repair (▶ **Video 21.1**).

21.3.2 Deciding on Graft Size (▶ Fig. 21.1)

The graft length in the anteroposterior direction is determined to be exactly the same as the length of the defect without partial repair of the torn tendon. In the mediolateral direction, the graft should be 15 mm longer than the distance from the superior glenoid to the lateral edge of the greater tuberosity to make a 10 mm footprint on the superior glenoid and allow for 5 mm of latitude in graft size. A biomechanical study has indicated that the appropriate graft thickness for SCR using the fascia lata is 6 to 8 mm.[2] Therefore, the amount of fascia lata that we need to harvest will be at least double the estimated graft length or width.

21.3.3 Harvesting the Fascia Lata and Making the Autograft (▶ Fig. 21.2, ▶ Fig. 21.3)

Fascia lata is harvested beginning at the tip of the greater trochanter, with care to include the posterior, thicker tissue. The average thickness of a single layer of autologous fascia lata is 1 to 3 mm. Therefore, a graft thickness of 6 to 8 mm is achieved by folding the fascia lata two or three times. Also, the fascia lata includes an intermuscular septum that consists of the tissues of two tendons and connects the fascia lata to the femur. To make a thicker graft, this intermuscular septum should be included in the graft. The fascia lata is mostly thinner at its anterior aspect than posteriorly; therefore, to make a flat graft of even thickness, the intermuscular septum is usually sutured to the anterior surface of the fascia lata after being completely detached from it. All fatty tissue should be removed from the graft. Finally, the layers of fascia lata are united very closely with nonabsorbable sutures to prevent delamination after surgery.

21.3.4 Treatment of Associated Lesions

Subscapularis tears should be repaired. Treatment of biceps is not necessary when SCR is performed. Preoperative biceps symptom is completely relieved without tenodesis or tenotomy after SCR. In my clinical experience, more than 95% of SCR were performed without biceps tenodesis or tenotomy and provided satisfactory results after surgery. In case of biceps dislocation, biceps tenodesis was performed.

21.3.5 Acromioplasty

Acromioplasty makes improved visualization during SCR, improved control of bleeding in the subacromial space, and increased concentrations of growth factors in the subacromial space, potentially improving tendon healing.[3,4,5] The coracoacromial ligament and spurs on the anterior, lateral, or medial side should be resected to prevent subacromial impingement after surgery. Also, the inferior surface of the acromion is usually made flat. A biomechanical study showed that acromioplasty decreased contact area between the graft and undersurface of acromion, suggesting that acromioplasty may help to decrease the postoperative risk of abrasion and tearing of the graft beneath the acromion when SCR is performed for irreparable rotator cuff tears.[6] Although acromioplasty is performed in all cases of SCR, we have had no cases of postoperative superior dislocation of the humeral head (▶ Video 21.2).

21.3.6 Anchor Placement on the Superior Glenoid

All soft tissue on the footprint of the superior glenoid should be removed to give a good bone bed before insertion of the suture anchors. Excessive resection of the cortical bone may lead to anchor pullout after surgery. Two 4.5-mm Corkscrew FT (Arthrex, Naples, FL) anchors are inserted, at the 10 or 11 o'clock and 11 or 12 o'clock positions on the glenoid of the right shoulder, and at the 12 or 1 o'clock and 1 or 2 o'clock positions on the left shoulder. Even for massive rotator cuff tears, two 4.5 mm Corkscrews are enough to prevent suture anchor pullout or graft tear on the glenoid (▶ Video 21.3).

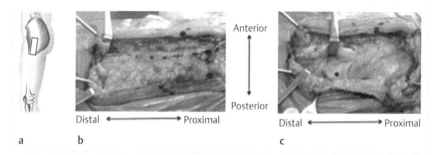

Fig. 21.2 Harvesting the fascia lata. **(a)** Fascia lata is harvested beginning at the tip of the greater trochanter. **(b)** Fascia lata is cut along the proximal, anterior, and distal marks. **(c)** After that, the fascia lata is flipped over. The fascia lata includes an intermuscular septum (asterisk) that consists of the tissues of two tendons and connects the fascia lata and the femur. To make a thicker graft, this intermuscular septum should be included in the graft.

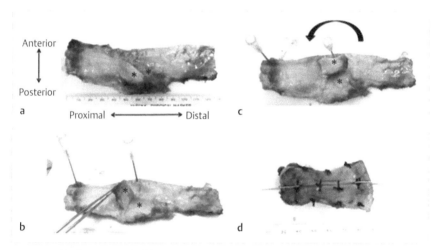

Fig. 21.3 **(a)** The reverse side of the harvested fascia lata. The fascia lata tends to be thinner anteriorly. **(b, c)** Therefore, to make a flat graft of even thickness, the intermuscular septum (*asterisk*) is usually sutured to the anterior surface of the fascia lata after being detached from it. Then the fascia lata is folded. **(d)** Finally, the layers of fascia lata are united by using nonabsorbable sutures.

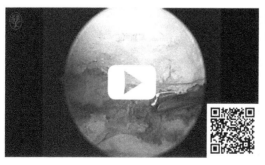

Video 21.2 Surgical demonstration of acromioplasty.

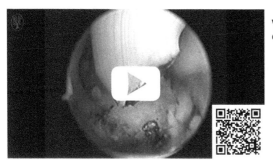

Video 21.3 Surgical demonstration of Glenoid anchor insertion.

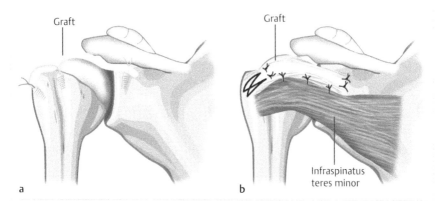

Fig. 21.4 Superior capsule reconstruction. The graft is attached medially to the superior glenoid and laterally to the greater tuberosity. This is followed by side-to-side suturing between the graft and the infraspinatus or teres minor tendon. **(a)** Compression double-row repair technique, and **(b)** SpeedBridge (Arthrex, Naples, FL) repair technique.

21.3.7 Anchor Placement on the Medial Footprint

All soft tissue on the footprint of the greater tuberosity should be removed. Excessive resection of the cortical bone, which may lead to anchor pullout after surgery, is not recommended for SCR. Two 4.75-mm SwiveLock (Arthrex) anchors with Fiber-Tape (Arthrex) are inserted on the medial footprint of the greater tuberosity to make a SpeedBridge (Arthrex) (▶ **Fig. 21.4**). Alternatively, when we fix the graft to the greater tuberosity by using a compression double-row repair technique, two 4.5-mm Corkscrew FT anchors are inserted on the medial footprint (▶ **Fig. 21.4**, ▶ **Video 21.4**).

21.3.8 Insertion of Fascia Lata into the Subacromial Space (▶ Fig. 21.5)

A 10 cc syringe is used as a cannula. FiberWire (Arthrex) from the superior glenoid suture anchors is placed through the fascia lata in a mattress fashion when the graft is still outside

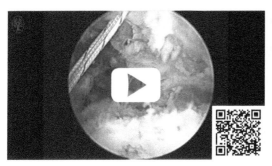

Video 21.4 Surgical demonstration of Greater Tuberosity anchor insertion.

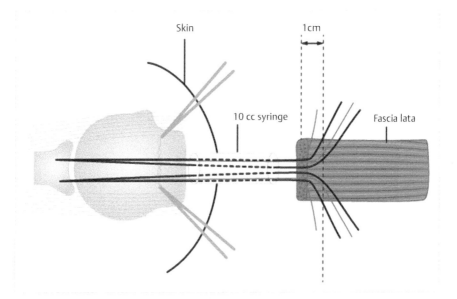

Fig. 21.5 Insertion of fascia lata into the subacromial space. A 10-cc syringe is used as a cannula. FiberWires (Arthrex, Naples, FL) from the superior glenoid suture anchors are placed through the fascia lata in a mattress fashion when the graft is still outside the body. After all FiberWires have been placed through the fascia lata, one FiberWire is tied while the graft is pushed into the subacromial space. The graft can then be inserted into its appropriate place on the glenoid. All sutures are tied in the subacromial space.

the body. After all FiberWires have been placed through the fascia lata, the graft is inserted in its appropriate place on the glenoid. All sutures are then tied in the subacromial space (▶ **Video 21.5**).

21.3.9 Attachment to the Greater Tuberosity

To complete the SpeedBridge fixation, the additional two 4.75-mm SwiveLock anchors are inserted at 5 mm distal to the lateral footprint of the greater tuberosity. I recommend making additional medial mattress suturing using FiberWire from two SwiveLock anchors,

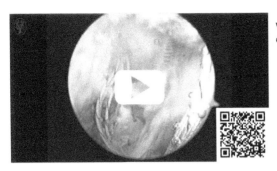

Video 21.5 Surgical demonstration of Graft insertion and fixation.

which had been inserted on the medial footprint of the greater tuberosity. For compression double-row repair, two 4.5-mm Corkscrew FT anchors are inserted at 5 mm distal to the lateral footprint of the greater tuberosity.

21.3.10 Side-to-Side Suturing between the Graft and the Infraspinatus Tendon or Teres Minor

In a dynamic observational study of cadaveric biomechanics,[7] four of seven shoulders had posterosuperior subluxation during external (ER) and internal rotations (IR) in the absence of side-to-side suturing; after the addition of posterior side-to-side suturing, the glenohumeral joint was secure and stable, and posterosuperior subluxation did not occur. Therefore, two or three sutures for posterior side-to-side suturing should be placed between the graft and the infraspinatus tendon or teres minor to increase superior shoulder stability and to prevent posterosuperior subluxation. Side-to-side suturing both anteriorly and posteriorly may cause postoperative shoulder stiffness, so anterior side-to-side suturing in SCR using the fascia lata is not recommended.

21.4 Surgeon Tips and Tricks

Deciding on the correct graft size is the most important step in this surgery. If the graft tears after surgery because it is too small or too thin, the clinical results will be poor. In our cases, postoperative clinical outcome scores (American Shoulder and Elbow Surgeons [ASES] standard shoulder assessment scores) and active elevation at final follow-up were significantly better in healed patients (ASES, 96.0; active elevation, 157° ± 22°) than in unhealed patients suffering from graft tear or re-tear of the repaired rotator cuff tendon (ASES, 77.1; active elevation, 100° ± 44°).[1]

In case of irreparable tear of subscapularis tendon as well as superoposterior tendons, SCR without subscapularis repair is performed. This surgery improves active shoulder elevation although IR strength is a little weaker than the contralateral shoulder. IR lag sign is eliminated after SCR without repairing the subscapularis tendon.

Patients with irreparable tear of teres minor tendon as well as supraspinatus and infraspinatus tendons have severely decreased ER strength (positive ER lag sign and positive Hornblower's sign). SCR with posterior side-to-side suturing between the graft and posteroinferior capsule increases shoulder ER strength and makes ER lag sign and Hornblower's sign negative, although ER strength is still weaker than the contralateral shoulder.

21.5 Pitfalls/Complications

The advantage of SCR is the relatively low rate of complications (graft tear 10/311, 3.2%; infection and severe synovitis 7/311, 2.3%; anchor pullout 4/311, 1.3%; severe stiffness 3/311, 1.0%: re-tear of the repaired infraspinatus tendon 3/311, 1.0%). To decrease the rate of graft tear, a "thick" and "stiff" graft (6 to 8 mm thick) should be made by carefully determining the correct graft size. Three of seven patients with postoperative severe synovitis had *Propionibacterium acnes*, while four patients had negative culture. In the case of postoperative shoulder infection, a couple of arthroscopic irrigation and debridement with removal of some sutures or anchors are necessary. However, the graft should not be removed to get a good clinical outcome. Even after deep infection in the shoulder joint, excellent or good outcome can be expected if the graft heals. All of our instances of anchor pullout occurred on the greater tuberosity side and were caused by poor bone quality, as is often seen in chronic rotator cuff tears. The use of screw-type suture anchors prevents pullout from the glenoid. To decrease the risk of postoperative shoulder stiffness, we recommend that the shoulder abduction angle used when fixing the graft should be 20° to 30°; moreover, anterior side-to-side sutures (i.e., rotator interval closure) should not be added. (For SCR using dermal graft, anterior side-to-side sutures are recommended because the elastic material makes low risk of postoperative shoulder stiffness.) To determine the graft size, the anteroposterior length of the defect should be measured without partial repair of the infraspinatus tendon. In our early cases, we performed partial repair of the torn tendons before SCR. In that series, we experienced postoperative re-tear of the repaired infraspinatus tendon even when the fascia lata graft had not been torn. The clinical results in such cases of partial re-tear are acceptable (approximately 50% to 70% of the degree of recovery that is achieved in cases where there is no re-tear), but not excellent. For this reason, we now omit the partial repair before measurement. Instead of doing a partial repair, a bigger graft should be placed as described earlier, to obtain consistently good outcomes. Degenerated (e.g., thin and weak) tendon tissue is also removed before measurement of the defect size, because postoperative tear of the degenerated rotator cuff tendon worsens the postoperative outcome even when the reconstructed superior capsule remains intact.

21.6 Rehabilitation

Postoperative physical therapy is essential to improve shoulder function after SCR. An abduction brace (Block Shoulder Abduction Sling, Nagano Prosthetics & Orthotics, Osaka, Japan) is used for 4 weeks after SCR. After the immobilization period, passive and active-assisted exercises are initiated to promote scaption (scapular plane elevation). Eight weeks after surgery, patients begin to perform exercises to strengthen the rotator cuff and the scapular stabilizers. Physical therapists have assisted all of our patients.

21.7 Rationale and Evidence for Fascia Lata SCR

In 2007, we developed SCR (▶ Fig. 21.6, ▶ Fig. 21.7) for the treatment of irreparable rotator cuff tears. The clinical outcomes of the first 24 shoulders in 23 consecutive patients with irreparable rotator cuff tears (11 large tears, 13 massive tears) that underwent arthroscopic SCR were first reported in 2013.[1] Mean active elevation increased

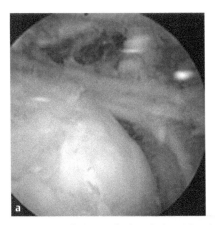
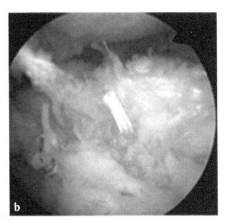

Fig. 21.6 Arthroscopic findings before (a) and after superior capsule reconstruction (b).

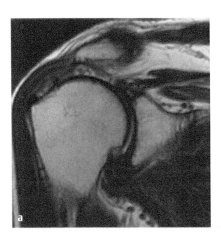
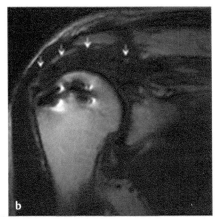

Fig. 21.7 Magnetic resonance imaging findings before and after superior capsule reconstruction (a) before surgery. The torn supraspinatus tendon is severely retracted, and the supraspinatus muscle is severely atrophied and infiltrated with fat. (b) One year after surgery.

significantly from 84° to 148° ($P < 0.001$) and ER increased from 26° to 40° ($P < 0.01$). Acromiohumeral distance increased from 4.6 mm preoperatively to 8.7 mm postoperatively ($P < 0.0001$) (▶ **Fig. 21.8**). The mean ASES score improved from 23.5 to 92.9 points ($P < 0.0001$).

The biomechanical role of SCR has been confirmed by a cadaveric study.[8] In that study, superior translation and subacromial contact pressure were significantly greater in simulated irreparable rotator cuff tears than in the intact condition (normal rotator cuff). After SCR using a fascia lata allograft, superior translation and subacromial contact pressure were completely normalized to the intact level. Side-to-side sutures between the graft and residual rotator cuff tendons improve force coupling in the shoulder joint. Restoration of shoulder stability after SCR improves deltoid function, resulting in increased active shoulder range of motion (especially elevation).

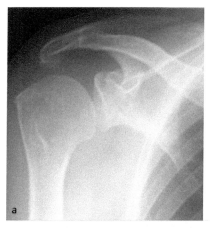 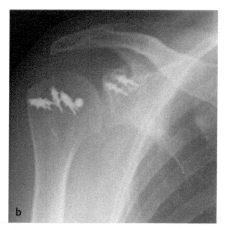

Fig. 21.8 X-ray findings before and after superior capsule reconstruction **(a)** before surgery. Acromiohumeral distance was 4 mm (Hamada grade 2). **(b)** One year after surgery. Acromiohumeral distance increased to 11 mm.

Patient suitability for SCR is determined by preoperative magnetic resonance imaging. Goutallier grades 3 and 4 (fatty infiltration equal to, or more than, muscle volume) are absolute indications. In Goutallier grade 2, if the torn tendon is severely retracted, degenerated, and thin, we also recommend SCR.

Irreparable rotator cuff tears of Hamada grades 1 to 3 are an absolute indication for SCR. Whereas young patients with Hamada grade 4 are recommended for SCR, elderly patients with Hamada grade 4 and all patients with Hamada grade 5 should have total shoulder arthroplasty with SCR.

During arthroscopy, the quality and mobility of the torn tendon are examined. If the torn tendon cannot be made to reach the original footprint (i.e., if the tear is irreducible), a preoperative decision is made to perform SCR alone. If the torn tendon can reach the original footprint after mobilization (i.e., if the tear is reducible), SCR followed by rotator cuff repair over the reconstructed superior capsule is recommended.

When patients already have severe deltoid atrophy and weakness from concomitant cervical spinal palsy (at the C5 level) or axillary nerve palsy, we do not recommend SCR because we cannot expect functional improvement after surgery, even when the graft is healed. If shoulder function does not recover after SCR, the cervical spine should be examined. Those patients may have cervical radiculopathy.

References

[1] Mihata T, Lee TQ, Watanabe C, et al. Clinical results of arthroscopic superior capsule reconstruction for irreparable rotator cuff tears. Arthroscopy. 2013; 29(3):459–470

[2] Mihata T, McGarry MH, Kahn T, Goldberg I, Neo M, Lee TQ. Biomechanical effect of thickness and tension of fascia lata graft on glenohumeral stability for superior capsule reconstruction in irreparable supraspinatus tears. Arthroscopy. 2016; 32(3):418–426

[3] Frank JM, Chahal J, Frank RM, Cole BJ, Verma NN, Romeo AA. The role of acromioplasty for rotator cuff problems. Orthop Clin North Am. 2014; 45(2):219–224

[4] Galliera E, Randelli P, Dogliotti G, et al. Matrix metalloproteases MMP-2 and MMP-9: are they early biomarkers of bone remodelling and healing after arthroscopic acromioplasty? Injury. 2010; 41(11):1204–1207

[5] Randelli P, Margheritini F, Cabitza P, Dogliotti G, Corsi MM. Release of growth factors after arthroscopic acromioplasty. Knee Surg Sports Traumatol Arthrosc. 2009; 17(1):98–101

[6] Mihata T, McGarry MH, Kahn T, Goldberg I, Neo M, Lee TQ. Biomechanical effects of Acromioplasty on superior capsule reconstruction for irreparable supraspinatus tendon tears. Am J Sports Med. 2016; 44(1):191–197

[7] Mihata T, McGarry MH, Kahn T, Goldberg I, Neo M, Lee TQ. Biomechanical role of capsular continuity in superior capsule reconstruction for irreparable tears of the supraspinatus tendon. Am J Sports Med. 2016; 44(6): 1423–1430

[8] Mihata T, McGarry MH, Pirolo JM, Kinoshita M, Lee TQ. Superior capsule reconstruction to restore superior stability in irreparable rotator cuff tears: a biomechanical cadaveric study. Am J Sports Med. 2012; 40(10): 2248–2255

22 Superior Capsular Reconstruction with Allograft

David M. Dines, Michael C. Fu, and Joshua S. Dines

Summary

Irreparable rotator cuff tears in the setting of minimal glenohumeral arthropathy is a challenging clinical problem, especially in young active patients. Reverse shoulder arthroplasty has been considered in these patients despite the absence of glenohumeral arthritis; however, concerns persist regarding implant longevity and activity limitations. Alternatively, superior capsular reconstruction (SCR) has emerged as a method of reconstructing the superior capsule and rotator cuff arthroscopically. Originally described in 2013, utilizing a fascia lata autograft, we have adopted a similar SCR technique but with a dermal allograft, which has higher tensile strength with decreased operative time and donor site morbidity. In this article, we describe our SCR technique with an accompanying video demonstration.

Keywords: dermal allograft, irreparable, massive, rotator cuff tear, shoulder arthroscopy, superior capsular reconstruction

22.1 Patient Positioning

At our institution, the vast majority of shoulder arthroscopy cases are performed with the use of regional anesthesia, if possible, for enhanced postoperative pain control. The patient is positioned in the beach chair position for superior capsular reconstruction (SCR), with the operative extremity secured to a pneumatic articulated arm holder. The back of the bed is elevated to approximately 60°, with the medial aspect of the scapula just lateral to the lateral edge of the bed. A kidney post and head holder are also used to secure the patient. We prefer the beach chair position because of ease of positioning, ability to dynamically position the arm intraoperatively, which is especially helpful in presenting the anterior and posterior aspects of the supraspinatus footprint to the arthroscopic field of view, and ease of conversion to open procedures if necessary.

22.2 Portal Placement

A standard posterior glenohumeral viewing portal is established first, followed by an anterior portal through the rotator interval. Typically, one or two lateral portals are used. Medial fixation on the glenoid is achieved with an anterior percutaneous portal just anterior to the acromion or the distal clavicle, and a posterior percutaneous portal, either through the Neviaser Portal or just posterior to the scapular spine.

22.3 Surgical Technique

Following induction of anesthesia and patient positioning, diagnostic arthroscopy is first performed through the posterior glenohumeral viewing portal along with an anterior portal through the rotator interval (▶ **Video 22.1**). Particular attention is directed

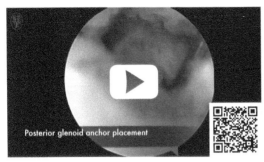

Video 22.1 Accompanying video of our preferred superior capsular reconstruction technique with dermal allograft. Individual surgical steps are detailed in the video captions.

toward the integrity of the subscapularis, which must be repaired if torn. If there is irreparable insufficiency of the subscapularis and/or infraspinatus, alternative treatment options such as reverse shoulder arthroplasty should be considered. There is also a high incidence of concomitant biceps pathology in patients undergoing SCR, and biceps tenodesis is performed in most cases.

Attention is then directed toward the subacromial space, first by establishing a lateral working portal. A 10-mm flexible cannula (PassPort Cannula, Arthrex, Naples, FL) is placed in the lateral portal to facilitate later graft passage and suture management. A limited subacromial decompression is performed in the standard fashion. The remaining supraspinatus tendon is carefully dissected from any attachments to the internal deltoid fascia, and an intraoperative determination is made whether to attempt rotator cuff repair or to proceed with SCR based on tissue quality and excursion.

After deciding to proceed with SCR, the bone beds medial to the superior glenoid labrum and over the humeral greater tuberosity are prepared with a shaver. Two single-loaded 3.0-mm biocomposite SutureTak anchors (Arthrex) are placed in the superior glenoid neck, at about the 2o'clock and 10o'clock positions. Then, two threaded 4.75-mm biocomposite SwiveLock(Arthrex) suture anchors preloaded with FiberTape(Arthrex) sutures are placed at the medial aspect of the greater tuberosity footprint just lateral to the articular margin, for the medial row of a double-row technique.

The distances between the anchors are measured arthroscopically using a calibrated probe. The positions of the anchors are marked accordingly on a 3.0-mm acellular dermal allograft (ArthroFlex, Arthrex). We typically add 5–10 mm of tissue on each of the four sides to reduce the chance of sutures cutting out. All sutures are retrieved through the lateral cannula, and the greater tuberosity sutures are passed through their respective holes in the graft. For the sutures from the medial glenoid anchors, each limb is passed individually through the graft, approximately 2 mm anterior and 2 mm posterior to the anchor marks on the graft. Therefore, there are four passes through the medial aspect of the graft. In the middle of the graft, one suture limb from each of the medial anchors are then tied to each other over a drill guide or a switching stick. By pulling on the two remaining outside sutures from the glenoid anchors, a double-pulley technique in combination with a tissue grasper are used to deliver the graft into the joint. Once the graft is docked onto the superior glenoid, the two remaining sutures from the glenoid anchor are then tied to each other in a static knot. In many cases, we may also augment the glenoid neck fixation with a previously placed FiberWire suture (Arthrex) at the center position on the graft, which is then fixed at the 12 O'clock position of the glenoid with a PushLock anchor (Arthrex).

Attention is then turned toward lateral fixation of the graft in a double-row fashion. One limb from each of the previously passed FiberTape sutures are retrieved in a criss-crossed fashion and secured at the lateral row using two unloaded 4.75-mm SwiveLock anchors. At this point, additional glenoid anchors may be placed for added fixation if necessary. Finally, the graft is repaired posteriorly to the infraspinatus with side-to-side sutures.

22.4 Surgeon Tips and Tricks

- Thorough bursectomy should be performed to view the entire rotator cuff defect to the glenoid surface.
- The medial glenoid anchors can be placed either through the NeviaserPortal, anterior to the acromion or distal clavicle, or posterior to the scapular spine, whichever allows for the best angle of approach.
- If a biceps tenodesis with an interference screw is placed at the edge of the bicipital groove, this anchor may be preloaded with FiberTape to serve as the anteromedial anchor for lateral graft fixation.
- All sutures should be passed through the graft outside of the body, with an assistant maintaining gentle constant tension to minimize the risk of sutures getting tangled.
- Using a tissue grasper to help in delivering the graft through the cannula and into the joint reduces the risk of the glenoid anchors pulling out when performing the double-pulley technique.
- Prior to completing the lateral fixation, redundancy in the FiberTape can be eliminated by pushing a retriever down each suture to reduce the graft onto the tuberosity bed, while tensioning the suture. The arm is placed at 30° of abduction during the lateral reconstruction.
- Perform margin convergence anteriorly if there is adequate tissue; however, care must be taken to not overconstrain the shoulder.

22.5 Pitfalls/Complications

- The suprascapular nerve may be injured during bursectomy or placement of anchors into the glenoid. Stay at least 5 mm lateral to the base of the scapular spine to avoid damage to the suprascapular nerve.
- Inadequate suture management will lead to tangling of the sutures.
- Inaccurate measurement of the distances between the anchors will result in a graft that is either too large or too small. A graft that is too small may result in postoperative stiffness, increased risk of re-tear, and overtightening of the sutures. Conversely, a graft that is too large may result in joint instability and dog-ear formation.

22.6 Rehabilitation

Postoperative rehabilitation following SCR is carried out rather slowly and cautiously to protect the reconstruction. To allow for adequate graft incorporation and healing, patients are typically immobilized with a shoulder immobilizer with limited motion allowed for the first 6 weeks. Gentle motion is then allowed, with progression to more aggressive mobilization and strengthening at 12–14 weeks.

22.7 Rationale and/or Evidence for Approach

In a cadaveric biomechanical study, Mihata et al[1] compared shoulders with intact rotator cuffs, shoulders with absent supraspinatus, and shoulders following SCR with a fascia lata allograft.[2] The authors found that relative to the intact condition, absence of the supraspinatus tendon resulted in significantly increased superior humeral translation, subacromial contact pressure, and significantly decreased glenohumeral contact force. Following SCR, superior translation and subacromial contact forces were fully restored. They also demonstrated that SCR with medial graft fixation to the glenoid was biomechanically superior to grafts that were medially repaired to remnant supraspinatus tendon.[2] Furthermore, in a separate cadaveric biomechanical study, Mihata et al[1] showed that performing acromioplasty concurrently with SCR reduced the subacromial contact area, which may reduce subacromial abrasion and tearing of the graft.[3] Finally, in the largest clinical series to date, Mihata et al[1] reported on the clinical outcomes of 23 patients that underwent SCR with fascia lata autograft. At an average follow-up of 34.1 months (24–51 months), all patients had an improved American Shoulder and Elbow Surgeons score from an average preoperative score of 23.5 to 92.9 postoperatively. Active elevation also improved from 84° to 148°. In terms of radiographic outcomes, the acromiohumeral distance increased from 4.6 mm to 8.7 mm, and 83% of patients had intact reconstructions without progression of muscle atrophy in postoperative magnetic resonance imaging.

References

[1] Mihata T, Lee TQ, Watanabe C, et al. Clinical results of arthroscopic superior capsule reconstruction for irreparable rotator cuff tears. Arthroscopy. 2013; 29(3):459–470

[2] Mihata T, McGarry MH, Pirolo JM, Kinoshita M, Lee TQ. Superior capsule reconstruction to restore superior stability in irreparable rotator cuff tears: a biomechanical cadaveric study. Am J Sports Med. 2012; 40(10): 2248–2255

[3] Mihata T, McGarry MH, Kahn T, Goldberg I, Neo M, Lee TQ. Biomechanical effects of acromioplasty on superior capsule reconstruction for irreparable supraspinatus tendon tears. Am J Sports Med. 2016; 44(1):191–197

23 Superior Capsular Reconstruction with Porcine Xenograft

Ruth A. Delaney and Daniel B.L. Garcia

Summary

Outcomes are variable with current nonarthroplasty techniques for treating massive, irreparable rotator cuff tears. Reverse shoulder arthroplasty may be a more reliable option but high complication rates in younger patients and in revision reverse arthroplasty are cause for concern. Superior capsular reconstruction (SCR) recreates superior stability, thereby restoring the glenohumeral fulcrum. In some countries, human allograft tissue is not readily available, therefore we use porcine xenograft. In this chapter, we describe our surgical technique for SCR using the DX Matrix xenograft. Technical pearls for portal placement, graft passage, and suture management are discussed. We also report clinical outcome data on our first 20 cases: 14 males, 6 females, mean age 60.8 years, mean follow-up 12.2 months, range 6–25 months. Seven patients were pseudoparalytic preoperatively; in five, the pseudoparalysis was reversed postoperatively. In one patient, the graft failed at the glenoid on magnetic resonance imaging at 15 months. Overall, mean visual analog scale improved from 5 preoperatively to 1.4 postoperatively, $p = 0.0013$; American Shoulder and Elbow Surgeons (ASES) score from 46.85 to 76.34, $p = 0.004$; and subjective shoulder value from 46% to 72%, $p = 0.018$. There was a significant difference in postoperative ASES scores ($p = 0.034$) and active forward elevation ($p = 0.002$) in patients who were pseudoparalytic preoperatively compared to those who were not.

Keywords: massive rotator cuff tear, porcine xenograft, pseudoparalysis, superior capsular reconstruction

23.1 Patient Positioning

We prefer to perform the superior capsular reconstruction (SCR) in the beach chair position, but it can also be performed in the lateral decubitus position. An iodine-impregnated adhesive drape is used to cover the skin, so that the allograft does not come into contact with skin flora prior to insertion.

23.2 Portal Placement

A standard posterior viewing portal and anterosuperior instrumentation portal are created to start. Thereafter, two lateral portals are created to allow for graft and suture passage as well as viewing from lateral. This does not differ from the typical approach to rotator cuff repair. Additional portals are created for insertion of the glenoid anchors, using an outside-in technique with a spinal needle. A separate portal is required for each glenoid anchor, anterior and posterior (▶ **Video 23.1**).

23.3 Surgical Technique

As with any arthroscopic procedure, visualization and preparation are critical. A mean arterial blood pressure of less than 80 mmHg is typically required, with a pump

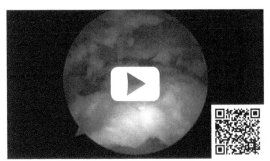

Video 23.1 Preparatory steps and anchor placement.

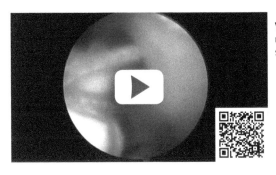

Video 23.2 Graft placement, lateral row fixation and posterior side to side repair.

pressure of 40 mmHg. A higher pump pressure can be used, but we prefer to do as much of the case as possible before increasing the pressure, as the resultant swelling can make the lateral row anchors difficult to visualize well for insertion on the humerus. The SCR becomes essentially a double-row cuff repair with a side-to-side posterior repair, once you have placed the glenoid anchors and passed the graft.

23.3.1 Key Steps (Steps 1–5, ▶ Video 23.1; Steps 6–15, ▶ Video 23.2)

- Prepare superior glenoid and rotator cuff footprint. The long head of biceps, if present, is usually tenotomized or tenodesed, depending on patient age, activity level, and body habitus; therefore, the superior labrum can be completely debrided to give access to a good bony surface for healing of the graft to the superior glenoid.
- Insert an anterior and a posterior anchor into the superior glenoid. We use 2.9-mm SutureTak anchors. These do not need to be double-loaded. If they are, then pull out one suture from each. It is a good idea to have a color-coding system, so have the blue suture in the posterior anchor and the white suture in the anterior anchor.
- Insert a cannula into the anterior of the two lateral portals. A 10-mm PassPort cannula facilitates graft passage without taking up too much space. A 12 mm cannula is also available if needed.
- Place medial row anchors in the humerus at the margin of the articular cartilage. Again, color code these so that the SwiveLock with blue FiberTape is posterior and white anterior. We do not typically use the safety suture in the reconstruction, but pull it out and use it later as a free suture for the side-to-side repair. It is also possible

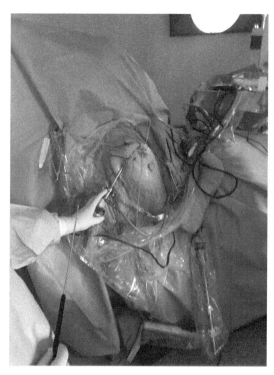

Fig. 23.1 Suture management is critical. All sutures and tapes are retrieved out the lateral PassPort portal and clipped to the drapes in a configuration that corresponds to their respective anchors.

to use it for a medial double pulley on the graft at this stage, but we have not found that to add to the reconstruction, and it tends to complicate suture management.

- Bring all sutures and tapes out through the PassPort cannula laterally (► **Fig. 23.1**).
- Measure the distance between the anchors on all four sides, while an assistant draws out the shape and writes down the measurements on the back table. Take care to measure as accurately as possible. There is a disposable measuring device (as seen in ► **Fig. 23.1**) or a reusable instrument available.
- Measure out the graft, add 5 mm on each side, mark suture placement, and double the graft over (► **Fig. 23.2**, ► **Fig. 23.3**). The porcine xenograft, DX Matrix, is licensed for use as a reinforcement of large rotator cuff repairs. When using it for SCR, it is recommended to double the graft over.
- Pass a traction suture through the middle of the glenoid end of the graft (► **Fig. 23.4**). We have found that the Scorpion device is the easiest instrument for passing all sutures and tapes through the graft, and leaves a smaller hole in the graft. Bring the graft over to the operative field. Pass the traction stitch in through one of the lateral portals (usually the more anterior one) and retrieve it out through the Neviaser portal created for the posterior glenoid anchor. Clip the traction stitch to the drapes while the remainder of the sutures are being passed.
- Pass two limbs of one suture from each glenoid anchor through the graft, therefore, four passes along the medial end of the graft. (See below for a modification to the glenoid suture configuration to reduce the risk of graft failure at the medial side.)
- Pass the tapes from each medial row humeral anchor through the graft. This can be done at this stage, or the graft can be passed first and then the humeral side tapes passed.

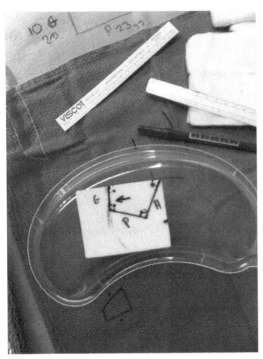

Fig. 23.2 The graft is measured, cut, and marked for orientation.

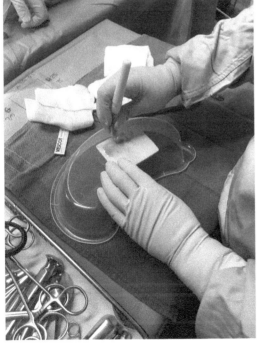

Fig. 23.3 Skin glue is used to double the graft over and fix the two layers.

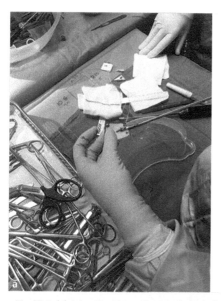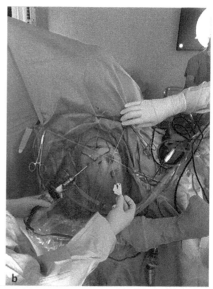

Fig. 23.4 (a) A traction suture is passed through the medial end of the graft to facilitate graft passage. **(b)** This suture is retrieved out the Neviaser portal.

- Tie one limb from each glenoid anchor together for a pulley, test all four limbs of the knot for security, and then cut the ends above the knot. Suture management is critical throughout the procedure, especially when ready to pass the graft (▸ **Fig. 23.5**).
- Shuttle graft into joint by pulling the other two sutures and the traction stitch. The glenoid sutures will run through the glenoid anchor, thereby pulling the graft into the joint. The traction suture is very helpful by providing tension in the correct vector to pull the graft medially toward the glenoid. Once the graft is seated in the shoulder, the traction suture can be removed.
- Complete the lateral row repair. This is exactly the same as for a standard rotator cuff repair. The joined FiberTapes from each anchor are cut to separate them. One tape from each medial row anchor is passed through a knotless anchor. One knotless anchor is placed anterior and one posterior, with the arm at 30° abduction for insertion and tensioning.
- Suture the graft to any remaining posterior cuff in a side-to-side fashion. There is almost always some remaining posterior cuff. A thorough bursectomy will help when only the teres minor is left and the tendon is quite posterior. This step is important to maximize the humeral head-depressing effect as well as to help with active external rotation (▸ **Fig. 23.6**).
- Check the reconstruction from an intraarticular view before leaving. This should be done for any rotator cuff repair. If the shoulder is swollen and it is difficult to reenter the joint from the posterior portal, use the anterosuperior portal in the rotator interval to get an intraarticular view.

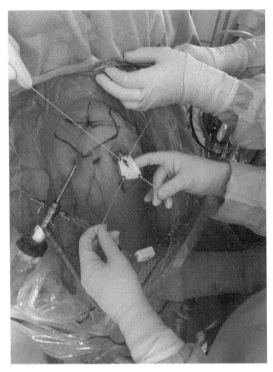

Fig. 23.5 All sutures have been passed through the graft, which is now ready to pass.

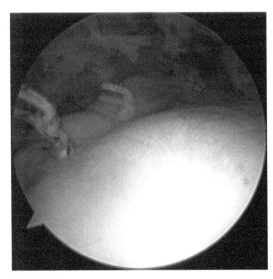

Fig. 23.6 The remaining posterior rotator cuff is sutured to the graft.

23.3.2 Tips and Tricks

- Preparation is key: make sure to take the time to do a thorough subacromial bursectomy and to prepare the superior glenoid.

- Acromioplasty: it is important that the graft not be abraded against the acromion, which is a particular risk with type II or III acromial morphology.
- The glenoid anchors can be inserted from a Neviaser portal for the posterior anchor and either another, more anterior Neviaser portal or a portal just anterior to the clavicle. With these portals, the tendency is to aim slightly lateral, which risks glenoid cartilage perforation. Another option is to place the glenoid anchors from the lateral portals. This gives a safer vector for aiming the drill and anchor, but is only possible if the patient's acromion is not very wide, as the angle will be too flat in patients with a larger acromion because of the longer distance from the lateral portal to the glenoid.
- Particularly when placing the glenoid anchors from Neviaser portals, watch the glenoid cartilage closely while the assistant is drilling for glenoid anchors, so that any potential perforation can be anticipated and stopped. A slightly more medial starting point for these anchors will also protect from cartilage perforation.
- The porcine allograft needs to be doubled over to be thick enough for SCR. We have found that using skin glue, Dermabond, is a quick way of securing the two layers of graft together and saves time compared to whipstitching the graft layers together. In addition, the dried Dermabond seems to add toughness to the graft. It does make it a little more difficult to pass the graft, but the traction suture helps overcome this problem.
- Rather than marking out anterior, posterior, medial/glenoid, and lateral/humerus on the graft, which can lead to a lot of marks close together and potential confusion, a simple arrow on the graft for orientation is best. We draw an arrow on the graft pointing toward the glenoid end of the graft.
- Inserting a traction stitch on the medial side of graft, which is retrieved out through the Neviaser portal prior to passage of the graft, allows for the graft to be pulled into the joint from medial as well as pushed in from lateral. We have found this extremely helpful.
- Glenoid side failure of the graft has been a concern. Using a lasso loop configuration rather than a simple shuttle means that fixation is not dependent on only two knots, one of which is tied arthroscopically, but rather on four knots and two lasso loops (▶ **Fig. 23.7**).
- Cut out the inner membrane on the PassPort cannula to make graft passage easier.
- If you wait until the graft is passed to pass the tapes through the graft, you need fewer assistants to manage the sutures and tapes during graft passage and can do it with only one assistant and the scrub nurse or tech.
- I find a suture shuttle device more versatile for the side-to-side repair to teres minor/infra.

23.4 Pitfalls, Complications

- SutureTaks pulling out of glenoid: insert 5 mm corkscrews with capital C (anchor brand name).
- Graft too small: sometimes if you cut rather than fold it and rotate the shape, then you are still able to double it over without having to open a second graft, which saves greatly on cost.
- Medial fixation: lasso loop technique on glenoid suture. Insert the four glenoid suture limbs (two from each anchor) into the graft in the following configuration: simple, lasso, lasso, simple (▶ **Fig. 23.7**). Then pull on the two simple suture limbs to shuttle

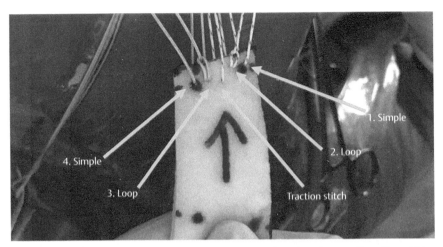

Fig. 23.7 An alternative method of medial suture passage using a lasso loop configuration, which may lead to stronger glenoid fixation of the graft.

the graft into the joint (while also pulling on the traction suture and pushing the graft in through the lateral cannula using a grasper). Tie these two simple sutures together once the graft is seated. Then tie each simple suture to a lasso loop suture (▶ **Fig. 23.7**).

- Sutures and tapes tangling: this is usually a result of the lateral tapes in the graft pulling into the shoulder with the graft and looping around the sutures from the glenoid anchors. To avoid this, either make sure the assistant holding those humeral tapes understands to keep pulling them out of the graft as you pass it, or alternatively just wait until after graft passage to pass the tapes (which can also be advantageous in terms of setting the correct mediolateral graft tension). It can also be helpful to use the SwiveLock handle to punch bigger holes on the humeral end of the graft to facilitate tape passage through the graft.

23.5 Rehabilitation

There are three key principles of rehabilitation that need to be considered for a patient following SCR. These are: optimize graft healing as part of a conservative rehabilitation approach; deltoid re-education; and collaborative working between the surgeon, therapist and patient. Rehabilitation is split into four main phases, over a 12-month period.

23.5.1 Phase 1

Protective phase, weeks zero to six post-op. Six weeks are spent in a shoulder immobilizer, with an abduction pillow. No active range of motion. Passive range of motion may commence before 6 weeks post-op, depending on the individual case, particularly if the patient was stiff preoperatively. This phase coincides with the initial inflammatory phase of healing of the graft.

23.5.2 Phase 2

Intermediate phase, 6 weeks to 3 months post-op, coincides with graft incorporation and revascularization. Goals are to establish basic rotator cuff and scapular neuromuscular control within a pain-free range, and to restore functional active range of movement. No bands, heavy lifting, or weights to be used for the first 12 weeks. No specific rotator cuff strengthening exercises for the first 12 weeks. Anterior deltoid reeducation is commenced during phase 2. Pool sessions are encouraged: supervised hydrotherapy or self-directed passive range of motion in the pool.

23.5.3 Phase 3

Strengthening phase, 3 to 6 months post-op, coincides with the remodeling phase of healing where collagen fibers are laid down to achieve the overall tensile strength of the graft. Goals are to design a structured and progressive strengthening program for the deltoid, remaining rotator cuff, and scapular stabilizers. Patients return to more physically demanding work and leisure activities toward the end of this phase.

23.5.4 Phase 4

Advanced rehabilitation, 6 to 12 months post-op. Goals are to motivate our patients to continue exercising up to 12 months postoperatively and beyond, and to design an individualized rehabilitation program for enhanced functional use of the upper extremities. This phase includes advanced strengthening exercises for return to full functional activities, as well as an advanced proprioceptive and neuromuscular control program. Patients are contacted via email using the Surgical Outcomes System program at 12 and 24 months post-op for patient-reported outcome measures.

23.6 Rationale and Evidence

23.6.1 Outcomes—Unpublished Data

The following are the current outcomes data on our first 20 cases: 14 males and six females, with a mean age 60.8 years. Mean follow-up, so far, is 12.2 months, range 6 to 25 months. Seven patients were pseudoparalytic preoperatively; in five, the pseudoparalysis was reversed postoperatively. In one patient, the graft failed at the glenoid on magnetic resonance imaging at 15 months. Overall, mean visual analog scale for pain improved from five preoperatively to 1.4 postoperatively, $p = 0.0013$; mean American Shoulder and Elbow Surgeons (ASES) score increased from 46.85 to 76.34, $p = 0.004$; and the mean subjective shoulder value improved from 46% preoperatively to 72% postoperatively, $p = 0.018$. There was a significant difference in postoperative ASES scores ($p = 0.034$) and active forward elevation ($p = 0.002$) in patients who were pseudoparalytic preoperatively compared to those who were not pseudoparalytic, with those patients whose main preoperative complaint was pain rather than pseudoparalysis tending to achieve better ASES scores and better active forward elevation. There was no difference in the other outcome parameters.

23.6.2 SCR Data

The SCR technique was originally described by Dr. Teruhisa Mihata, using a fascia lata autograft to restore glenohumeral kinematics.[1] His group's clinical results are similar to ours, with longer follow-up.[2] He has also studied the biomechanical rationale for the importance of the acromioplasty in the context of the SCR procedure.[3]

23.6.3 DX Matrix Graft

Based on biomechanical testing done by Arthrex, the doubled-over DX Matrix porcine allograft fails at 440N, compared to fascia lata failure at 180N and Arthroflex (the human dermal allograft) failure at 550N. The longest follow-up of SCR procedures is Mihata's series, which uses a fascia lata autograft, and based on the biomechanical figures above, we felt comfortable extrapolating to SCR with the porcine allograft. We continue to track our outcomes closely.

23.6.4 Evidence Supporting our Rehabilitation Protocol

The timing of the rehabilitation phases is based largely on a combination of known principles of rotator cuff repair and reverse shoulder arthroplasty rehabilitation,[4] as well as the biology of dermal allograft healing and integration.[5,6] Our rehabilitation protocol was developed by senior physiotherapist, Fiona Noonan-Taylor.[7]

References

[1] Mihata T, McGarry MH, Pirolo JM, Kinoshita M, Lee TQ. Superior capsule reconstruction to restore superior stability in irreparable rotator cuff tears: a biomechanical cadaveric study. Am J Sports Med. 2012; 40(10): 2248–2255

[2] Mihata T, Lee TQ, Watanabe C, et al. Clinical results of arthroscopic superior capsule reconstruction for irreparable rotator cuff tears. Am J Sports Med. 2012; 40(10):2248–2255

[3] Mihata T, McGarry MH, Kahn T, Goldberg I, Neo M, Lee TQ. Biomechanical effects of acromioplasty on superior capsular reconstruction for irreparable supraspinatus tendon tears. Am J Sports Med. 2016; 44(1):191–197

[4] Boudreau S, Boudreau ED, Higgins LD, Wilcox RB, III. Rehabilitation following reverse total shoulder arthroplasty. J Orthop Sports Phys Ther. 2007; 37(12):734–743

[5] Valentin JE, Badylak JS, McCabe GP, Badylak SF. Extracellular matrix bioscaffolds for orthopaedic applications. A comparative histologic study. J Bone Joint Surg Am. 2006; 88(12):2673–2686

[6] Hackett ES, Harilal D, Bowley C, Hawes M, Turner AS, Goldman SM. Evaluation of porcine hydrated dermis augmented repair in a fascial defect model. J Biomed Mater Res B Appl Biomater. 2011; 96(1):134–138

[7] Noonan-Taylor F, Langford C, O'Leary H, Kingston R, Delaney RA. Superior capsule reconstruction (SCR) of the shoulder: Clinical relevance and current perceptions in the post-operative rehabilitation. [unpublished thesis]. Limerick, Ireland: MSc Advanced Healthcare Practice, University of Limerick; 2017

24 All-Arthroscopic Superior Capsular Reconstruction with Dermal Allograft

Sriram Sankaranarayanan, Frances Cuomo, and Konrad I. Gruson

Summary

Superior capsular reconstruction using human acellular dermal allograft has emerged as a promising surgical treatment option for massive irreparable rotator cuff tears. The reconstructed superior capsule acts as a restraint to superior humeral migration during active shoulder abduction. It also helps to balance the force couples necessary for overhead shoulder function. In this chapter, we describe our all-arthroscopic surgical technique for performing a superior capsular reconstruction utilizing a dermal allograft. We find the superior capsular reconstruction most useful in relatively younger, symptomatic patients with chronic massive irreparable rotator cuff tears who are deemed not to be candidates for a reverse total shoulder arthroplasty. Furthermore, we reserve this procedure for those patients with an intact or repairable subscapularis tendon, in addition to Hamada 1 or 2 changes to the glenohumeral joint.

Keywords: dermal allograft, massive irreparable cuff tear, superior capsular reconstruction

24.1 Patient Positioning

- The patient is positioned in the beach chair position.
- All the bony prominences are adequately padded.
- A pneumatic arm holder is utilized during the procedure.

24.2 Portal Placement

The procedure can be performed with standard anterior, posterior, and lateral subacromial portals. Percutaneous stab incisions are utilized for anchor insertion as well as for docking sutures. Specifically, the Neviaser portal can be useful for placement of the glenoid anchors.

24.3 Surgical Technique

- The shoulder joint is entered via a standard midglenoid posterior portal. A diagnostic arthroscopy is performed. We typically release the long head biceps tendon at its insertion on the glenoid with a biter and perform a subpectoral biceps tenodesis. The subscapularis is repaired if it is torn. All other intraarticular pathology is addressed as needed.
- The subacromial space is then initially entered from the posterior portal. A midlateral portal is then established. A subacromial decompression is performed. Bursal- and articular-sided releases of the rotator cuff are performed. The mobility of the cuff is evaluated after the releases are performed. We make every effort to repair the native rotator cuff if possible.

- If the tear is determined to be irreparable, we proceed to perform a superior capsular reconstruction. Even in this case, we make every effort to balance the joint and minimize the amount of graft required by repairing the posterior rotator cuff using standard anchor repair techniques.
- The superior glenoid neck immediately medial to the labrum is prepared. We elect not to resect the superior labrum, but to create a bleeding bony bed medially using cautery and a burr. Care is taken not to go more than 1 cm medial to the glenoid edge to avoid injury to the suprascapular nerve.
- Two 3-mm glenoid anchors bio-composite or PEEK (Suture-Tak, Arthrex, Naples, FL) are inserted either through the standard anterior, posterior, or Neviaser portals. Alternatively, knotless Suture-Tak anchors may be utilized to reduce the risk of suture entanglement. Care is taken to direct the anchors away from the glenoid to avoid inadvertent penetration into the joint.
- The greater tuberosity is prepared in a standard fashion using a burr. Two 4.75 mm anchors (SwiveLock anchors with FiberTape sutures, Arthrex) are inserted through stab incisions into the medial aspect of the rotator cuff footprint on the greater tuberosity. It is critical to place the anchor as anteriorly as possible to maximize the coverage of the humeral head and reduce the risk for humeral superior escape. The anterior anchor is inserted just posterior to the biceps groove. The posterior anchor is inserted close to the infraspinatus insertion.
- A measuring device is utilized to measure the medial-to-lateral as well as anterior-to-posterior distances between each of the sets of anchors. Prior to measurement, the shoulder should be placed in 20-30 degrees of abduction, neutral flexion and neutral rotation to appropriately tension the graft.
- A 10 mm cannula (PassPort, Arthrex) is inserted through the midlateral portal.
- The sutures from the four anchors are brought out through the midlateral portal. The sutures are held separately and clamped to avoid tangling.
- The graft (ArthroFLEXacellular dermal allograft, Arthrex, 3 mm thickness) is prepared on the back table. The distances previously measured are marked on the graft material using a marking pen. The dimensions are extended by 5 mm over the medial, anterior, and posterior aspects to prevent suture cut-through. The dimension is extended 10-15 mm over the lateral aspect to recreate the anatomical lateral footprint. The graft is then cut based on these dimensions.
- Utilizing a suture passer device, the sutures limbs from the anchors are passed through the graft. This can be facilitated by using the empty anchor driver for the SwiveLock anchor (Arthrex, Naples, FL) to punch the holes in the graft.
- A double-pulley technique is then utilized. One limb from each of the glenoid anchors is tied over a switching stick. The leading edge of the graft is grasped with a tissue grasper. The graft is advanced into the lateral cannula by pulling on the two untied suture ends from the glenoid anchor and by pushing it in through the cannula with a grasper. Tension is held on the remaining sutures as the graft is shuttled into the cannula.
- Viewing from the posterior portal, a switching stick is inserted through the lateral portal to flatten out the graft.
- The sutures from the individual medial greater tuberosity anchors are retrieved via their respective stab incisions through which they were initially inserted. This reduces the risk for suture entanglement.
- The remaining sutures from the two glenoid anchors are tied down to secure the medial edge of the graft.

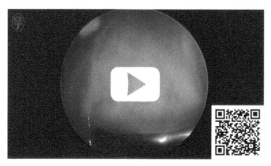

Video 24.1 Surgical demonstration of all-arthroscopic superior capsular reconstruction with dermal allograft.

- A extraneousness-equivalent technique is then utilized to secure the graft to the greater tuberosity.
- The suture limbs from the medial tuberosity anchors are tied in a double-pulley fashion to further secure the graft to the medial aspect of the greater tuberosity. Alternatively, these sutures may be used to close the respective intervals between the graft material and the native intact rotator cuff.
- Side-to-side sutures are placed between the posterior aspect of the graft and the remaining infraspinatus and tied down. Similarly, the interval between the graft material and the subscapularis tendon should be closed (▶ **Video 24.1**).

24.4 Surgeon Tips and Tricks

- Care should be taken during preparation of the glenoid to prevent injury to the suprascapular nerve.
- Care should be taken while inserting the glenoid anchors to prevent inadvertent penetration into the joint.
- During retrieval of glenoid and medial tuberosity sutures through the lateral cannula as well as during the passage of the graft into the shoulder, the suture limbs are held separately and clamped. This prevents tangling of the sutures.
- Anchor pull-out can sometimes be encountered during this procedure especially during the passage of the graft. Care is taken to be gentle during graft insertion.

24.5 Rehabilitation

- An abduction sling is utilized in the postoperative period.
- Initial rehabilitation focuses on protected range of motion (ROM) with an aim to prevent stiffness and to improve glenohumeral and scapulothoracic biomechanics.
- Progressive active and active-assisted ROM from the supine position is begun at 6 weeks postoperatively.
- Progressive strengthening is started at 3 months postoperatively.

24.6 Rationale and Evidence for Approach

- The first biomechanical studies on the superior capsule of the shoulder were performed by Ishihara et al[1] They found that sectioning of the superior capsule resulted in increased humeral translation in all directions.

- Mihata et al[2] in their biomechanical studies found that reconstructing the superior capsule of the shoulder resulted in complete restoration of the superior translation of the humerus.
- These studies formed the basis of performing superior capsular reconstruction in patients with massive irreparable rotator cuff tears. The reconstructed superior capsule was believed to act as a superior restraint to the humerus in these patients.
- Mihata et al[3] reported their clinical findings on 24 patients treated with a superior capsular reconstruction with an average follow-up period of 34 months. The mean age of the patients in their study was 65 years. They found that forward elevation in their patients increased from 84°to 148°. External rotation increased from 26° to 40°. The American Shoulder and Elbow Surgeons scores increased from 23 to 92.
- Other studies[4,5,6,7,8] on superior capsular reconstruction with acellular dermal allograft showed similar results at 2- to 4-year follow-up with significant improvement in patient-reported outcome measures, decrease in pain, as well as improvement in ROM. More recent clinical studies have focused on the patient-related factors such as the degree of glenohumeral arthritis that can adversely affect clinical outcomes.[9]
- Histological studies performed by Snyder et al[10] suggest that there was host cellular infiltration as well as organization of new tissue along the margins of the graft in the postoperative period. This forms the basis of performing a margin convergence of the native infraspinatus to the edge of the graft.
- Mihata et al[11] determined the effect of acromioplasty on superior capsular reconstruction in their biomechanical studies. They found that performing an acromioplasty in the superior capsular reconstruction decreased the subacromial contact area and had no effect on the subacromial contact pressures. They concluded that acromioplasty may help to decrease the postoperative risk of abrasion and tearing of the graft beneath the acromion. Hence, acromioplasty can be safely performed in patients undergoing a superior capsular reconstruction.
- Recent cadaveric studies have reported on the use of 3 glenoid-sided anchors to reduce the ultimate load-to-failure of the graft on the glenoid.[12]
- In conclusion, superior capsular reconstruction can be utilized as an option for relatively younger patients with symptomatic massive irreparable cuff tears who are deemed not to be candidates for a reverse total shoulder arthroplasty.

References

[1] Ishihara Y, Mihata T, Tamboli M, et al. Role of the superior shoulder capsule in passive stability of the gleno-humeral joint. J Shoulder Elbow Surg. 2014; 23(5):642–648

[2] Mihata T, McGarry MH, Pirolo JM, Kinoshita M, Lee TQ. Superior capsule reconstruction to restore superior stability in irreparable rotator cuff tears: a biomechanical cadaveric study. Am J Sports Med. 2012; 40(10): 2248–2255

[3] Mihata T, Lee TQ, Watanabe C, et al. Clinical results of arthroscopic superior capsule reconstruction for irreparable rotator cuff tears. Arthroscopy. 2013; 29(3):459–470

[4] Bond JL, Dopirak RM, Higgins J, Burns J, Snyder SJ. Arthroscopic replacement of massive, irreparable rotator cuff tears using a GraftJacket allograft: technique and preliminary results. Arthroscopy. 2008; 24(4): 403–409.e1

[5] Gupta AK, Hug K, Berkoff DJ, et al. Dermal tissue allograft for the repair of massive irreparable rotator cuff tears. Am J Sports Med. 2012; 40(1):141–147

[6] Wong I, Burns J, Snyder S. Arthroscopic GraftJacket repair of rotator cuff tears. J Shoulder Elbow Surg. 2010; 19(2) Suppl:104–109

[7] Modi A, Singh HP, Pandey R, Armstrong A. Management of irreparable rotator cuff tears with the GraftJacket allograft as an interpositional graft. Shoulder Elbow. 2013; 5:188–194

[8] Petri M, Greenspoon JA, Moulton SG, Millett PJ. Patch-augmented rotator cuff repair and superior capsule reconstruction. Open Orthop J. 2016; 10:315–323

[9] Denard PJ, Brady PC, Adams CR, Tokish JM, Burkhart SS. Preliminary results of arthroscopic superior capsule reconstruction with dermal allograft. Arthroscopy. 2018;34(1):93–99

[10] Snyder SJ, Arnoczky SP, Bond JL, Dopirak R. Histologic evaluation of a biopsy specimen obtained 3 months after rotator cuff augmentation with GraftJacket Matrix. Arthroscopy. 2009; 25(3):329–333

[11] Mihata T, McGarry MH, Kahn T, Goldberg I, Neo M, Lee TQ. Biomechanical effects of acromioplasty on superior capsule reconstruction for irreparable supraspinatus tendon tears. Am J Sports Med. 2016; 44(1):191–197

[12] Pogorzelski J, Muckenhirn KJ, Mitchell JJ, et al. Biomechanical comparison of 3 glenoid-side fixation techniques for superior capsular reconstruction. Am J Sports Med. 2018;46(4):801–808

25 Subpectoral Biceps Tenodesis

Jacob M. Kirsch and Michael T. Freehill

Summary

Subpectoral biceps tenodesis is a safe, reliable, and efficient procedure for managing various pathologies of the long head of the biceps (LHB) tendon. The LHB tendon is a common source of shoulder pain and generally occurs concomitantly with rotator cuff disease and labral injuries. A number of strategies exist to address the LHB including tenotomy and multiple tenodesis techniques. Subpectoral biceps tenodesis offers a distinct advantage by removing all diseased tissue from the bicipital groove. This potentially reduces the incidence of persistent pain, which otherwise may be left unaddressed with more proximally based techniques. Additionally, subpectoral biceps tenodesis may better restore the anatomic resting length and tension of the LHB, thereby providing a more cosmetic result with a decreased likelihood of biceps cramping. The all-suture double-loaded anchor utilizes a smaller osseous pilot hole and the benefit of unicortical intramedullary fixation. A small self-retrieving suture device (Accupass Direct, Smith & Nephew, London, UK)allows for smaller diameter soft tissue penetration while performing a double-lasso-loop configuration, resulting in a circumferential capture of the tendon. This subpectoral biceps tenodesis technique offers reliable pain relief, high patient satisfaction rates, and low rates of complications.

Keywords: biceps tendonitis/tenosynovitis, biceps tenodesis, SLAP, all-suture anchor

25.1 Patient Positioning and Planning the Surgical Approach

- Beach chair position with extremity in pneumatic arm holder (Spider2, Smith & Nephew).
- Abduct arm to identify and mark the inferior border of the pectoralis major tendon.
- Adduct arm to identify a crease to be utilized for skin incision.
- Roughly a 3 cm incision in marked axillary skin crease.

25.2 Surgical Technique

25.2.1 Surgical Exposure

- Abduct and slightly externally rotate the arm to expose axillary crease.
- 3 cm skin incision with No. 15 blade knife.
- Curved Metzenbaum scissors to bluntly dissect, exposing the interval between the pectoralis major tendon inferior border and the conjoined tendon critical plane to avoid neurovascular injury.
- A sharp Hohmann retractor placed deep to the pectoralis major tendon and over the lateral humeral cortex exposing the long head of the biceps (LHB) tendon.

- A blunt Hohmann retractor can be placed anterior (lateral) to the conjoined tendon to retract, helping visualization and to isolate the LHB; no retractive force is placed here. Hold the retractor straight to the bone.
- Once the LHB is confirmed, the blunt Hohmann is repositioned to reflect the LHB medially and expose the bicipital groove.
- A small Cobb elevator is used to roughen the periosteum of the bicipital groove at the planned tenodesis site.

25.2.2 Placing the Suture Anchor

The drill guide is placed at the planned tenodesis site and a unicortical pilot hole is made using a 2.8 mm drill. It is critical to stay perpendicular to the bicipital groove to avoid an eccentric hole and increased humeral stress riser.

The 2.8-mm,double-loaded all-suture anchor is then placed into the pilot hole and deployed.

The blunt Hohmann retractor is used to assist with visualization of the LHB.

A right-angle clamp is used to secure the LHB proximal to the planned tenodesis site.

Using a small diameter suture shuttle device, one of the suture limbs is passed through the LHB at the same level as the anchor. This suture will function as a post and provides an anatomic in situ position for the tenodesis for theoretical appropriate tensioning and symmetry.

25.2.3 Arthroscopic Portal Placement

Standard arthroscopic posterior and anterior portals are made following passing the initial suture though the LHB tendon.

25.2.4 Initiate Shoulder Arthroscopy

- Diagnostic arthroscopy.
- Tenotomy of the LHB is performed with an arthroscopic cutter or radiofrequency device.
- A stump of tissue is left to ensure the superior labrum is not breached. After the tenotomy, the remaining stump is gently debrided with a motorized shaver to recontour the superior labrum.

25.2.5 Completing the Tenodesis

- Returning to the surgical incision in the axilla, the sharp Hohmann retractor is replaced and the LHB is pulled from the shoulder into the wound.
- Using the opposite limb of the suture that was initially passed through the LHB as the post, a circumferential double-lassoloop is performed using the following steps:
  - Pierce the LHB, retrieve the suture limb (nonpost), and pull part way through the tendon such that a loop is formed.
  - Place the suture passer through this suture loop and then around one side of the LHB to retrieve the same suture tail and pull through. This completes half of the circumferential tenodesis for that suture limb.
  - Complete the 360° circumferential tenodesis by repeating the above two steps; however, this time, pass around the other side of the LHB to retrieve the suture tail.

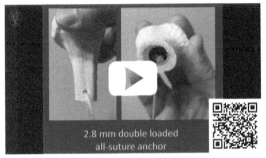

Video 25.1 Surgical demonstration of a subpectoral biceps tenodesis with an all-suture double-loaded anchor.

- Once the circumferential tenodesis is complete for the first suture, the second suture in the double-loaded all-suture anchor is passed.
- As before, one limb is initially passed through the tendon in its entirety. This functions as another post.
- Using the opposing limb of this second suture, the circumferential tenodesis is completed using the steps described above.
- Once both sutures have been passed, the two suture limbs, which are posts of both sutures, are pulled delivering the tendon into the wound and down to the suture anchor against the periosteum.
- Each suture set is then tied and cut.
- The biceps tendon is then cut a minimum of 1 cm above the tenodesis site to avoid loss of suture fixation.

25.2.6 Wound Closure

- The wound is copiously irrigated.
- A layered closure is performed with 2–0 Vicryland a subcuticular running 3–0 Monocryl.
- Skin glue is optional, but is our preferred approach.
- A sterile nonadherent dressing strip is placed over the wound and then covered with a sterile dressing (▶ **Video 25.1**).

25.3 Tips and Tricks

- Establishing the plane between the pectoralis and the conjoined tendon is critical to avoid neurovascular injury.
- Retractor placement under the pectoralis and over the lateral humerus is essential for adequate exposure.
- In situ tenodesis helps approximate anatomic biceps length and tension.
- The all-suture double-loaded anchor utilizes a smaller osseous pilot hole and the benefit of unicortical intramedullary fixation.
- Double-lasso-loop configuration results in circumferential capture of the tendon for better definitive fixation.

25.4 Pitfalls and Complications

- Dissection beneath the conjoined tendon on initial dissection may lead to iatrogenic neurovascular injury.

- Avoid aggressive retraction of the conjoined tendon to minimize likelihood of iatrogenic neurovascular injury.
- The pilot drill hole should be perpendicular to the bicipital groove to avoid an eccentric stress riser, which could lead to fracture.

25.5 Rehabilitation

- Phase I: Passive range of motion (PROM) (starts 1 week post-op).
  - Non-weight-bearing (NWB), sling at all times.
  - PROM at the elbow (flexion/extension and forearm supination/pronation) to minimize activity of biceps.
- Phase II: Active range of motion (AROM) (starts 4 weeks post-op).
  - NWB, wean from sling.
  - Progress shoulder PROM to active assisted range of motion (AAROM) and AROM all planes to tolerance.
- Phase III: Strengthening (starts 6–8 weeks post-op).
  - No heavy lifting at this time.
  - Initiate biceps curls and supination/pronation with light resistance, progress as tolerated.
- Phase IV: Advanced strengthening (starts 10 weeks post-op).
  - Return to full strenuous work/recreational activities.
  - Avoid military press and wide grip bench press.

25.6 Rationale for Approach

- The LHB tendon is a common source of shoulder pain.[1,2,3,4,5,6,7]
- Subpectoral biceps tenodesis.[8]
  - Reduces pain.
  - High patient satisfaction.
  - Removes all diseased tissue from the bicipital groove.
  - Low complication rate.
  - Aesthetically pleasing.
- All-suture anchor uses a small unicortical pilot hole theoretically decreasing the likelihood of iatrogenic fracture.
- In situ tenodesis may better restore the anatomic resting length and tension of the LHB, resulting in more predictable symmetric contour of the biceps and lower incidence of biceps cramping.

References

[1] Friedman DJ, Dunn JC, Higgins LD, Warner JJ. Proximal biceps tendon: injuries and management. Sports Med Arthrosc Rev. 2008; 16(3):162–169

[2] Werner BC, Pehlivan HC, Hart JM, et al. Increased incidence of postoperative stiffness after arthroscopic compared with open biceps tenodesis. Arthroscopy. 2014; 30(9):1075–1084

[3] Moon SC, Cho NS, Rhee YG. Analysis of "hidden lesions" of the extra-articular biceps after subpectoral biceps tenodesis: the subpectoral portion as the optimal tenodesis site. Am J Sports Med. 2015; 43(1):63–68

[4] Werner BC, Lyons ML, Evans CL, et al. Arthroscopic suprapectoral and open subpectoral biceps tenodesis: a comparison of restoration of length-tension and mechanical strength between techniques. Arthroscopy. 2015; 31(4):620–627

[5] Szabó I, Boileau P, Walch G. The proximal biceps as a pain generator and results of tenotomy. Sports Med Arthrosc Rev. 2008; 16(3):180–186

[6] Carr RM, Shishani Y, Gobezie R. How accurate are we in detecting biceps tendinopathy? Clin Sports Med. 2016; 35(1):47–55

[7] Elser F, Braun S, Dewing CB, Giphart JE, Millett PJ. Anatomy, function, injuries, and treatment of the long head of the biceps brachii tendon. Arthroscopy. 2011; 27(4):581–592

[8] Nho SJ, Reiff SN, Verma NN, Slabaugh MA, Mazzocca AD, Romeo AA. Complications associated with subpectoral biceps tenodesis: low rates of incidence following surgery. J Shoulder Elbow Surg. 2010; 19(5):764–768

26 Identifying and Exposing the Proximal Biceps in Its Groove: The "Slit" Technique

Mark R. Wilson, Eric D. Field, and Larry D. Field

Summary

Proximal biceps tendon pathology is a common source of shoulder symptoms. Thus, visualization of the entire extent of the biceps tendon is often required for both diagnostic and therapeutic purposes. Accurately recognizing the presence and extent of biceps pathology intraoperatively is made more difficult, however, due to the extraarticular location of a significant portion of the biceps tendon as it courses within the bicipital groove. Unfortunately, identification of the biceps groove in the subacromial space is often challenging due to the lack of visual and tactile landmarks. A technique coined the "slit" technique that facilitates efficient and reliable bicipital groove identification and biceps tendon visualization along its entire course within the groove is presented.

Keywords: biceps exposure, biceps tendonitis, biceps tenodesis, slit technique, SLAP tear

26.1 Patient Positioning

Both beach chair and lateral decubitus positions are acceptable.

26.2 Portal Placement

- Standard posterior portal placed initially for diagnostic arthroscopic evaluation.
- Anterosuperior glenohumeral portal and subsequently a subacromial lateral portal is created.
- Anterior and posterior subacromial accessory portals are created as needed.

26.3 Surgical Technique

- The patient is positioned in the beach chair position and prepped and draped in usual sterile fashion.
- A standard posterior glenohumeral joint–viewing portal is created initially, and a 30° arthroscope is used.
- Next, a standard anterosuperior working portal that is centered within the rotator interval is made. A thorough diagnostic arthroscopy is then completed.
- The biceps tendon is carefully evaluated by probing the superior labrum and proximal origin of the biceps tendon and by palpating the biceps tendon.[1] Also, as much of the biceps tendon as possible is pulled into the glenohumeral joint using this probe in an effort to assess the tendon for fraying, tearing, synovial reaction, and instability.[1]
- If the entire proximal biceps tendon requires visualization, either because of concern about pathology within the more distal portion of the biceps tendon that cannot be visualized by pulling the tendon into the glenohumeral joint or when a suprapectoral tenodesis is planned, the authors' "slit" technique is routinely employed.[2]

- This technique simply and reliably exposes the location and vertical orientation of the bicipital groove while still allowing the arthroscope to remain within the glenohumeral joint using standard arthroscopic equipment.
- First, an 18-gauge spinal needle is inserted into the anterior shoulder approximately 3 cm lateral to the previously placed anterosuperior portal cannula and advanced until the spinal needle is arthroscopically identified within the bicipital groove at the location where the biceps exits the glenohumeral joint (▶ **Fig. 26.1**).
- This spinal needle location and trajectory are then used as a guide to allow the surgeon to direct a percutaneously placed standard knife handle loaded with a #11 scalpel blade through the skin. It then advances through the anterior soft tissues in a parallel path until the tip of the scalpel blade is identified as it perforates the proximal aspect of the transverse humeral ligament overlying the bicipital groove (▶ **Fig. 26.2**).

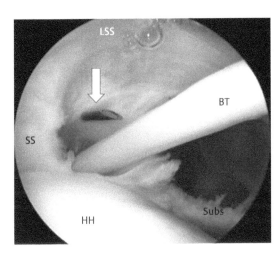

Fig. 26.1 An 18-gauge spinal needle (*white arrow*) is seen percutaneously localizing the biceps tendon(BT) in this left shoulder in the beach chair position as viewed from the posterior portal. This spinal needle penetrates the most proximal aspect of the tissue overlying tendon as it enters the bicipital groove. SS, supraspinatus; HH, humeral head; SubS, subscapularis; white arrow, 18-gauge spinal needle.

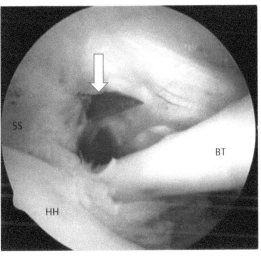

Fig. 26.2 The tip of the #11 scalpel blade (*white arrow*) is advanced through the tissue overlying the proximal aspect of the bicipital groove in a left shoulder in the beach chair position as viewed from the posterior portal. SS, supraspinatus; HH, humeral head; BT, biceps tendon; white arrow, #11 scalpel blade.

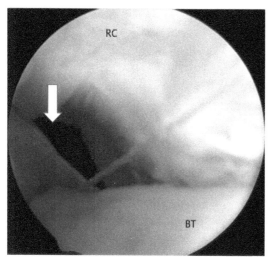

Fig. 26.3 The incised tissue or "slit" (*white arrow*) in the proximal aspect of the transverse humeral ligament overlying the bicipital groove is seen in a left shoulder in the beach chair position as viewed from the posterior portal. RC, rotator cuff; BT, biceps tendon; white arrow, slit in the transverse humeral ligament overlying the biceps.

- This scalpel blade is then directed distally, while viewing arthroscopically from the posterior portal, following the course of the biceps tendon to create a split or "slit" in the transverse humeral ligament. Also, care is taken to avoid damage to the biceps tendon as this slit is created and enlarged. Slight forward flexion of the shoulder can sometimes improve visualization within the biceps groove as the incision proceeds more distally.
- Typically, 2–3 cm of the overlying transverse humeral ligament is easily incised (▶ **Fig. 26.3**). Care should be taken to minimize iatrogenic damage to the underlying biceps tendon as the slit is extended.[3,4]
- This incision in the transverse humeral ligament will then be easily and reliably identified arthroscopically once the arthroscope is subsequently redirected into the subacromial space.
- When arthroscopic suprapectoral biceps tenodesis is to be carried out, the authors generally employ suture anchor fixation by impacting a suture anchor into the abraded bicipital groove while viewing from the subacromial space. However, prior to transferring the arthroscope to the subacromial space, the most proximal aspect of the biceps tendon is released from its origin at the superior glenoid except for a very small, residual portion of the biceps tendon that is left intact (▶ **Fig. 26.4**) until the suture anchor sutures are passed through the biceps tendon and tied.
- Following arthroscopic knot tying, detachment of this small residual intact portion of the biceps tendon is completed, often with a gentle distal tug on the tendon using a standard arthroscopic grasper. These few fibers of the proximal biceps are intentionally left intact by the authors so as to preserve anatomic biceps length until the tenodesis is completed.
- Following completing this partial release of the proximal biceps tendon, the arthroscope is then transferred to the standard posterior subacromial portal site.
- Next, a lateral subacromial working portal is created and used to accomplish a thorough subacromial bursectomy. The arthroscope is then moved to this lateral subacromial portal site and, with slight external rotation of the glenohumeral joint, the previously placed "slit" incision in the transverse humeral ligament along with the exposed biceps tendon can be clearly visualized (▶ **Fig. 26.5**).

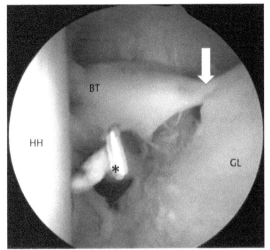

Fig. 26.4 The proximal biceps tendon(BT) is nearly, but not completely, released prior to biceps tenodesis as seen in a left shoulder in the beach chair position viewing from the posterior portal. Leaving a very limited amount of residual tendinous tissue intact (*white arrow*) ensures that the anatomic length of the biceps is preserved during tenodesis using a suture anchor technique at the bicipital groove. Following completion of the tenodesis, the remaining tendon is then freed usually by simply tugging on the biceps. GL, glenoid/labrum; HH, humeral head; *arthroscopic suture scissors.

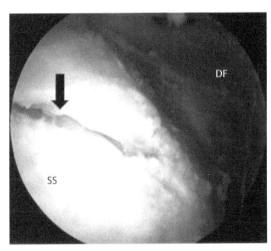

Fig. 26.5 The slit (*black arrow*) is easily located while viewing from the lateral portal in the subacromial space after a standard bursectomy is performed in a left shoulder in the beach chair position. SS, supraspinatus; DF, deltoid fascia; black arrow, slit created over the biceps tendon.

- The #11 blade scalpel (▶ **Fig. 26.6**) or an arthroscopic shaver blade can then be used to incise the more distal portion of the transverse humeral ligament and other tissue overlying the biceps tendon so as to expose them along the length of the biceps.
- A probe can then be used to manipulate the biceps and further assess it for synovial reaction, fraying, or partial tearing (▶ **Fig. 26.7**).
- Once the biceps tendon has been thoroughly evaluated, the surgeon can then proceed with suprapectoral tenodesis, if indicated, using the fixation method of choice.
- Again, the authors' preferred tenodesis technique usually utilizes a double- or triple-loaded suture anchor(Healicoil Regenesorb 4.5 mm, Smith & Nephew) inserted into the bicipital groove followed by passage of these sutures through the biceps tendon using a locking-loop construct (▶ **Fig. 26.8**, ▶ **Video 26.1**).

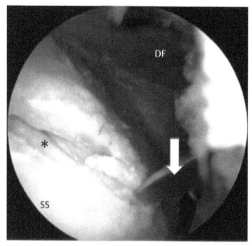

Fig. 26.6 While viewing from the lateral portal in the subacromial space in a left shoulder in the beach chair position, the #11 blade(*white arrow*) is used to incise the more distal tissue overlying the biceps(*) until the tendon is completely unroofed and exposed. SS, supraspinatus; DF, deltoid fascia; white arrow, #11 scalpel blade; *biceps tendon below the slit.

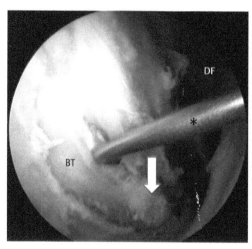

Fig. 26.7 Visualizing and probing (*) the entire biceps tendon (BT) is carried out after the incision of the tissue overlying the biceps is completed. Note the significant fraying (*white arrow*) of the very distal aspect of the biceps tendon that was not able to be identified when visualized intraarticular. This image is taken of a left shoulder in the beach chair position while viewing from the lateral portal in the subacromial space. DF, deltoid fascia, *arthroscopic probe; white arrow, frayed/degenerative biceps tendon.

26.4 Surgeon Tips and Tricks

- Near complete, but not complete, sectioning of the biceps from its attachment on the superior labrum helps keep accurate tension when performing tenodesis.
- Accurate trajectory of the spinal needle in all planes is key for both creating a good "slit" and for creating an accessory portal that provides maximum access to the biceps groove.
- Slight forward flexion of the arm can help visualization while extending the slit distally when viewing from the joint in the posterior portal.

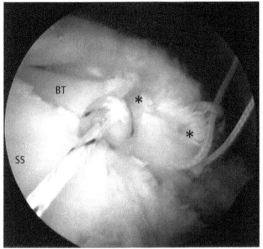

Fig. 26.8 This image is taken of a left shoulder in the beach chair position while viewing from the lateral portal in the subacromial space. The suture anchor sutures have been passed, but not yet tied, in a locking-loop pattern(*). Note that biceps tendon length and tension are maintained during this suture passage phase. BT, biceps tendon; SS, supraspinatus.

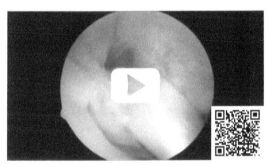

Video 26.1 Surgical demonstration of identifying and exposing the proximal biceps in its groove: the "slit" technique.

26.5 Pitfalls/Complications

- There is a risk of iatrogenic damage to biceps or surrounding structures when percutaneously inserting the #11 scalpel blade or when advancing this blade distally through the transverse ligament in close proximity to the parallel biceps tendon.
- The scalpel blade could potentially become dislodged from the knife handle.

26.6 Rehabilitation

- Limit active biceps activity for 4 weeks postoperatively.
- Rehabilitation regimen is tailored to any additional procedures performed at the time of biceps surgery (rotator cuff repair, labral repair).

26.7 Rationale and/or Evidence for Approach

- Visualization of the entire biceps is often necessary when biceps tendon pathology is suspected and when an arthroscopic tenodesis is to be carried out.
- Complete exposure of the biceps is important as research has shown that extensive release of the biceps tendon, carried out at the time of tenodesis, has been associated with lower revision rates.[5]
- Identification and exposure of the biceps tendon within the bicipital groove can be challenging because of the difficulty in sometimes identifying this groove within the subacromial space and also in recognizing its anatomic direction and orientation. This "slit" technique obviates the need to find the bicipital groove and biceps within the subacromial space since the biceps has been unroofed and exposed by the slit created before the arthroscope and other arthroscopic instruments are even inserted into the subacromial space.

References

[1] Nho SJ, Strauss EJ, Lenart BA, et al. Long head of the biceps tendinopathy: diagnosis and management. J Am Acad Orthop Surg. 2010; 18(11):645–656

[2] Abraham VT, Tan BH, Kumar VP. Systematic review of biceps tenodesis: Arthroscopic versus open. Arthroscopy. 2016; 32(2):365–371

[3] Boileau P, Krishnan SG, Coste JS, Walch G. Arthroscopic biceps tenodesis: a new technique using bioabsorbable interference screw fixation. Arthroscopy. 2002; 18(9):1002–1012

[4] Mazzocca AD, Romero AA. Arthroscopic biceps tenodesis in the beach chair position. Oper Tech Sports Med. 2003; 11:6–14

[5] Sanders B, Lavery KP, Pennington S, Warner JJ. Clinical success of biceps tenodesis with and without release of the transverse humeral ligament. J Shoulder Elbow Surg. 2012; 21(1):66–71

27 Arthroscopic Suprapectoral Biceps Tenodesis with Lasso Loop

Kyle A. Borque and Jon J.P. Warner

Summary

Arthroscopic suprapectoral biceps tenodesis is a good option for surgeons that are looking for a minimally invasive alternative to open tenodesis. To prevent post-operative bicipital groove pain, the entire groove needs to be released. The below technique provides surgeons a reproducible method to achieve this.

Keywords: Biceps tenodesis, biceps, shoulder pain, biceps tendonitis

27.1 Patient Positioning

- Beach chair.

27.2 Portal Placement

- Standard posterior viewing portal and anterior working portal. Lateral and anterolateral (AL) portals made under direct visualization.

27.3 Surgical Technique (step-by-step approach)

Diagnostic scope with posterior portal and created anterior portal:

Step 1: Interval exposure: Probe through anterior portal and hook overtop of the biceps and pull it inferiorly toward the subscapularis. This tensions the biceps pully and allows access toward the groove.

Step 2: AL portal: Needle localization through the interval (most AL position) directly onto biceps. Use coablation through this portal to tease the biceps out and resect the interval. Proceed until subacromial space is exposed including the coracoacromial ligament.

Step 3: Tag biceps with suture: Clever hook (R for left shoulder; L for right shoulder) to pierce biceps. Retrieve out anterior portal.

Step 4: Subacromial exposure. Posterior portal with trochar through to anterior portal and back to central. Use (or create) lateral portal and resect bursa with coablation. Switch to lateral viewing portal when biceps are clearly visible and ready to complete preparation.

Step 5: Finish biceps preparation. Identify tag suture. Pull up externally and tease remaining tissue off biceps and expose the groove. Shaver to stimulate bleeding in the groove.

Step 6: Helicoil anchor placement. Pull biceps out of groove with traction stitch and punch/tap/anchor. Retrieve all four sutures out of the posterior portal.

Step 7: Biceps suturing. Retriever to take one limb (blue) and advance inline with the biceps into the glenohumeral joint. Clever hook: to pierce biceps, grab suture, pull just out of biceps remaining intraarticular. Now release suture and pass through the loop created and grab the *same* suture from below the tendon. Repeat with white suture. Next take the second limb of each suture and pierce biceps with the clever hook and grab both.

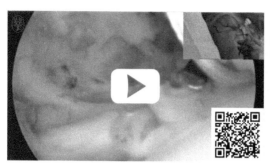

Video 27.1 Surgical demonstration of Arthroscopic Suprapectoral Biceps Tenodesis with Lasso Loop.

Step 8: Tenotomy. Retrieve all sutures through AL portal, then ablate the tendon 1 cm proximal to most proximal suture.

Step 9: Prepare for tying (cannula to avoid soft tissue bridging). Retrieve all four limbs through the posterior portal. Remove cannula from the anterior portal and place in the AL portal directly over the tenodesis site. Retrieve two like sutures at a time.

Step 10: Tie down and pull on each suture limb. One will tighten in cinch fashion. The other will loosen the construct. Use the tightening limb as the post (two same-direction half-hitches; three alternating). Repeat for the second suture.

27.4 Surgeon Tips and Tricks

- Clever hook is useful for shuttling sutures through the biceps.
- Make sure to "park" the sutures intraarticularly when performing the lasso loop to make them easier to grab.
- Can externally rotate arm to allow better visualization of the groove.

27.5 Pitfalls/Complications

- Must make sure the entire groove is released to prevent post-op pain in the bicipital groove.

27.6 Rehabilitation

- Phase 1: Passive range of motion (about 4 weeks).
- Phase 2: Active range of motion (starts about 4 weeks post-op).
- Phase 3: Strengthening (starts between 6 and 8 weeks post-op).

27.7 For the Rationale and/or Evidence for the Approach

- See Sanders et al[1] and Millet et al (▶ Video 27.1).[2]

References

[1] Sanders B, Lavery KP, Pennington S, Warner JJ. Clinical success of biceps tenodesis with and without release of the transverse humeral ligament. J Shoulder Elbow Surg. 2012; 21(1):66–71
[2] Millett PJ, Sanders B, Gobezie R, Braun S, Warner JJ. Interference screw vs. suture anchor fixation for open subpectoral biceps tenodesis: does it matter? BMC Musculoskelet Disord. 2008; 9:121

28 Transosseous Arthroscopic Biceps Tenodesis

Brett Sanders

Summary

Transosseous tendon repair techniques have been established as safe and effective in the rotator cuff. Tenodesis in the suprapectoral location is believed to yield the same pain relief as other tenodesis methods and locations, without the risk of a subpectoral wound complication. This chapter presents a fully transosseous biceps tenodesis in the suprapectoral location utilizing tendon grasping suture techniques with multi-point fixation. This technique can be used during cuff repair to perform biceps tenodesis at physiologic length and tension while decreasing hardware cost.

Keywords: biceps, tenodesis, transosseous biceps tenodesis, suprapectoral

28.1 Patient Positioning

Beach chair position with mechanical arm holder.

28.2 Portal Placement

The previously described midlateral is used for viewing and the anteroinferolateralportal is used for instrumentation.

28.3 Surgical Technique

- The biceps sheath is released with an ablator just above (▶ **Video 28.1**) the anterior circumflex humeral artery.
- A posterior grasper is introduced to bring the biceps out to the physiological length tension relationship.
- Two medial awl tunnels are made in the biceps groove in the suprapectoral location. The bone here is usually of excellent quality.
- The tunneler is used to create the inferior tunnel, leaving the suture doubled.

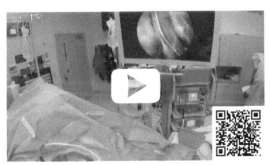

Video 28.1 Arthroscopic Transosseous Biceps tenodesis is demonstrated in the right shoulder in beach chair position. The biceps is secured with multi-point cerclage suture fixation in the suprapectoral location at physiologic length and tension in anchorless fashion.

- A low inferomedial and anterior portal is used to retrieve the suture through the biceps tendon in a retrograde fashion and create a locking loop, grasping the lateral limb through the loop. The sutures are then retrieved and tied through the infero anterolateral portal.
- The superior tunnel passing suture is then deployed in a similar fashion, and the same inferomedial portal is used to retrieve the double loop through the biceps tendon, leaving the loop long.
- A grasper is placed through the anterior portal, through the loop, and it is used to stabilize the biceps tendon in its physiologic location proximally. A posterior grasper is then used to bring the loop over the end of the biceps, creating a circumferential suture.
- The inferomedial portal is then used again to retropass a suture through the circumferential loop, and this suture is used to tie to the lateral post.
- The remaining biceps is then transected and the tendon ends are annealed with the ablator.

28.4 Tips and Tricks

- Forward flexing the arm aids in visualization under the deltoid.
- Internal rotation once the tunneling device is introduced allows easier tunnel creation.
- The tensor TransOs Tunneler is utilized to arthroscopically create reproducible tunnels with strong compact bone tunnels.

28.5 Pearls and Pitfalls

The anterior circumflex humeral artery is at risk for injury and can create bleeding intraoperatively. Occasionally a subchondral cyst may exist under the biceps groove; however, the tunnel can be created through it in the standard fashion.

28.6 Rehabilitation

No active elbow flexion or forearm supination is allowed for 4 weeks. Gravity extension and pendulums only.

28.7 Rationale

Multiple different biceps tenodesis techniques may be used to create the same clinical pain relief, including suprapectoral tenodesis. It has been suggested that releasing the biceps sheath is beneficial to remove the pain-generating elements of the synovium or other neural elements. The described technique avoids a separate incision in the axilla, which can be prone to infection or dehiscence, and also avoids the extra expense of another bone anchor.[1] Multiple fixation points are achieved in the hardest bone of the humerus, and tendon-grasping sutures allow a high strength construct that may be tightened independently. The technique is all arthroscopic with no extra instrumentation and does allow formal release of the entire biceps sheath.

Reference

[1] Sanders B, Lavery KP, Pennington S, Warner JJP. Clinical success of biceps tenodesis with and without release of the transverse humeral ligament. J Shoulder Elbow Surg. 2012; 21(1):66–71

29 Revision Rotator Cuff Repair and Techniques for Mobilization

Joseph N. Liu, Anirudh K. Gowd, Brandon C. Cabarcas, Grant H. Garcia, and Nikhil N. Verma

Summary
Failed rotator cuff repairs are a challenging problem for the sports medicine surgeon. The initial approach involves identifying reasons for failure of the index repair such as diagnostic and/or technical errors, surgical complications, and patient intrinsic factors leading to nonhealing including advanced age and smoking. A systematic investigation of other causes of shoulder pain should also be exhausted before proceeding with revision repair. Imaging to assess the quality of the remaining tendon, presence of fatty infiltration or muscle atrophy, presence of underlying glenohumeral arthritis or humeral head migration should be obtained. Revision rotator cuff repair may be indicated particularly in the acute traumatic setting in the physiologically young, active patient. The preferred technique of the authors is an all-arthroscopic technique performed in the beach chair position. Complete visualization is of paramount importance to characterize the recurrent tear pattern to perform an optimal repair with the goal of restoring the length–tension relationship of the musculotendinous unit. Mobilization of the tendon can be facilitated with anterior and/or posterior slides as needed. Finally, biologic augmentation may be considered particularly in the presence of poor patient intrinsic factors.

Keywords: massive rotator cuff tear, revision rotator cuff repair, mobilization, shoulder arthroscopy

29.1 Patient Positioning

- Both beach chair and lateral positioning can be used; however, we prefer a beach chair position for rotator cuff repairs.
- Patient is brought to the edge of the bed and safely secured with the head and neck in a neutral position.
- An articulated arm-holding device can be used to facilitate arm position during the case (Spider2 Limb Positioner, Smith & Nephew, Andover, MA) (▶ **Fig. 29.1**).

29.2 Portal Placement

- Prior portals can be used if they are in the appropriate position.
- Standard posterior used for diagnostic arthroscopy.
- Anterior portal created in rotator interval just lateral to coracoid after spinal needle localization.
- Additional accessory lateral portals created during visualization of subacromial space can be used for suture anchor placement and suture management (▶ **Fig. 29.2**).

29.3 Surgical Technique (Step-by-Step Approach)

- Examination under anesthesia to determine range of motion and pattern of capsular contracture.

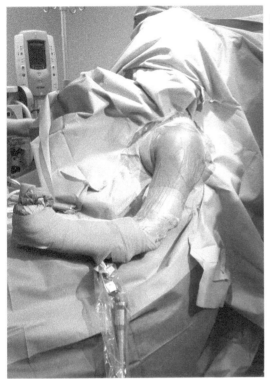

Fig. 29.1 Modified beach chair position.

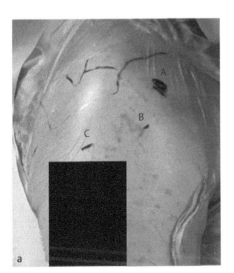

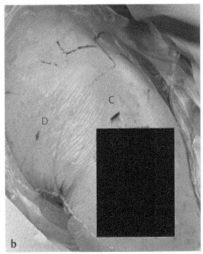

Fig. 29.2 (a, b) Portal placement for Rotator Cuff Repair. A: Anterior portal, B: Accessory Anterolateral Portal, C: Direct Lateral Portal, D: Posterior Portal

- Diagnostic arthroscopy through the standard posterior portal with particular attention to the biceps tendon as it may be a source of pain if not previously treated at the index procedure.
  – Low threshold to perform tenotomy or tenodesis if signs of tendonitis or tearing.
- Perform glenohumeral intraarticular work (e.g., biceps tenotomy, labral debridement, and/or chondroplasty, capsular release, subscapularis repair).
  – Recreate space that is typically present above glenoid labrum between the undersurface of the rotator cuff to facilitate tendon mobilization.
- Enter subacromial space.
  – Establish lateral/accessory lateral portals under direct visualization.
  – Find plane between acromion and rotator cuff in adhesed tendons.
  – Lateral viewing portal, posterior working portal.
  – Bounce off scapular spine and push laterally through scar.
  – Subacromial debridement including clearing up anterior, lateral, and posterior gutters to release adhesions between deltoid/acromion and rotator cuff.
  – Thorough bursectomy to ensure appropriate visualization.
  – Acromioplasty as needed (if not previously performed).
  – Expose scapular spine down to the base, be careful of the suprascapular nerve when working close to fat.
  – Spine excellent guide for identifying supraspinatus and infraspinatus, to lead toward anatomic repair.
- Rotator cuff repair.
  – Tendon mobilization.
  – Anterior Interval slide.
- Dissect plane between supraspinatus and subscapularis from the bursal then articular side, but leave lateral tissues intact.
- Palpate coracoid with radiofrequency wand, once you know where the bone is, can be liberal in fully exposing the base. You are safe as long as you stay lateral to coracoid.
  – Posterior interval slide.
- Traction stitches placed in supraspinatus and infraspinatus.
- Use scapular spine as a guideline for plane between supraspinatus and infraspinatus.
- Thickened tissue is the plane of dissection.
- Use arthroscopic Metzenbaum tissue to cut in intervals.
- When you get to the adipose tissue, sign that you may be close to the nerve.
- As you get more medial, complete dissection bluntly to avoid damaging the nerve.
  – Preparation of tendon footprint.
  – Prepare entirety of footprint even if doing a medialized repair.
  – Can medialize footprint 5–7 mm without changing biomechanics.
  – Microfracture of lateral aspect of greater tuberosity to create better bony bleeding.
  – Tendon repair.
  – Infraspinatus repair.
- Begin repair by bringing infraspinatus above equator to lateral margin of tuberosity and place first anchor.
- Augmented suturing technique with triple-loaded anchor(Healicoil Suture Anchor, Smith & Nephew).
  – Pass first stitch (ACCU-PASS, Smith & Nephew) in mattress suture (stay out of musculotendinous junction); around mattress stitch, place separate simple suture to create mason allen equivalent; finally, third suture is another simple suture at the lateral margin (tied first) to hold the tendon in reduced fashion.

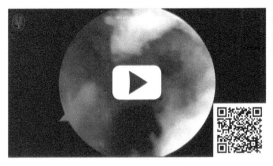

Video 29.1 Surgical demonstration of revision rotator cuff repair and techniques for mobilization.

- Infraspinatus tied down first to give reference for repairing supraspinatus.
  – Supraspinatus repair.
- Using more posterior suture anchor, pass mattress stitches (ACCU-PASS) through infra and supraspinatus to help close the defect between supraspinatus and infraspinatus (Healicoil Suture Anchor).
- Anterior suture anchor can be passed in the same augmented fashion as the infraspinatus repair.
- Augment reduction by holding tendon in place during knot tying to reduce tension on knot during tying (▶ **Video 29.1**).

29.4 Surgeon Tips and Tricks (Use of Specific Instrumentation)

- Can use same suture anchor sites if prior anchors were nonmetal.
- Stay out of musculotendinous junction when passing sutures through the rotator cuff.
- Prefer using penetrating device as these devices allow more precise passage of suture through the tendon.

29.5 Pitfalls/Complications

- Pitfalls.
  – Avoid high-tension double-row repairs as they are at higher risk of failure. Prefer medialized single-row repair to get low-tension repair compared to high-tension double-row repair.
  – Failure to recognize significant tears of the subscapularis tendon as a source of pain and/or dysfunction.
  – Failure to adequately mobilize the rotator cuff tendons during surgery, which would lead to high-tension repair.
- Complications.
  – Failure of the rotator cuff tear to heal.
  – Hardware-related complications: greater tuberosity fracture, loose body, anchor or suture pull out or dislodgement, hypersensitivity reaction to suture anchors.
  – Adhesive capsulitis.
  – Infection (use of allograft patch).
  – Deltoid insufficiency (open repairs).

29.6 Rehabilitation

- Sling for 6 weeks with no motion of shoulder.
- Passive, active assist until 8 weeks.
- Out of sling at 8 weeks.
- No strengthening until 14–16 weeks.

29.7 Rationale and/or Evidence for Approach

- Initial evaluation of a patient for revision rotator cuff repair first involves identification of patient- or surgeon-specific factors resulting in a symptomatic failed rotator cuff repair.
  - Patient factors include smoking,[1] diabetes,[2,3] and osteoporosis.[2]
- A failed rotator cuff resulting in patient dissatisfaction can be from pain, weakness, stiffness, loss of function, or a combination.
- Patient should be carefully interviewed to delineate cause of failure.
  - Shoulder pain persistent following surgery may be due to incorrect diagnosis, failure to address all pain generators at time of surgery (e.g., failure to recognize subscapularis tear or biceps tenosynovitis), postoperative synovitis/capsulitis, or perioperative rotator cuff failure.
  - Shoulder pain following an interval of symptom improvement may be due to a traumatic acute retear.
  - Insidious shoulder pain after surgery may be due to a chronic recurrent tear.
- Physical exam should help delineate cervical pathology, evaluate rotator cuff/deltoid atrophy, and/or scapular dyskinesia.
  - Special tests for impingement (Neer's, Hawkin's), massive cuff tears (external rotation lag sign, horn blower sign), AC joint pathology (cross-arm adduction), biceps pathology (O'Briens, Speed's, Yergason's) should be performed to identify additional pathology that needs to be addressed at the time of surgery.
- Plain films should be repeated as they are the most reliable method for identifying prior metallic implants, proximal humeral migration, and assessment of glenohumeral arthritis.
- Advanced imaging includes repeat magnetic resonance imaging should be obtained to review the status of the remaining rotator cuff tendons, quality of tissue, presence of fatty infiltration, tendon retraction, presence of biceps subluxation, and/or subscapularis tendon tears if present.
- In low-demand older patients, a trial of nonoperative therapy with anti-inflammatories, injections, and physical therapy, may be sufficient for pain relief and regaining strength and function.
- Younger patients and those who fail nonoperative treatment may be indicated for surgery.
  - Advanced age, fatty infiltration (Goutallier stage > 2),[4] chronic massive rotator cuff tears, and severe arthropathy have a relative contraindication to revision rotator cuff repair.[5,6,7,8]
- Transosseous equivalent has superior contact pressure at cuff footprint and greater load to failure compared to double-row repair.[9]
  - However, medialized single-row low-tension repair may be beneficial compared to double-row repairs[10] when anatomic bone-to-tendon repair is difficult due to excessive tension of the repaired tendon or tendon unable to reach anatomic insertion.

- Microfracture of the lateral aspect of the greater tuberosity may be helpful in recreating healing environment at anatomic footprint to release marrow aspects.[11]
- Other biologics may be considered to augment repair particularly in the setting of poor patient intrinsic factors (advanced age, diabetes, osteoporosis).
  - Platelet-rich plasma has controversial clinical results[12]; however, the majority of randomized trials are under powered.
  - Animal studies using mesenchymal stem cells (e.g., bone marrow aspirate concentrate) have shown promise[13,14,15]; however, clinical studies are limited[16] to demonstrate definitive benefit.
- Patch grafts have been used both as augmentation and bridging in the setting of massive rotator cuff tears.[17]
  - May be used in larger tears and in patients with poor underlying healing potential such as those with brittle diabetes, poor tissue quality, with relatively high levels of success assuming low-tension repair.
- Adjunct procedures such as suprascapular nerve release, biceps tenodesis, and subacromial decompression may be of significant value in treatment of auxillary pain generators.

References

[1] Mallon WJ, Misamore G, Snead DS, Denton P. The impact of preoperative smoking habits on the results of rotator cuff repair. J Shoulder Elbow Surg. 2004; 13(2):129–132

[2] Chung SW, Oh JH, Gong HS, Kim JY, Kim SH. Factors affecting rotator cuff healing after arthroscopic repair: osteoporosis as one of the independent risk factors. Am J Sports Med. 2011; 39(10):2099–2107

[3] Clement ND, Hallett A, MacDonald D, Howie C, McBirnie J. Does diabetes affect outcome after arthroscopic repair of the rotator cuff? J Bone Joint Surg Br. 2010; 92(8):1112–1117

[4] Goutallier D, Postel JM, Bernageau J, Lavau L, Voisin MC. Fatty muscle degeneration in cuff ruptures. Pre- and postoperative evaluation by CT scan. Clin Orthop Relat Res. 1994(304):78–83

[5] Dwyer T, Razmjou H, Henry P, Gosselin-Fournier S, Holtby R. Association between pre-operative magnetic resonance imaging and reparability of large and massive rotator cuff tears. Knee Surg Sports Traumatol Arthrosc. 2015; 23(2):415–422

[6] Yoo JC, Ahn JH, Yang JH, Koh KH, Choi SH, Yoon YC. Correlation of arthroscopic repairability of large to massive rotator cuff tears with preoperative magnetic resonance imaging scans. Arthroscopy. 2009; 25(6): 573–582

[7] Goutallier D, Postel JM, Radier C, Bernageau J, Zilber S. Long-term functional and structural outcome in patients with intact repairs 1 year after open transosseous rotator cuff repair. J Shoulder Elbow Surg. 2009; 18 (4):521–528

[8] Meyer DC, Wieser K, Farshad M, Gerber C. Retraction of supraspinatus muscle and tendon as predictors of success of rotator cuff repair. Am J Sports Med. 2012; 40(10):2242–2247

[9] Park MC, ElAttrache NS, Tibone JE, Ahmad CS, Jun BJ, Lee TQ. Part I: Footprint contact characteristics for a transosseous-equivalent rotator cuff repair technique compared with a double-row repair technique. J Shoulder Elbow Surg. 2007; 16(4):461–468

[10] Kim Y-K, Jung KH, Won JS, Cho SH. Medialized repair for retracted rotator cuff tears. J Shoulder Elbow Surg. 2017; 26(8):1432–1440

[11] Milano G, Saccomanno MF, Careri S, Taccardo G, De Vitis R, Fabbriciani C. Efficacy of marrow-stimulating technique in arthroscopic rotator cuff repair: a prospective randomized study. Arthroscopy. 2013; 29(5): 802–810

[12] Greenspoon JA, Moulton SG, Millett PJ, Petri M. The role of platelet rich plasma (PRP) and other biologics for rotator cuff repair. Open Orthop J. 2016; 10:309–314

[13] Gulotta LV, Kovacevic D, Ehteshami JR, Dagher E, Packer JD, Rodeo SA. Application of bone marrow-derived mesenchymal stem cells in a rotator cuff repair model. Am J Sports Med. 2009; 37(11):2126–2133

[14] Kida Y, Morihara T, Matsuda K, et al. Bone marrow-derived cells from the footprint infiltrate into the repaired rotator cuff. J Shoulder Elbow Surg. 2013; 22(2):197–205

[15] Oh JH, Shin SJ, McGarry MH, Scott JH, Heckmann N, Lee TQ. Biomechanical effects of humeral neck-shaft angle and subscapularis integrity in reverse total shoulder arthroplasty. J Shoulder Elbow Surg. 2014; 23(8): 1091–1098

[16] Ellera Gomes JL, da Silva RC, Silla LM, Abreu MR, Pellanda R. Conventional rotator cuff repair complemented by the aid of mononuclear autologous stem cells. Knee Surg Sports Traumatol Arthrosc. 2012; 20(2):373–377

[17] Ono Y, Dávalos Herrera DA, Woodmass JM, Boorman RS, Thornton GM, Lo IK. Graft augmentation versus bridging for large to massive rotator cuff tears: A systematic review. Arthroscopy. 2017; 33(3):673–680

30 Arthroscopic Transosseous Revision Rotator Cuff Repair

Jeremy Smalley and Uma Srikumaran

Summary

This chapter describes a revision rotator cuff repair using an arthroscopic transosseous technique with a dedicated transosseous tunneling device. We discuss and demonstrate the use of arthroscopically placed tunnels with large numbers of suture to provide load spreading and compression for repair of a large complex recurrent cuff tear. The positioning, portal placement, and post-op rehabilitation timeline are addressed. The relevant supporting literature is discussed.

Keywords: arthroscopic osseous repair, revision rotator cuff repair, rotator cuff repair, rotator cuff tear

30.1 Patient Positioning

- Following intubation, the patient is positioned supine on the beachchair positioner.
- The head support height and patient adjustment is corrected to keep the back support below the level posterior glenohumeral portal incision. The facemask is then placed with no pressure on the eyes.
- The leg elevator pillow is placed under the patient's legs, with heels and other prominences padded.
- The patient is elevated to 60° in the beach chair positioner, and the head and neck immediately adjusted for optimal neck position and tension cooperatively by the surgeon and the anesthesiologist, using the adjustment knobs.
- The well arm is supported in the arm holder.
- The patient's operative shoulder is examined under anesthesia for range of motion and ligamentous laxity.
- The operative arm is prepped in its entirety with chloraprep and allowed the appropriate time to dry. A sterile impervious stockinette is placed from the hand past the elbow. Impervious blue U-drapes are placed medially, tails up then down, with a shoulder arthroscopy drape. The arm is placed into a padded Smith & Nephew Spider arm positioner, then overwrapped with Coban proximal to the elbow.

30.2 Portal Placement

- The bony landmarks are traced at the margins of the clavicle, acromion, and scapular spine. The acromioclavicular (AC) joint is marked.
- The posterior midglenoid portal is placed based on AC joint position and humeral head ballotment. A small longitudinal stab incision through the skin only is made with a #11 knife. The arthroscopic cannula with a tapered-tip obturator is placed through the subcutaneous tissue, muscle, and to the medial humeral head, then through the posterior capsule into the glenohumeral joint.
- The anterior midglenoid portal is typically established with the outside-in technique with the spinal needle technique under direct visualization from the posterior portal,

with incision along Langer's lines and a clear threaded operating cannula placed over a blunt trocar.

- The lateral subacromial portals are placed under direct visualization with spinal needle guidance in the subacromial space. The initial lateral portal is typically made 3–4 cm lateral to the anterolateral edge of the acromion. If needed for a large or massive tear, a second is typically made posterior to this, with the goal of placing the portals and cannulas at the anterior third of the cuff tear, and the middle-third-posterior third junction.

30.3 Surgical Technique (See accompanying ▶ Video 30.1)

30.3.1 Diagnostic Arthroscopy

- Diagnostic arthroscopy of the shoulder is performed, primarily from the posterior portal. In a revision cuff repair, particular attention is paid to checking the inferior pouch and lateral subacromial space for debris, and for locating prior sutures for removal.

30.3.2 Bursectomy, Debridement, Removal of Loose Implants, Footprint Preparation, Cuff Mobilization (if Needed)

- In the glenohumeral position, any procedures indicated for noncuff structures, such as biceps tenotomy, labral debridement, or anterior capsular release, are performed prior to cuff repair.
- The scope is repositioned to the subacromial bursa space through the posterior portal, and the anterolateral subacromial portal is established with an outside-in technique.
- An extensive bursectomy is performed with shaver and ablator, with the soft tissue removed from the underside of the acromion, and the bursal curtain debrided medially and laterally, with attention to exposure of the lateral greater tuberosity (GT) without damaging the deltoid muscle fascia. Subacromial decompression with a bur is performed if indicated by bony morphology.
- The footprint of the GT is debrided with shaver and ablator in the case of a revision cuff repair.

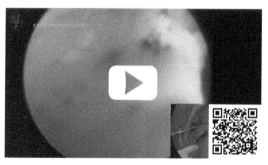

Video 30.1 Arthroscopic transosseous revision rotator cuff repair.

- During revision cuff repair, in the course of the two steps above, all sutures and other loose debris from the failed repair are removed with a combination of shaver and graspers. The previously placed anchors are left in place if stable.
- The frayed edges of the cuff tear are debrided with a shaver, and if the cuff is significantly retracted and adherent to the superior glenoid, cuff release is performed off the glenoid and/or acromion with ablator, elevator, and lateral traction of the cuff with a grasper. This is performed with the scope in the posterior portal and/or lateral portal as needed.

30.3.3 Tunneling and Suture Shuttling

- The medial tunnel sites are punched at the medial GT articular margin with a round tapered awl through a lateral portal. This is performed with the arm in adduction to make the medial side of the tunnel as "vertical," or parallel to the lateral cortex of the GT, if possible (▶ **Fig. 30.1**).
- The arthroscopic tunneler instrument (in this demonstration, the Tensor TransOs) is then placed into the joint through the lateral portal, and the capture hook tip fully inserted into the punched medial tunnel. The hook is typically most easily introduced into the subacromial space in an inverted position, then rotated into position for tunnel insertion. This maneuver is reminiscent of the way an anterior cruciate ligament tibial tunnel guide is typically introduced and positioned in the knee.
- Placement of the protector sleeve down to bone is directly visualized with the arthroscope in the subacromial space.
- The punch needle is then loaded with a small guagehigh-strength shuttle suture, and placed through the soft tissue sleeve to the bone, and advanced with a series of gentle taps with a mallet. The punch needle is then retracted and the capture hook extracted from the medial tunnel with the shuttle suture captured (▶ **Fig. 30.1**).
- The shuttle suture is then used to pull several fixation sutures or tapes through the tunnel.
- Additional tunnels are created and sutures shuttled as needed depending on the size of the cuff tear.
- In this demonstration, four sutures per tunnel are used (▶ **Fig. 30.2**).

30.3.4 Suture Passage Through the Cuff

- A cannula is inserted into the superolateral portal for suture passage. A loop grasper is used to shuttle the desired medial suture limb into the cannula. Alternatively, passage can be performed without a cannula.

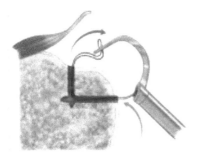

Fig. 30.1 Suture passage with the transosseoustunneler.

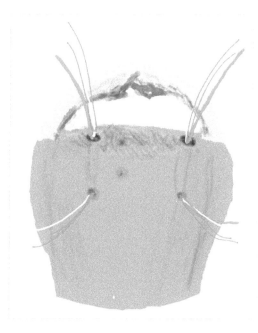

Fig. 30.2 Sutures shuttled through tunnels.

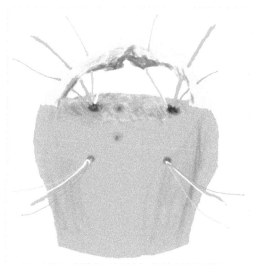

Fig. 30.3 Sutures passed through the cuff.

- Nonworking suture limbs may be shuttled to the anterior or other lateral portal to minimize risk of tangles.
- Lateral suture limbs are left out the lateral portals until needed for tying.
- A retrograde suture passer, in this demonstration a Smith & Nephew FIRSTPASS, is used to pass sutures through the cuff. Typically, and as demonstrated here, a single pass and subsequent simple suture knot is performed with transosseous tunnels, to spread load and optimize compression (▶ **Fig. 30.3**).

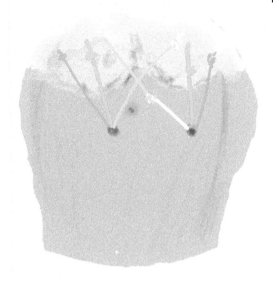

Fig. 30.4 Sutures tied, cuff reduced.

30.3.5 Suture Tying

- Medial suture and associated lateral suture tails are selected with loop grasper and shuttled through the cannula.
- Sutures are tied using a sliding knot and a knot pusher through a cannula, with backup half-hitches. A Duncan slider is used in this demonstration but other typical sliding knots may be used according to surgeon preference and experience.
- In the center of the cuff tear, suture tails from the posterior and anterior tunnels are typically cross-tied to optimize central tear compression, as demonstrated (▶ **Fig. 30.4**).
- Knots are generally tied anterior to posterior with the arthroscope in the posterior portal.
- The large number of simple sutures distributes the fixation load through the cuff and in revision repairs allows accommodation for tendon edge irregularity to optimize tension and footprint compression.

30.4 Surgeon Tips and Tricks

- Perform sufficient lateral bursectomy to facilitate lateral tunnel placement and associated suture passage and management.
- Place lateral tunnel as inferiorly as possible from the GT edge to engage stronger bone; target 2 cm from the GT edge.
- Limit abduction torque on transosseous tunneler capture hook when in medial bone to avoid bending it.
- The relatively large number of available sutures facilitates use of single pass medially with simple suture tying and optimized compression of the lateral part of the tendon to the footprint.

- To mitigate "suture madness," pass sutures though tunnels with a snap on lateral limbs, then separate pair with medial limbs as each medial limb is passed through the cuff tendon.
- During debridement in a revision cuff repair, an "alligator roll" maneuver with a grasper locked on the suture may facilitate unthreading a suture remnant from an anchor in a controlled and efficient manner.
- Marrow bleeding occurs from tunnels, so there is no need for additional punch or burring for marrow access.

30.5 Pitfalls/Complications

- Early learning curve of new technology.
- Tunneler instrumentation required but largely reusable.
- More extensive lateral bursectomy may be needed versus cuff repair with anchors.
- Increased suture management complexity due to the large number of initially passed sutures.

30.6 Rehabilitation

- 0–6 weeks: Passive range of motion, consistent sling wear.
- 6–12 weeks: Active range of motion per progressive protocol, D/C sling.
- 3–9 months: progressive strengthening, activities of daily living, weight and strain limits.
- 9 months: unrestricted activity.

30.7 Rationale and Evidence of Approach

- Tunneling allows placement flexibility around prior anchors (adjacent, medial, or lateral, with tunnel path often deep to anchors).
- Plentiful suture availability for spreading cuff fixation load.[1]
- Sequential tying for optimal cuff reduction and tension balancing versus all-at-once knotless lateral row.
- Footprint compression.[2]
- Less medial tendon stress concentration versus a mattress suture medial row.
- Better failure mechanism.[3]
- Intrinsic bone marrow access.
- Implant cost savings.[4]

References

[1] Jost PW, Khair MM, Chen DX, Wright TM, Kelly AM, Rodeo SA. Suture number determines strength of rotator cuff repair. J Bone Joint Surg Am. 2012; 94(14):e100

[2] Park MC, Cadet ER, Levine WN, Bigliani LU, Ahmad CS. Tendon-to-bone pressure distributions at a repaired rotator cuff footprint using transosseous suture and suture anchor fixation techniques. Am J Sports Med. 2005; 33(8):1154–1159

[3] Kilcoyne KG, Guillaume SG, Hannan CV, Langdale ER, Belkoff SM, Srikumaran U. Anchored transosseous-equivalent versus anchorless transosseous rotator cuff repair: A biomechanical analysis in a cadaveric model. Am J Sports Med. 2017; 45(10):2364–2371

[4] Black EM, Austin LS, Narzikul A, Seidl AJ, Martens K, Lazarus MD. Comparison of implant cost and surgical time in arthroscopic transosseous and transosseous equivalent rotator cuff repair. J Shoulder Elbow Surg. 2016; 25(9):1449–1456

Suggested Readings

Bishop J, Klepps S, Lo IK, Bird J, Gladstone JN, Flatow EL. Cuff integrity after arthroscopic versus open rotator cuff repair: a prospective study. J Shoulder Elbow Surg. 2006; 15(3):290–299

Kummer FJ, Hahn M, Day M, Meislin RJ, Jazrawi LM. A laboratory comparison of a new arthroscopic transosseous rotator cuff repair to a double row transosseous equivalent rotator cuff repair using suture anchors. Bull Hosp Jt Dis (2013). 2013; 71(2):128–131

Tashjian RZ, Deloach J, Green A, Porucznik CA, Powell AP. Minimal clinically important differences in ASES and simple shoulder test scores after nonoperative treatment of rotator cuff disease. J Bone Joint Surg Am. 2010; 92(2): 296–303

31 Biological Augmentation of Rotator Cuff Repair with Platelet-Rich Plasma and Multiple Channeling

Paul Shinil Kim and Chris Hyunchul Jo

Summary

Several augmentation strategies have been described to enhance rotator cuff tendon healing after surgical repair. We discuss two techniques: 1) platelet-rich plasma augmentation and 2) multiple channeling (bone marrow stimulation) to improve structural integrity after repair.

Keywords: rotator cuff, platelet-rich plasma, biological augmentation

31.1 Patient Positioning

- Lateral decubitus position.
  - Maintain stability with the beanbag.
  - Shoulder traction with the Spider Limb Positioner (Tenet Medical Products, Smith & Nephew, Andover, MA).
  - Tilting the table ~20–30° posteriorly.

31.2 Portal Placement

31.2.1 Posterior Portal

- 2 cm medial and 3 cm distal to the posterolateral tip of the acromion.
- Soft spot in the triangular region between the acromion, glenoid, and humeral head.

31.2.2 Anterior Portal

- Halfway between the acromioclavicular (AC) joint and the lateral aspect of the coracoids.
- Intraarticular space border: superolaterally by the biceps tendon, inferiorly by the subscapularis tendon, and medially by the anterosuperior portion of the glenoid.

31.2.3 Lateral Portal (50-Yard Line View)

- 3 cm lateral to lateral border of the acromion, in line with the posterior edge of the AC joint.
- Used for subacromial decompression, and ultimately provides a working portal for rotator cuff repair.

31.2.4 Posterolateral Portal (Grand Canyon View)

- Just lateral to the posterolateral edge of the acromion.
- Better visualization of rotator cuff pathology.

31.3 Surgical Technique (Step-by-Step Approach)

31.3.1 Exploration for the Glenohumeral Joint

- Biceps tendon and superior labrum.
  - The biceps tendon anchor at the superior glenoid serves as an obvious anatomic landmark for orientation in the joint.
- Posterior labrum.
- Glenoid surface and humeral head cartilage.
- Inferior capsule and axillary recess.
  - For evidence of loose bodies or synovitis.
- Supraspinatus tendon articular side.
- Superior glenohumeral ligament (SGHL) and middle glenohumeral ligament (MGHL).
  - Draped obliquely over the deep surface of the subscapularis tendon and becomes taut with external rotation.
  - In most cases, the MGHL can be identified at its origin from the anterosuperior labrum.
- Subscapularis tendon.
  - Insertion of the subscapularis tendon can be inspected during internal rotation and posteriorly translation of the humeral head.

31.3.2 Management of the Biceps Tendon[1]

- Depending on the patient's age, activity level, symptoms, rehabilitation, and degree of subscapularis tear.
  - Biceps tenotomy should be considered if the patients are more than ~55–60 years old, female, low demand for physical activity, within repairing the torn cuff tendon, and not doing passive range of motion (ROM) exercise for postoperative rehabilitation.
  - Biceps tenodesis are preferred for male and younger patients (< 50 years) or the patients of any age involved in heavy labor.

31.3.3 Preparation for the Tendon Repair[2]

- Debride the bursal tissue, subacromial, and distal clavicle osteophytes minimally.
- Extensive acromioplasty to flatten the hooked or curved acromion are rarely performed.
  - Debride the frayed and atrophied tendons of torn end minimally so the structural fibers of the tendon are preserved.
  - Evaluation of the rotator cuff tear: anteroposterior dimension, mediolateral retraction, and the numbers of involved tendons.
  - Tendon mobility is evaluated by grasping the tendon and gently pulling it laterally. This determines the position of the tendon edge relative to the repair site on the greater tuberosity.
  - Excursion can be increased, when necessary, with superior capsulotomy, release of the coracohumeral ligament, and medialization of the greater tuberosity.
  - The footprint of the greater tuberosity is debrided to achieve complete clearance of the remnant soft tissue with preservation of the calcified fibrocartilage of the insertion.

31.3.4 Arthroscopic Repair

- Insert the medial anchors at the medial border of the rotator cuff footprint.
- Placing sutures through the torn end of the rotator cuff.
  - The medial row sutures are tied using the slippage-proof knot[3,4] if necessary.
  - The lateral row is secured using suture anchors, and the sutures are cut.

31.4 Surgeon Tips and Tricks (Use of Specific Instrumentation)

31.4.1 Platelet-Rich Plasma Augmentation[5,6,7,8,9,10]

- Especially for the large to massive tears, biological augmentation with platelet-rich plasma (PRP) could enhance the quality of the structural integrity after repair.
- PRP is prepared using a platelet pheresis system with a leuko-reduction set and a standard collection program 1 day before surgery.
- To produce a gel from PRP, 0.3 mL of 10% calcium gluconate is added to 3 mL of PRP.
- Threading No.1 polydioxanone (PDS II) suture to the posterior rotator cuff using a suture hook near the footprint. Opposite end of the PDS suture is retrieved through the lateral portal and then PRP gels are threaded consecutively to the PDS suture.
- The PRP gels are introduced into the 5.5 mm cannula and a knot pusher pushed the gels to reach to the repair site.
- While blocking the outer opening of the cannula with a finger, a suture retriever passes through the anterior rotator cuff and brings PDS suture back out to the anterior portal.
- With the PRP gels in place, medial row sutures are tied and the lateral row is secured using suture anchors, and the sutures are cut.

31.4.2 Multiple Channeling[11,12,13,14,15]

- The multiple channeling procedure is a kind of bone marrow stimulation technique.
- A bone punch with a thin and long tip is preferred to create channels.
- Make multiple channels from immediately adjacent to the articular cartilage of the humeral head to the lateral ridge of the greater tuberosity.
- By internally and externally rotating the arm, holes are made over the greater tuberosity. Usually, the holes are 4 to 5 mm apart and 10 mm deep. This procedure usually takes 10 min for any tear size.
- After multiple channeling, suture anchors are placed in the usual manner. See accompanying ▶ **Video 31.1**.

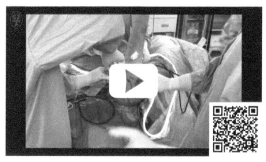

Video 31.1 Video of rotator cuff repair with microchanneling and PRP augmentation.

31.5 Pitfalls/Complications

- In the application of PRP, there are several techniques are introduced and it is important to choose the proper technique of arthroscopic application of PRP before the surgery and practices should be needed.
- Create the multiple channels with a thinner and longer bone punch rather than a thicker and shorter awl for microfracturing, which might cause the fracture of greater tuberosity and may not be enough to reach the bone marrow.

31.6 Rehabilitation

- Same as the conventional arthroscopic rotator cuff repair in both procedures.
- The shoulders are immobilized for 4–6 weeks using an abduction brace.
- Shrugging, protraction, and retraction of shoulder girdles and intermittent exercise of the elbow, wrist, and hand are encouraged immediately after surgery as tolerated.
- However, no passive motion is allowed for patients with a massive tear until6 weeks after surgery.
- Passive ROM exercise is allowed after gradual weaning off the abduction brace from 4 to 6 weeks after surgery.
- Beginning strengthening exercise after 3 months.
- Full return to sports is allowed after 6 months according to the individual recovery.

References

[1] Hsu AR, Ghodadra NS, Provencher MT, Lewis PB, Bach BR. Biceps tenotomy versus tenodesis: a review of clinical outcomes and biomechanical results. J Shoulder Elbow Surg. 2011; 20(2):326–332

[2] Jo CH, Kim JE, Yoon KS, et al. Does platelet-rich plasma accelerate recovery after rotator cuff repair? A prospective cohort study. Am J Sports Med. 2011; 39(10):2082–2090

[3] Jo CH, Lee J-H, Kang S-B, et al. Optimal configuration of arthroscopic sliding knots backed up with multiple half-hitches. Knee Surg Sports Traumatol Arthrosc. 2008; 16(8):787–793

[4] Clark RR, Dierckman B, Sampatacos N, Snyder S. Biomechanical performance of traditional arthroscopic knots versus slippage-proof knots. Arthroscopy. 2013; 29(7):1175–1181

[5] Jo CH. Arthroscopic rotator cuff repair with platelet-rich plasma (PRP) gel: a technical note. Acta Orthop Belg. 2011; 77(5):676–679

[6] Jo CH, Shin JS, Shin WH, Lee SY, Yoon KS, Shin S. Platelet-rich plasma for arthroscopic repair of medium to large rotator cuff tears: a randomized controlled trial. Am J Sports Med. 2015; 43(9):2102–2110

[7] Charousset C, Zaoui A, Bellaïche L, Piterman M. Does autologous leukocyte-platelet-rich plasma improve tendon healing in arthroscopic repair of large or massive rotator cuff tears? Arthroscopy. 2014; 30(4): 428–435

[8] McCarrel T, Fortier L. Temporal growth factor release from platelet-rich plasma, trehalose lyophilized platelets, and bone marrow aspirate and their effect on tendon and ligament gene expression. J Orthop Res. 2009; 27(8):1033–1042

[9] Zargar Baboldashti N, Poulsen RC, Franklin SL, Thompson MS, Hulley PA. Platelet-rich plasma protects tenocytes from adverse side effects of dexamethasone and ciprofloxacin. Am J Sports Med. 2011; 39(9): 1929–1935

[10] Jo CH, Lee SY, Yoon KS, Shin S. Effects of Platelet-rich plasma with concomitant use of a corticosteroid on tenocytes from degenerative rotator cuff tears in interleukin 1β-induced tendinopathic conditions. Am J Sports Med. 2017; 45(5):1141–1150

[11] Jo CH, Shin JS, Park IW, Kim H, Lee SY. Multiple channeling improves the structural integrity of rotator cuff repair. Am J Sports Med. 2013; 41(11):2650–2657

[12] Jo CH, Yoon KS, Lee JH, et al. The effect of multiple channeling on the structural integrity of repaired rotator cuff. Knee Surg Sports Traumatol Arthrosc. 2011; 19(12):2098–2107

[13] Kida Y, Morihara T, Matsuda K, et al. Bone marrow-derived cells from the footprint infiltrate into the repaired rotator cuff. J Shoulder Elbow Surg. 2013; 22(2):197–205

[14] Milano G, Saccomanno MF, Careri S, Taccardo G, De Vitis R, Fabbriciani C. Efficacy of marrow-stimulating technique in arthroscopic rotator cuff repair: a prospective randomized study. Arthroscopy. 2013; 29(5): 802–810

[15] Taniguchi N, Suenaga N, Oizumi N, et al. Bone marrow stimulation at the footprint of arthroscopic surface-holding repair advances cuff repair integrity. J Shoulder Elbow Surg. 2015; 24(6):860–866

32 Load-Sharing Rip-Stop and Knotless Rip-Stop Repairs for Massive Rotator Cuff Tears

Matthew P. Noyes and Patrick J. Denard

Summary

Massive rotator cuff tears associated with poor tendon quality remains a challenging condition. While double-row suturing bridging repairs have improved biomechanical strength, this technique may not be possible in the setting of tendon loss or limited tendon mobility. Single-row repairs are frequently performed in these settings, but re-tear rates have been reported up to 94% in massive rotator cuff tears. Therefore, alternative repair constructs must be sought. A loading–sharing rip-stop (LSRS) suture technique combines the advantages of a rip-stop suture tape and load-sharing properties of a double-row repair. Biomechanically, the LSRS construct has superior properties compared to a single-row repair, and clinically the repair has demonstrated promising initial results. A variation of this technique is to perform a knotless rip-stop (KRS) repair with only two suture anchors. This technique eliminates knot tying and decreases the anchor burden, while still maintaining the benefit of 2-mm suture tape. This chapter describes the authors' technique for the LSRS and KRS repair for massive rotator cuff-tears in which a double-row repair is not achievable.

Keywords: knotless rip-stop, load-sharing rip-stop, rotator cuff, single-row

32.1 Patient Positioning

- The patient is placed in the lateral decubitus position and secured with a beanbag. An axillary role is used to protect the brachial plexus. Pillows are placed underneath the fibular head of the down leg to protect the peroneal nerve and between the legs.
- The arm is held in 20° to 30° of abduction combined with 20° forward flexion utilizing an articulated electrically powered arm holder (Spider2, Smith & Nephew, Memphis, TN).
- An arthroscopic pump (Arthrex, Naples, FL) is used starting at 40 mm Hg and using fluid with added epinephrine to each bag to minimize bleeding, utilizing a standard dose (1 mg epinephrine per 3-Lsaline bag).

32.2 Portal Placement

32.2.1 Posterior Portal

A posterior glenohumeral viewing portal is established in the posterior "soft spot." We palpate the "soft spot" created by the glenoid medially and humeral head laterally.

32.2.2 Anterosuperolateral Portal

An anterosuperolateral portal is established 1–2 cm lateral and distal to the anterolateral corner of the acromion with a 5°–10° angle of approach to the lesser tuberosity.

A threaded cannula is placed in this portal. Biceps tenodesis, subscapularis repair, and coracoplasty (if indicated) are performed through this working portal. Note that the repair of the subscapularis must precede repair of the posterosuperior rotator cuff to have success in repair of massive rotator cuff tears. Then, the scope is redirected from the joint into the subacromial space.

32.2.3 Lateral Portal

A lateral portal is established in the mid tuberosity, approximately 3–4 cm lateral to the acromion. A limited subacromial decompression that preserves the coracoacromial arch is performed through this portal. After the decompression, bony landmarks (scapular spine and undersurface of acromioclavicular [AC] joint) are dissected so that they are fully visualized. Good visualization of the scapular spine is particularly important to see the raphe between the supraspinatus and the infraspinatus. Every effort is made to obtain a complete repair of the cuff, including careful excavation of the cuff, excision of bursal leaders, and interval slides when indicated. During this phase of the procedure, we have found that a 70° arthroscope is particularly useful because of the expanded field of view that it offers. Once mobilization is complete, a threaded cannula is placed in this portal for suture placement and lateral anchor placement.

32.2.4 Percutaneous Portals

Percutaneous portals are used as necessary for placement of anchors. These are established as 5–10 mm stab incisions just off the lateral edge of the acromion and are used for placement of anchors placed adjacent to the articular margin.

32.3 Surgical Technique

32.3.1 Load-Sharing Rip-Stop

- An antegrade suture passer is used to pass a 2-mm suture (FiberTape, Arthrex) through the rotator cuff as an inverted mattress stitch; the suture is placed 5–10 mm lateral to the tendon edge depending on remaining tendon length.
- If the tear has a large anterior-to-posterior dimension, then a second FiberTape may be placed in similar fashion. These rip-stop suture tapes must not be tensioned and repaired to bone until after the sutures from the medial anchors have been passed.
- Next, two double-loaded 5.5 mm anchors (Bio Composite Corkscrew, Arthrex)are placed anteromedially and posteromedially, along the articular margin. Beginning posteriorly, the sutures are passed from the medial anchors as simple stiches that penetrate the rotator cuff about 1 mm medial to the rip-stop suture.
- Once the medial sutures are passed, the FiberTape rip-stop sutures are retrieved from an accessory portal and secured laterally with two knotless suture anchors, making sure they encircle the sutures from the medial anchors.
- Finally, simple sutures from the medial anchors are retrieved and static knots are tied (▶ Fig. 32.1, ▶ Video 32.1).

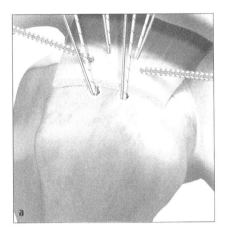
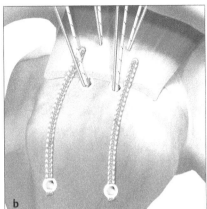
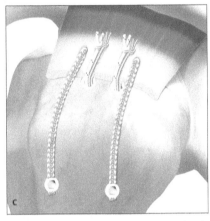

Fig. 32.1 Schematic illustrations of an anchor-based rip-stop rotator cuff repair for a rotator cuff tear with lateral tendon loss. **(a)** A FiberTape (Arthrex, Naples, FL) suture has been placed as an inverted mattress stitch in the rotator cuff. Two medial anchors (Bio Composite Corkscrew, Arthrex) have also been placed and sutures from these anchors are passed medial to the rip-stop stitch. **(b)** Prior to tying the sutures from the medial Corkscrew anchors, the rip-stop stitch is secured to bone with two lateral Bio Composite SwiveLock C anchors (Arthrex). **(c)** Tying the suture limbs from the Corkscrew anchors completes the repair.(Reprinted with permission from Burkhart et al 2012.)

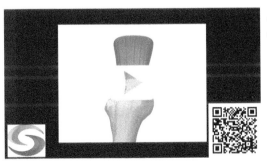

Video 32.1 Surgical demonstration of load sharing rip-stop.

32.3.2 Knotless Rip-Stop

- In the knotless rip-stop (KRS) repair, two knotless constructs are created. This technique is similar in concept to the loading–sharing rip-stop (LSRS) repair but is simpler to perform.
- As in the LSRS repair, this repair begins by placing a 2-mm suture tape (FiberTape, Arthrex) as an inverted mattress stitch in the rotator cuff, 5–10 mm medial to the lateral tendon edge. The suture is passed with 1 cm of spacing between the suture limbs.
- Next, a #2 suture with a free end on one end and a loop on the other end (FiberLink; Arthrex) is passed just medial to the mattress suture. The free end is passed through the loop to create a cinch stitch.
- A second KRS construct is then placed.
- A small punch is used to create bone vents adjacent to the articular margin to open the marrow elements and facilitate healing of the tendon to bone.
- Each KRS construct is secured in the lateral greater tuberosity with a knotless anchor (5.5 mm Bio Composite SwiveLock C, Arthrex) for a total of two anchors.
- Beginning posteriorly, the suture limbs of one construct are retrieved out the lateral portal cannula. The free limbs of the sutures are threaded through the eyelet of the knotless anchor, slack is removed, the anchor is placed in a pre-placed bone socket, and the suture limbs are cut to complete the KRS.
- The anterior construct is then secured in an identical fashion (▶ Fig. 32.2, ▶ Video 32.2).

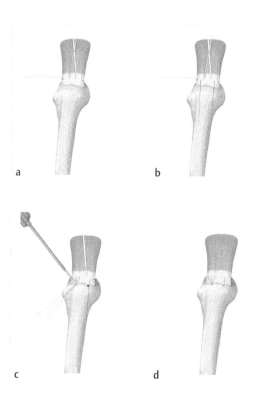

a

b

c

d

Fig. 32.2 Schematic illustrations of a knotless rip-stop technique. **(a)** Two 2-mm suture tapes (FiberTape, Arthrex, Naples, FL) are placed as an inverted mattress stitches in the rotator cuff, 1 cm medial to the lateral tendon edge. **(b)** Next, a cinch suture (FiberLink, Arthrex) is passed just medial to the inverted mattress suture tape. **(c)** Each suture tape/cinch loop construct is secured independently with two knotless anchors (5.5 mm Bio Composite SwiveLock C, Arthrex). **(d)** Final illustration demonstrating knotless rip-stop repair.

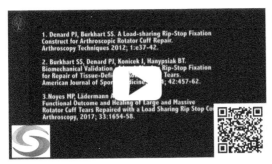

1. Denard PJ, Burkhart SS. A Load-sharing Rip-Stop Fixation Construct for Arthroscopic Rotator Cuff Repair. Arthroscopy Techniques 2012; 1:e37-42.

2. Burkhart SS, Denard PJ, Konicek J, Hanypsiak BT. Biomechanical Validation [...] Rip-Stop Fixation for Repair of Tissue-Defi[...] [...] Tears. American Journal of Spor[...] [...]icine[...]; 42:457-62.

3.Noyes MP, Lädermann [...] Functional Outcome and Healing of Large and Massive Rotator Cuff Tears Repaired with a Load Sharing Rip Stop Co[...] Arthroscopy, 2017; 33:1654-58.

Video 32.2 Surgical demonstration of knotless rip-stop.

32.4 Tips and Tricks

- We routinely use a 70° scope during the rotator cuff repair portion of the procedure, which we have found particularly useful for the expanded field of view that it offers. Use of this scope from the posterior portal facilitates triangulation with a lateral working portal and also makes lateral row anchor placement easier.
- 8.25 or 8.5 threaded mm cannulas are routinely placed in the anterosuperolateral and lateral portals and are used as the main working portals during the procedure.
- Accessory percutaneous portals are created as needed for anchor placement or suture management.
- An antegrade suture passer that is self-retrieving (Scorpion FastPass, Arthrex) facilitates suture passage.
- For the LSRS, it is important to delay knot tying until after the rip-stop stitch is secured laterally for two reasons. First, it is important to have a firm, taut rip-stop. Second, the FiberTape serves to unload the medial sutures as the rip-stop construct is secured laterally to an anchor.
- Suture management during the LSRS is facilitated by retrieving sutures from the medial anchors out of the same percutaneous portals used for anchor placement; this is done after each pass.
- For the KRS, the anchors are placed in the tuberosity, positioned in the same location normally used for the lateral row of a double-row repair, which is about 1 cm lateral to the tuberosity edge. This placement drapes the tendon over the bone vents in the tuberosity. However, as such, it is important to not overtension the rotator cuff when securing the construct.
- We try to take advantage of biology. In the LSRS, the medial anchors are cannulated and vented. In the KRS construct, bone vents are used medially to encourage healing (i.e., reverse "crimson duvet").
- Rehabilitation after this type of repair should be slow given the poor-quality tissue. We avoid motion until 6 weeks and delay strengthening until 12 weeks.

32.5 Complications

- Anchor failure is uncommon with threaded anchors. But we have seen pullout with smaller anchors (4.5 or 4.75 mm) in these types of repairs and only use larger anchors laterally (5.5 mm) given that many of these patients have poor bone quality.
- Re-tear is lowered with these types of repairs but can still occur. Our healing rates are outlined in the literature.[1]

32.6 Rehabilitation

Postoperatively, patients undergo immobilization in a sling for 6 weeks with basic hand, elbow, and wrist exercises started immediately. If a concomitant subscapularis repair is performed, we limit external rotation to neutral. Otherwise, if no repair was performed, external rotation to 30° is allowed. After 6 weeks, the sling is discontinued and passive forward elevation along with table slides are allowed. At 3 months postoperatively, strengthening is initiated.

32.7 Literature

Rip-stop sutures are used to limit tendon cut through given that the majority of rotator cuff failures occur at the suture–tendon interface. Ma et al demonstrated that a rip-stop suture with a double-loaded anchor had load to failure equivalent to a modified Mason–Allen stitch.[2] This construct is particularly useful for cases in which there is limited medial tendon that precludes a standard double-row repair.

The LSRS technique was first reported by Denard and Burkhart.[3] This technique combines the advantages of a wide rip-stop suture tape and load-sharing properties of a double-row repair. A biomechanical study performed by Burkhart et al compared the LSRS to a standard single-row repair.[4] The mean load to failure for LSRS was nearly twice that for a single-row repair construct(616 N vs. 371 N; P =0.031). Notably, in the single-row group, four of six failures occurred at the suture tendon interface (suture cutout) versus only one failure in the LSRS group. In a recent clinical study, Noyes et al evaluated the functional outcomes and healing rates for large and massive rotator cuff tears repaired with an LSRS construct.[5] Postoperative ultrasound evaluation demonstrated complete healing in 53% and partial healing in 29% of the cohort. Mean supraspinatus strength improved by one grade and 82% of patients were satisfied at their final follow-up. These results are promising considering the difficult patient population.

We are not aware of any clinical data on the KRS at this time. We performed a biomechanical investigation comparing the KRS to a single-row repair with triple-loaded anchors (submitted). The mean load to failure for triple-loaded anchors compared to KRS was equivalent (438 N vs. 457 N; P = 0.582). Interestingly, the triple-loaded anchor group had two tendon tears (type 1 failures) as a mode of failure while the KRS group had no tendon tears.

References

[1] Galatz LM, Ball CM, Teefey SA, Middleton WD, Yamaguchi K. The outcome and repair integrity of completely arthroscopically repaired large and massive rotator cuff tears. J Bone Joint Surg Am. 2004; 86(2):219–224

[2] Ma CB, MacGillivray JD, Clabeaux J, Lee S, Otis JC. Biomechanical evaluation of arthroscopic rotator cuff stitches. J Bone Joint Surg Am. 2004; 86(6):1211–1216

[3] Denard PJ, Burkhart SS. A load-sharing rip-stop fixation construct for arthroscopic rotator cuff repair. Arthrosc Tech. 2012; 1(1):e37–e42

[4] Burkhart SS, Denard PJ, Konicek J, Hanypsiak BT. Biomechanical validation of load-sharing rip-stop fixation for the repair of tissue-deficient rotator cuff tears. Am J Sports Med. 2014; 42(2):457–462

[5] Noyes MP, Ladermann A, Denard PJ. Functional outcome and healing of large and massive rotator cuff tears repaired with a load-sharing rip-stop construct. Arthroscopy. 2017; 33(9):1654–1658

Suggested Reading

Burkhart SS, Lo IK, Brady PC, Denard PJ. The Cowboy's Companion. Philadelphia, PA: Lippincott Williams & Wilkins; 2012

33 Arthroscopically Assisted Lower Trapezius Transfer for Irreparable Posterosuperior Rotator Cuff Tears

Joaquin Sanchez-Sotelo and Bassem T. Elhassan

Summary

Posterosuperior rotator cuff tears may lead to substantial pain and weakness. Primary repair of posterosuperior cuff tears may not be feasible or reliable for very large, chronic tears with substantial atrophy, fatty infiltration, and poor tendon quality. Tendon transfers represent salvage procedures that may be considered in these circumstances. Direct transfer of the lower portion of the trapezius to the infraspinatus tendon was described as a successful surgical procedure to improve strength in external rotation for the paralytic shoulder. This procedure has been adapted to be performed as an indirect arthroscopically, assisted tendon transfer for irreparable posterosuperior cuff tears. The lower portion of the trapezius is harvested through a relatively small posterior exposure. A graft (typically an Achilles tendon allograft) is then delivered into the subacromial space from this posterior surgical site; the narrower end of the Achilles allograft is then fixed to the anterior portion of the greater tuberosity using arthroscopic anchors and techniques. The arm is placed in abduction and external rotation and the wider portion of the graft repaired to the lower trapezius (LT) with multiple nonabsorbable and absorbable sutures. The shoulder is immobilized in external rotation for 6 weeks. A few cadaveric studies have analyzed the biomechanical properties of transferring the LT. Early clinical results are promising, with improvement in pain, motion, and strength. Follow-up studies will be required to determine the long-term outcome of this reconstructive technique.

Keywords: allograft, fatty infiltration, rotator cuff tear, tendon transfer, trapezius

33.1 Introduction

Symptomatic posterosuperior rotator cuff tears that not amenable to surgical repair represent a substantial challenge. Multiple procedures have been considered for the salvage of these shoulders, including debridement, tendon transfers, reconstruction of the superior capsule, and reverse shoulder arthroplasty. Transferring the lower portion of the trapezius to the greater tuberosity has become our tendon transfer of choice for patients with massive irreparable posterosuperior cuff tears for no or minimal cartilage damage (▶ **Fig. 33.1**).

Transfer of the trapezius was initially described to improve external rotation and elevation motion and strength in paralytic shoulders.[1,2,3,4,5] A few cadaveric studies have analyzed the biomechanical properties of the LT transfer.[6,7] The outcome of open indirect transfer of the lower portion of the trapezius to the greater tuberosity using a intercalary Achilles tendon allograft has been reported to be satisfactory.[8] This initial open technique has been modified to be performed with arthroscopic assistance,[9] as detailed in this chapter.

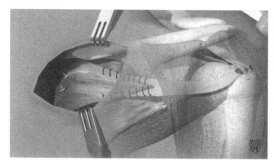

Fig. 33.1 Schematic representation of the final construct after indirect transfer of the lower trapezius to the greater tuberosity.

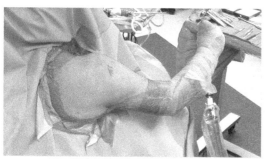

Fig. 33.2 Our preference is to perform this procedure with the patient in the beachchair position. The arm is placed in an articulated mechanical limb positioner. It is critical to confirm adequate draping of the surgical field to allow access several centimeters medial to the medial border of the scapula.

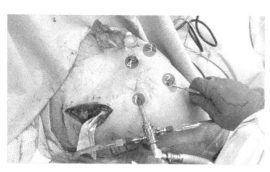

Fig. 33.3 Main portals used: posterolateral subacromial viewing portal (**1**), 50-yard-line subacromial portal (**2**), anterior subacromial portal to retrieve allograft leading end sutures (**3**), and anterosuperior subacromial portal for graft fixation (**4**).

33.2 Patient Positioning (▶ Fig. 33.2)

- High beachchair position (barber chair position)
- Articulated mechanical limb positioner
- Confirm unrestricted access to whole scapula
- Drape the arm free attached to the mechanical limb positioner
- Drape the surgical field to at least 5 cm medial to the medial border of the scapula

33.3 Portal Placement (▶ Fig. 33.3)

- Posterolateral subacromial portal as main viewing portal
- Two lateral subacromial portals
  - Centered in reference to the humeral head

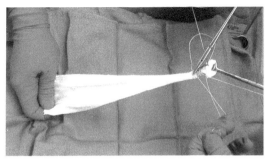

Fig. 33.4 An Achilles tendon allograft is prepared in the back-table to receive two heavy nonabsorbable sutures. Partially coloring the allograft will aid with orientation at the time of arthroscopic fixation.

   ◦ Working portal
   ◦ Viewing portal
  – Anterior for retrieval of allograft leading end sutures
• One anterosuperior subacromial portal for graft fixation

33.4 Surgical Technique

33.4.1 Partial Cuff Repair and Biceps Tenotomy/Tenodesis if Indicated

• Bursectomy, selective acromioplasty
• Biceps assessment, tenotomy/tenodesis if indicated
• Cuff tear pattern identification and release/mobilization if indicated
• Partial cuff repair
• Keep sutures after tying for augmentation of allograft fixation

33.4.2 Achilles Tendon Allograft Preparation (▶ Fig. 33.4)

• Narrow (calcaneal) end of the graft prepared for fixation to the tuberosity
  – Place two heavy nonabsorbable sutures (Fiberwire #2 by Arthrex, Naples, FL; Orthocord by DePuy, Warsaw, IN; or equivalent) at the end of the graft using running locked sutures, one on each side of the graft
  – Sutures of different color will make suture identification easier at the time of arthroscopic fixation
• A marking pen may be used to partially color one of the sides of the graft to aid with orientation of the graft at the time of arthroscopic fixation
• Depending on the fixation mode preferred to secure the graft to the transferred LT, nonabsorbable sutures may also be placed on the opposite (wider) side of the graft for later use

33.5 Lower Trapezius Tendon Harvesting and Mobilization

• Place a horizontal skin incision parallel to the spine of the scapula and slightly below the level of the spine, starting at the medial border of the body of the scapula and measuring approximately 8 cm (▶ **Fig. 33.5**a).

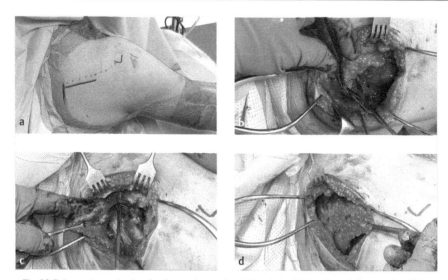

Fig. 33.5 Lower trapezius tendon harvesting and mobilization.x **(a)** Horizontal skin incision. **(b)** Identification of the inferior leading edge of the trapezius. **(c)** Trapezius tendon detachment off the scapular spine. **(d)** Mobilized lower trapezius.

- Carefully mobilize subcutaneous skin flaps avoiding inadvertent damage to the trapezius, very superficial on the posterior periscapular region.
- Identify the lower leading edge of the trapezius and develop the plane between the trapezius and the infraspinatus fascia (▶ **Fig. 33.5**b).
- Follow the lower edge of the trapezius laterally to its insertion into the spine of the scapula.
- Detach the tendon of the LT subperiosteally off the spine of the scapula from lateral to medial until the medial edge of the scapular spine is reached (▶ **Fig. 33.5**c).
- Complete the mobilization deep to the trapezius and medial to the medial border of the scapula with extreme caution to avoid damage to the neurovascular pedicle of the LT, located approximately 2 cm medial to the medial border of the body of the scapula.
- Mobilize the trapezius further laterally by placing an atraumatic clamp at the lateral end of the tendon and dissecting subcutaneously (▶ **Fig. 33.5**d).

33.6 Allograft Passage and Fixation to the Greater Tuberosity

- Divide the fascia of the infraspinatus in line with its fibers to communicate the trapezius tendon harvest site with the subacromial space.
- Pass the narrow end of the Achilles tendon allograft from the trapezius tendon harvest site into the subacromial space using the sutures placed at the allograft (▶ **Fig. 33.6**a).
  - A large curve clamp may be inserted in an antegrade or retrograde fashion.
  - The sutures are retrieved into the more anterior lateral subacromial portal.

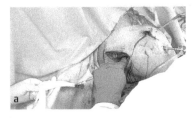
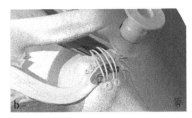
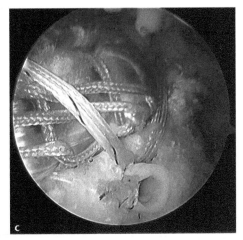

Fig. 33.6 Allograft passage and fixation. (a) Allograft passage. (b) Schematic of graft fixation. (c) Arthroscopic view of the fixed allograft.

- Anchor the sutures into the anterior aspect of the greater tuberosity using any of the commercially available lateral row anchors.
  - The two limbs of the first suture are anchored medial and superior, close to the partially repaired rotator cuff or margin of the articular cartilage.
  - The other two limbs of the second suture are anchored laterally, in line with the medial/superior anchor(▶ Fig. 33.6b, c).
- Use the sutures used for partial repair of the rotator cuff to further compress the graft to the greater tuberosity by placing them over the graft and anchoring them to the lateral cortex of the proximal humerus with lateral row anchors.

33.6.1 Trapezius to Allograft Repair

- Place the shoulder in abduction and external rotation with the assistance of the mechanical limb positioner (▶ Fig. 33.7a).
- Apply traction to the Achilles allograft medially and the LT tendon laterally.
- Repair the Achilles allograft to the LT with multiple absorbable and nonabsorbable sutures(▶ Fig. 33.7b).
  - Place the Achilles allograft deep to the trapezius.
  - Consider a Pulvertaft weave type of repair.
  - Consider use of a commercially available tendon protection device combining a porous matrix of cross-linked type I collagen and glycosaminoglycan (TenoGlide, Integra LifeSciences, NJ) (▶ Video 33.1).

33.7 Tips and Tricks

- If you know for sure that you will need to transfer the LT, consider harvesting the trapezius prior to arthroscopic bursectomy, biceps procedures, and partial cuff repair.
  - Benefit: The dissection is cleaner prior to arthroscopic fluid extravasation.

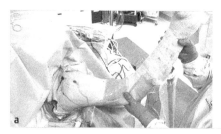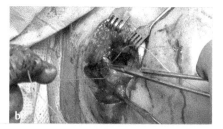

Fig. 33.7 Graft to lower trapezius fixation. (a) Arm placed in abduction and external rotation. (b) Repair.

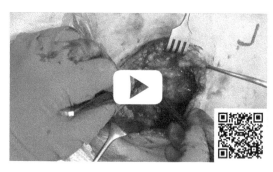

Video 33.1 Surgical demonstration of arthroscopically assisted lower trapezius transfer for irreparable posterosuperior rotator cuff repair.

- Downside:
  - If the cuff can be repaired better than expected, commitment to transfer has already been made when it may not be necessary.
  - Loss of fluid containment from the subacromial space into the tendon harvest site may compromise arthroscopic visualization during partial arthroscopic cuff repair.
- Remember to save the tied sutures used for partial repair of the rotator cuff to further compress the LT to the cuff footprint on the greater tuberosity.
- Mark graft with marking pen and use color coded sutures to facilitate orientation of the graft under arthroscopic visualization.
- Consider marking the overall expected location of the trapezius on the skin so that the location of the lower border can be easily identified at the time of harvest.
- Open the fascia of the infraspinatus prior to passage of the Achilles allograft from the harvest site into the subacromial space.

33.8 Pitfalls and Complications

- Damage of the trapezius tendon at the time of harvest.
- Injury to the neurovascular bundle of the trapezius due to excessive dissection deep to the muscle and more than 2 cm medial to the medial border of the scapular body.
- Poor fixation of the Achilles tendon allograft to the proximal humerus (poor orientation, suture entanglement, and poor anchor placement).
- Failure to tension the trapezius during allograft repair by not placing the arm in abduction and external rotation at the time of repair.
- Failure to protect the reconstruction by not immobilizing the shoulder in abduction and external rotation for 6 weeks or longer.

33.9 Rehabilitation

- Immediately after surgery the operative side is placed in an external rotation immobilizer or brace.
- Elbow, wrist, and hand exercises are initiated on postoperative day #1, but shoulder therapy is delayed for 6 to 8 weeks.
- Patients are specifically instructed to avoid letting their shoulder fall into internal rotation (avoid letting their hand rest on their belly) for the first 6 to 8 weeks after surgery.
- At week 6 to 8, passive and active assisted range of motion exercises are initiated.
- Isometrics are typically initiated at week 8 to 10, and strengthening with elastic bands at week 10 to 12.

33.10 Rationale and Evidence

- Basic science studies
  - Biomechanical analysis of various tendon transfers to restore external rotation of shoulder[6]
    - Six fresh-frozen cadaveric hemithoraces
    - Six experimental conditions assessing latissimus dorsi (LD), teres major (TM), and LT:
    - LD to greater tuberosity or humeral diaphysis
    - TM to greater tuberosity or humeral diaphysis
    - LT to infraspinatus or teres minor attachment site
    - Primary outcome: external rotation moment arm (ERMA)
    - At 0 degree of abduction, LT was superior to LD or TM
    - With increasing abduction, LD was superior to LT
  - Biomechanical comparison of transferring the LT or the LD[7]
    - Eight cadaveric shoulders
    - Testing performed a 0, 30, and 60 degrees of abduction
    - Transfer of the LT was superior to transfer of the LD in terms of
    - Restoration of external rotation in all angles of abduction
    - Restoration of joint compression forces in all angles of abduction
    - Partial reversal of superolateral shift of the humeral head apex
- Clinical studies
  - Outcome of open indirect LT transfer for massive irreparable posterosuperior cuff tears[8]
    - 33 shoulders
    - Pain, subjective shoulder value, and Disabilities of the Arm, Shoulder and Hand (DASH) scores improved in 32
    - Mean active elevation of 120 degrees
    - Mean active external rotation of 50 degrees
    - Better outcomes in patients with more than 60 degrees of flexion prior to the procedure
    - Outcome of arthroscopically assisted indirect LT transfer for massive irreparable rotator cuff tears
  - 41 shoulders
    - Pain, subjective shoulder value, and DASH improved in 37 shoulders (90%)
    - Mean active elevation of 133 degrees

- Mean active external rotation of 47 degrees
- Three shoulders progress to cuff-tear arthropathy, two revised to reverse shoulder arthroplasty
- Two shoulders suffered a traumatic disruption of the transfer
- Poor prognostic factors: symptoms for more than 2 years, arthropathy Hamada grade 3, and true pseudoparalysis.

33.11 Conclusion

- Direct transfer of the lower portion of the trapezius to the infraspinatus tendon has emerged as a successful surgical solution to provide active external rotation in paralytic shoulders.[1,2,3,4,5]
- Arthroscopically assisted indirect transfer of the LT was developed as a tendon transfer option for shoulders with massive irreparable posterosuperior cuff tears, both in the primary and revision setting.[9]
- Short-term results are promising in terms of both pain relief and improved strength in external rotation; gains in active elevation and the durability of the improvement prior to salvage with additional surgery remain unknown.[8,9]

References

[1] Mir-Bullo X, Hinarejos P, Mir-Batlle P, Busquets R, Carrera L, Navarro A. Trapezius transfer for shoulder paralysis: 6 patients with brachial plexus injuries followed for 1 year. Acta OrthopScand. 1998; 69(1):69–72
[2] Rühmann O, Gossé F, Wirth CJ. Trapezius-transfer for shoulder paralysis: 6 patients with brachial plexus injuries followed for 1 year. Acta OrthopScand. 1999; 70(4):407–408
[3] Bertelli JA. Lengthening of subscapularis and transfer of the lower trapezius in the correction of recurrent internal rotation contracture following obstetric brachial plexus palsy. J Bone Joint Surg Br. 2009; 91(7): 943–948
[4] Elhassan B, Bishop A, Shin A. Trapezius transfer to restore external rotation in a patient with a brachial plexus injury: a case report. J Bone Joint Surg Am. 2009; 91(4):939–944
[5] Bertelli JA. Upper and lower trapezius muscle transfer to restore shoulder abduction and external rotation in longstanding upper type palsies of the brachial plexus in adults. Microsurgery. 2011; 31(4):263–267
[6] Hartzler RU, Barlow JD, An KN, Elhassan BT. Biomechanical effectiveness of different types of tendon transfers to the shoulder for external rotation. J Shoulder Elbow Surg. 2012; 21(10):1370–1376
[7] Omid R, Heckmann N, Wang L, McGarry MH, Vangsness CT, Jr, Lee TQ. Biomechanical comparison between the trapezius transfer and latissimus transfer for irreparable posterosuperior rotator cuff tears. J Shoulder Elbow Surg. 2015; 24(10):1635–1643
[8] Elhassan BT, Wagner ER, Werthel JD. Outcome of lower trapezius transfer to reconstruct massive irreparable posterior-superior rotator cuff tear. J Shoulder Elbow Surg. 2016; 25(8):1346–1353
[9] Elhassan BT, Alentorn-Geli E, Assenmacher AT, Wagner ER. Arthroscopic-assisted lower trapezius tendon transfer for massive irreparable posterior-superior rotator cuff tears: surgical technique. Arthrosc Tech. 2016; 5(5):e981–e988

Suggested Reading

Elhassan BT, Sanchez-Sotelo J, Wagner ER: Outcome of arthroscopically assisted lower trapezius transfer to reconstruct massive irreparable posterior-superior rotator cuff tears. J Shoulder Elbow Surg 2020 Jun 9; S1058–2746(20)30229–9

34 Subacromial Balloon Spacer for Irreparable Cuff Tears

J. Gabriel Horneff III and Joseph A. Abboud

Summary

The massive irreparable rotator cuff repair is a difficult problem to treat in patients who are not suitable candidates for reverse shoulder arthroplasty. The subacromial balloon spacer is a newer technique designed to restore the relationship of the humeral head to the glenoid and allow patients to achieve improved function despite loss of their rotator cuff. This technique is relatively quick and easy to perform and affords patients the ability to regain functional use of their shoulder without jeopardizing the chance for any further surgeries in the future. The device is approved for use in the European Union and has undergone a Food and Drug Administration trial in the United States with promising results.

Keywords: balloon arthroplasty, irreparable cuff tear, massive cuff tear, proximal migration, subacromial spacer

34.1 Patient Positioning

- The patient is placed in the beach chair position. This allows for gravitational distraction of the humeral head and a more accurate depiction of the amount of subacromial space available without traction.
- The operative extremity is prepped and draped in the typical sterile fashion.
- A mechanical arm holder can be utilized to position the operative extremity in space.

34.2 Portal Placement

- A standard posterosuperior arthroscopic portal is initially created for placement of the arthroscope. This portal is utilized for the initial diagnostic arthroscopy of the glenohumeral joint and subacromial space.
- A lateral portal in line with the posterior border of the clavicle is created under spinal needle localization with arthroscope visualizing from the posterior portal. This portal is initially utilized for the debridement and decompression instruments prior to balloon insertion. Prior to balloon insertion, the lateral portal is utilized as the visualization portal for the remainder of the case.
- Alternative portal: an anterior portal just above the superior border of the subscapularis can be created under spinal needle localization if initial intraarticular pathology needs to be addressed prior to balloon implantation.

34.3 Surgical Technique (Step-by-Step Approach)

- Prior to incision, a surgical timeout should always be performed to correctly identify the patient, procedure, and correct operative limb (▸ **Video 34.1**).

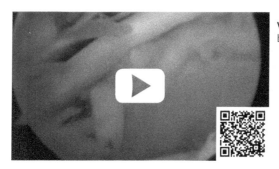

Video 34.1 Description of the balloon with arthroscopic placement.

- A standard posterior portal is created and the arthroscope is introduced into the glenohumeral joint. A diagnostic arthroscopy is performed to assess the rotator cuff, labrum, articular surface, and remaining structures.
- If the subscapularis tendon is torn, this should be repaired as best as possible by the surgeon's preferred technique.
- Once all intraarticular work is completed, the arthroscope should be redirected to the subacromial space.
- A lateral portal is created under spinal needle localization in line with the posterior border of the clavicle.
- A combination of arthroscopic shavers, burs, and electrocautery are used via the lateral portal to remove any debris from the undersurface of the acromion. Any large subacromial spurs can be smoothed to allow for unimpeded placement/inflation of the balloon.
- Once visualization is adequate, a calibrated probe is used to measure the defect left behind from the deficient rotator cuff tissue. This measurement is performed in the anterior-to-posterior plane (rotator interval to intact posterior cuff) as well as the medial-to-lateral plane (superior glenoid rim to greater tuberosity).
- The InSpace balloon (OrthoSpace, Caesarea, Israel) is available in three sizes: small (40 mm × 50 mm), medium (50 mm × 60 mm), and large (60 mm × 70 mm).
- Once the defect is measured, an arthroscopic switching stick is placed laterally to allow for placement of the arthroscope into the lateral portal in the subacromial space.
- Select an appropriately sized balloon and prepare it on the back table to ensure an efficient placement.
- A syringe is filled with sterile saline warmed to roughly 40 °C. Attach this syringe to the extension tubing. Ensure that there is no air within the syringe or tubing.
- Introduce the balloon insertion device into the posterior portal and position over the superior glenoid rim.
- Once the balloon is in the proper position, retract the protection sheath to expose the balloon.
- Attach the extension tubing to the insertion handle and advance the plunger of the syringe to fill the balloon under visualization. Refer to the balloon size reference guide for the proper volume of saline to be injected.
- When filling of the balloon is complete, deploy the red safety button and turn the green knob on the insertion handle to seal the balloon as the handle is removed.
- With the balloon in place, take the patient's shoulder through a range of motion to visualize that the balloon is stable without subluxation.

- Remove all instrumentation from the shoulder and close the portal sites with a nonabsorbable suture and dress with sterile dressings to preference.
- The patient is placed in a regular sling prior to awakening from anesthesia and then taken to the recovery room.

34.4 Surgeon Tips and Tricks

- One of the most important keys to success with interpositional balloon arthroplasty is proper patient selection. The following are criteria that we use to select patients:
  – Functioning deltoid muscle.
  – No history of infection.
  – No significant glenohumeral arthritis.
  – Intact or repairable subscapularis and posterior rotator cuff.
  – Ability to actively forward elevate to at least 90° prior to surgery.
- Perform a thorough subacromial bursectomy using an arthroscopic shaver and electrocautery. It is important to achieve hemostasis with electrocautery to maintain a good visual field for deployment of the balloon.
- Avoid an aggressive bursectomy medial to the face of the glenoid as this can lead to medial migration of the balloon and decrease its depressing force effect on the humeral head.
- We find the long head of the biceps tendon to be a pain generator in the shoulder and prefer either biceps tenodesis or tenotomy prior to balloon insertion.
- Be sure to take careful and thorough measurements with the probe to select the appropriate balloon size. If visualization for sizing is difficult with the arthroscope in the posterior portal, use a switching stick to place the arthroscope into the lateral portal to allow for a better perspective when measuring.
- We have found that placement of the balloon via the posterior portal with lateral visualization allows for more accurate placement of the balloon. This is in contrast to the manufacturer's recommendation of visualizing from the posterior portal and placing the balloon laterally.
- Avoid overinflation of the balloon as this can lead to rupture or possible subluxation of the device.
- Motion of the patient's arm with the arthroscope visualizing the inserted balloon is essential to ensure that there is no subluxation or displacement of the device.

34.5 Pitfalls/Complications

- Aside from the usual possible risks that come with arthroscopic shoulder surgery (i.e., infection, bleeding, wound healing, etc.), we have found minimal risks with the use of this device.
- The largest concern with the use of this device is the possible migration of balloon from out of the subacromial space. In our experience, this has happened only one time and was resolved with removal and replacement of the balloon.
- In the literature, four studies from Europe have had a combined 93 patients who have undergone the balloon arthroplasty procedure. Only one patient of those combined cohorts had a dislocation of the device.
- No other device-related complication has been reported in the literature.

- As the availability of this device becomes more widespread, the most concerning pitfall with its use is improper patient selection. We think it is important that patients retain active functional ability to raise their arms to at least 90° of elevation. This device should not be used for patients with true shoulder pseudoparalysis.
- The InSpace balloon is CE marked in Europe and available for use in the patient with a rotator cuff tear that is otherwise unfixable. Currently, in the United States, there is a Food and Drug Administration investigational device exemption (IDE) trial that randomized patients to either balloon placement or the best attempted rotator cuff repair, required at least 90 degrees of active forward elevation and no signs of glenohumeral arthritis.

34.6 Rehabilitation

- Weeks 0 to 4: Sling use for comfort. Patient is allowed to use the arm for light activity (eating, hygiene, writing, typing). Patient encouraged to move hand, wrist, and elbow to prevent joint stiffness.
- Weeks 4 to 8: Discontinuation of the sling. Patient can return to activities of daily living. Formal physical therapy (PT) is started with a concurrent home exercise program. The patient's PT begins with phase I and II stretching and early strengthening for up to 3 pounds.
- Weeks 8 to 12: The physical therapy regimen is advanced to full strengthening with transition to a home-based program. Strengthening can advance to 10–15 pounds.
- Weeks 12 and beyond: All restrictions are lifted and the patient can resume full activity.

34.7 Rationale and/or Evidence for Approach

- Patients with large irreparable rotator cuff tears develop proximal humeral migration as the compromised function of the torn cuff allows the deltoid muscle to create a superiorly directed shearing force at the glenohumeral interface.
- The biomechanical purpose of the subacromial balloon is to depress the humeral head and reduce subacromial friction for improved elevation and abduction.
- The first study published on this technique was by Senekovic et al in 2013 with 20 patients demonstrating improved Constant scores and range of motion as early as 6 weeks following their surgery. These improvements continued during the 3-year period of the study. Subjective pain and night pain also improved over the 3-year study period starting as early as 1 week out from surgery.[1]
- A follow up prospective study at 5 years for 21 patients for the InSpace technique found that 84.6% had a clinical improvement of at least 15 points with regard to Constant scores. In addition, 61.5% of those patients had at least 25 points of improvement. Scores improved as early as 3 months after surgery and lasted for 5 years.[2]
- Looking at all patients from published studies demonstrated only one device-related complication, which was a dislocation of the balloon that required replacement. The operative times for these same patients ranged from 2 to 30 minutes at an average time of 10 minutes.[1,2,3,4]

References

[1] Senekovic V, Poberaj B, Kovacic L, Mikek M, Adar E, Dekel A. Prospective clinical study of a novel biodegradable sub-acromial spacer in treatment of massive irreparable rotator cuff tears. Eur J Orthop Surg Traumatol. 2013; 23(3):311–316

[2] Senekovic V, Poberaj B, Kovacic L, et al. The biodegradable spacer as a novel treatment modality for massive rotator cuff tears: a prospective study with 5-year follow-up. Arch Orthop Trauma Surg. 2017; 137(1):95–103

[3] Deranlot J, Herisson O, Nourissat G, et al. Arthroscopic subacromial spacer implantation in patients with massive irreparable rotator cuff tears: Clinical and radiographic results in 39 retrospective cases. Arthroscopy. 2017; 33(9):1639–1644

[4] Gervasi E, Maman E, Dekel A, Cautero E. Fluoroscopy-guided biodegradable spacer implantation using local anesthesia: safety and efficacy study in patients with massive rotator cuff tears. Musculoskelet Surg. 2016; 100 Suppl 1:19–24

35 Acellular Human Dermal Allograft Rotator Cuff Reconstruction

Michael Bahk, Stephen Snyder, and J. Ryan Taylor

Summary

Large and massive rotator cuff tears with retraction present a challenge for adequate repair. We present the use of dermal allograft to assist with arthroscopic rotator cuff repair and reconstruction to the native footprint.

Keywords: dermal allograft, massive rotator cuff tear, arthroscopic repair

35.1 Patient Positioning

Please refer to the chapter 2 on SCOI Row Rotator Cuff Repair for patient positioning.

35.2 Portal Placement

Please refer to the chapter 2 on SCOI Row Rotator Cuff Repair for techniques in identifying bony landmarks and for portal placement. Sequence of portal placement is described in the surgical technique below.

35.3 Surgical Technique

35.3.1 Preoperative Preparation (Back Table)

- Tie 12 short-tailed interference knot (STIK) sutures using three different colors of #2 braided suture. The STIK knots are made by wrapping a suture once around a 2-mm metal rod (switching stick) and tying a bulky knot at the end. The small loop created near the knot will facilitate grasping of suture when retrieving for tying.
- Make a knotted measuring suture, spaced with 1 cm increments on a 0 braided suture with a STIK loop at one end. Color every other knot with a surgical marker with a total of five knots (5 cm). The knotted measuring suture is then loaded though a knot pusher with the free loop end held with the grasper for ease in measuring the defect via another portal.
- Hydrate the graft in room temperature saline if necessary once it is certain it will be used.

35.3.2 Shoulder Arthroscopic Evaluation, Debridement, Decompression, and Preparation

- Create a standard posterior midglenoid portal (PMGP) and anterior midglenoid portal (AMGP) and place a 7-mm docking cannula in each one (DryDoc 2 × 95 mm, Conmed/Linvatec, Largo, FL). These "docking" cannulas will remain in these portals for the entire case.

- Perform a 15-point arthroscopic evaluation of the shoulder, documenting the condition of the rotator cuff, biceps tendon, labrum, cartilage surfaces, subscapularis, and synovium.
- Debride the degenerative edges of the cuff and thickened bursal scar. Mobilize the medial stump of the rotator cuff by carefully releasing the scar and capsule at the level of the glenoid. If needed, repair any significant subscapularis or labral pathology.
- Continue preparation of the bursal space by smoothing the undersurface of the acromioclavicular(AC) joint. All remaining suture material or anchor should be removed if they are obstructing bone needed for graft placement. Use the motorized shaver to lightly debride the greater tuberosity and the biceps groove leaving the cortex intact to induce healing of tendon and graft to bone.
- Use a spinal needle 3–4 cm lateral from the acromial edge on the lateral deltoid to localize the midpoint of the cuff defect (this is not always at the midpoint of the acromion) to create the midlateral subacromial portal (MLSAP). Insert a larger, 8-mm docking cannula in this portal (8 × 75 mm "red" DryDoc cannula). If the cuff defect is found to be greater than 3.5 cm, then a 10-mm cannula with an external rubber diaphragm is recommended (Smith & Nephew, Andover, MA).
- Create a suprascapular portal by making a small stab incision though the skin at the soft spot of the suprascapular fossa, just posterior to the AC joint. A spinal needle is used to identify proper placement of the portal. The shaver is then used to remove soft tissue below the suprascapular notch for better visualization of the portal. This portal is used to retrieve and store free ends of medial STIK sutures after they are passed though the top of the cuff stump. This facilitates pulling the graft into the shoulder and lessens the chance of twisting sutures.

35.3.3 Placement of First Suture Anchor

- With the scope in the MLSAP at the 50-yard line of the tear, a spinal needle is used as a guide to identify the proper position of the first anchor.
- The ideal position is a few millimeters anterior to the posterior edge of the cuff stump and 5 mm lateral to the edge of the articular cartilage.
- Prior to inserting the anchor, a small 2-mm bone punch is used to create a starter hole, as well as five to nine "bone marrow vents" by puncturing the exposed bone of the lateral tuberosity (away from the anchor sites).
- Insert a triple-loaded suture anchor into the pilot hole using a medial "tent peg" angle, seating the anchor 2 mm below the surface of the cortex.
- Pass the medial limb of the posteriormost suture from the posterior anchor through the edge of the posterior cuff near the attachment site on the bone to accomplish a "partial cuff repair," taking care not to place any tension on sutures when they are tied.
- This can be accomplished using a suture shuttle technique, by first retrieving the medial limb of the posterior most suture into the AMGP. A crescent-shaped suture hook is used to pass the shuttling suture through the cuff stump via the posterior midglenoid (PMG) cannula. The shuttle suture is then retrieved into the anterior midglenoid (AMG) cannula with the grasper, and the suture is loaded and carried back through the cuff and out the PMG cannula. The suture is tied using a sliding-locking knot.
- Clamp the remaining sutures outside the skin to hold them snug.

35.3.4 Placement of Second Anchor and Performing the Biceps Tenodesis Using the ThRevo "Italian Loop" Method

- The curette and shaver are used to "freshen" the biceps groove by removing the cartilage and synovial tissue. Three bone marrow vents are created in the groove leaving 5 mm of bone between each hole.
- Use the spinal needle to guide placement of the anterior anchor. The anchor is placed 5 mm lateral to the articular cartilage and a few mm posterior to the biceps tendon.
- The most anteromedial suture limb is retrieved out the PMG cannula with the crochet hook.
- A suture hook is then used via the AMG cannula to traverse any substantial tissue from the rotator interval and pass through the center of the biceps tendon at the same level as the anchor. The shuttle is carried out the PMG portal, where the suture is loaded and carried back though the biceps and rotator interval tissue out the AMG cannula. The same suture is again retrieved out the PMG cannula. The same process is again repeated with the suture hook a few millimeters from the initial pass obtaining a second robust bite of tendon and using the shuttle to carry the same suture back out the AMG portal, completing the "Italian loop" stitch. A nonsliding Revo knot is then used to complete the biceps tenodesis.
- One of the remaining sutures can be used to suture the anteriormost edge of the supraspinatus tendon. The sutures are tied.
- The remaining suture from the anchor is clamped outside of the skin for later use.

35.3.5 Measuring the Defect in the Rotator Cuff

- Graft size is measured in both anterior-to-posterior and medial-to-lateral dimensions using a knotted measuring suture, spaced in 1 cm increments. The knotted measuring suture is loaded though the eye of a knot pusher such that the free loop is on the tip inserted into the anterior cannula.
- The knotted measuring suture is used to measure between the two lateral suture anchors from the center of the cuff tendon stump to the edge of the humeral head cartilage.
- The graft should be oversized by 3 mm per side to ensure coverage of the defect.
- The corresponding measurements are then drawn on a towel using a surgical pen to create a pattern for cutting the allograft.

35.3.6 Preparation of the Graft (Back Table)

- A surgical assistant prepares the graft on the back table.
- Press the moist graft into the pattern that was drawn on the towel to transfer the pattern to the graft.
- Dermal allografts have a basement membrane "smooth" side and a reticular "fuzzy" side. Dimensions are drawn and knots set on the basement membrane side, while the reticular side is oriented down over the tendon/bone.
- The graft is cut sharply over a metal surface to ensure no fabric fibers are introduced into the specimen.
- Draw a 1-cm centerline in the middle of the lateral edge to orient the graft.
- Mark dots for STIK suture placement 5 mm from the edge of the graft and 6 mm apart on the posterior, medial, and anterior boarders. Place a dot at the antero- and

posterolateral corners for placement of the remaining suture from the posterior and anterior anchors.
- Place a STIK suture at each anterior and posterior mark using a Keith needle so that the loop and knot are on the basement membrane (shiny) side. The two most lateral corners are left open.
- Use white suture for the medial STIK sutures, coloring every other suture with a surgical pen for easy identification when passing and tying.
- Alternate dark green and light green for the anterior and posterior STIK sutures.
- Ensure the graft remains hydrated with normal saline throughout the preparation process.

35.3.7 Attachment of the Graft to the Posteromedial Cuff

- Wrap a moistened surgical towel around the arm lateral to the MLSA cannula and secure it with a clamp. Orient the graft on the towel anatomically, rotated 45° posteriorly. Use an Alice clamp to secure the STIK suture tails to the towel in an orderly manner. This step is critical, as each successive suture must pass parallel and anterior to the previous suture. If any of the sutures twist or cross, the graft will twist when it is brought into the shoulder, making it extremely difficult to complete the case.
- To begin the graft passing process, first retrieve the medial limb of the center suture from the posterior anchor and out the MLSA cannula, ensuring the suture passes medial to the "suture stack" and between the suture anchors.
- Use a Keith needle to pass the retrieved medial suture through the graft from bottom to top at the posterolateral corner mark. Tie a STIK knot on the top of the graft to match the other previously placed STIK knots.
- Keep the remaining sutures from the posterior anchor taut outside of the skin with a hemostat clamp.
- Select and clamp the free end of the most posterolateral STIK suture from the graft, and clamp through an Alice clamp on the posterior aspect of the towel. This is referred to as "staging the suture"(i.e., preparing it to be next to pass).
- A crescent suture hook is then used to pass a shuttle suture though a healthy bite of posterior cuff, 6 mm medial to the posterior anchor. The suture is retrieved from the MLSA cannula anterior to the previously passed suture from the anchor and between the "suture stacks" from the remaining anchor sutures held outside the skin with hemostat clamps. Load the shuttle and carry it back though the cuff and though the PMG cannula.
- Repeat this process with the crescent suture hook, passing the STIKs along the posterior edge, toward the medial aspect of the cuff defect, spacing the sutures 6 mm apart. Store the ends of the sutures inside the posterior cannula.

35.3.8 Alternative Method—Direct Suture Passing

- The "direct pass" method via the lateral portal is preferred by some surgeons. This can be accomplished by passing the free ends of the STIK sutures sequentially, starting from the posterior aspect of the defect, moving to the medial stump and then to anterior, with a direct pass suture needle device. Great care must be taken not to cross the sutures during this process. When using the suture shuttle method, the needle is inserted into the PMAC and sutures are passed from posterior medial to anterior medial. As you progress medially along the cuff stump, use the appropriate suture needle with a shuttle, usually a 45° right or left hook and sometimes using a 60° or 90° hook needle. It is usually best to pass four medial sutures to ensure a firm hold of graft to cuff stump.

- The first medial suture is passed just posterior to the scapular spine, the second just anterior to the spine and the other two through a healthy bite of the supraspinatus tendon beneath the distal clavicle.
- The free ends of the white medial STIK sutures can be brought out of the suprascapular notch portal using a circle grasper to help avoid entanglement.

35.3.9 Attachment of the Graft to the Anterior Cuff and Biceps Tendon

- With the scope in the PMGP or accessory posterolateral portal, use an appropriately curved suture hook though the AMG cannula to continue progression from the medial to the anterior aspect of the cuff defect. Use the same method as was done posteriorly. Pass the suture hook anterior to the anchor "suture stack" and retrieve the shuttle with the grasper posterior to it, out of the MLSA cannula. Each suture is then shuttled though the cuff back out the AMG cannula. Each STIK suture should be passed with 6 mmof space between them. Often, the anterior edge defect requires incorporation of tissue from the coracohumeral ligament, rotator interval, and biceps tendon but seldom the superior edge of the subscapularis tendon.
- Remember to proceed carefully to not cross any suture, always retrieving the shuttle suture "anterior" and parallel to previously passed sutures.
- As you continue to progress along the anterior edge, incorporating rotator interval tissue (and biceps if needed). Leave the free end of the STIK sutures in the AMG cannula.
- Retrieve the medial end of the middle suture from the anterolateral anchor and carry it out the MLSA cannula, to any other sutures from the anchor, to avoid twisting. This suture is passed though the anterolateral corner of the graft from bottom to top using a Keith needle. A STIK loop is tied on top of the graft. Remove the slack from the suture and clamp the end outside the skin.

35.3.10 Deliver the Graft into the Shoulder Joint

- Orient the graft so the medial edge is directly adjacent the MLSA cannula. Pull the free ends of all the STIK knot sutures to ensure all of the sutures are free of slack and all equally tensioned in their respective portal/cannula.
- Roll the graft so that the knots are inside.
- Continue to gently pull on white and white/purple suture tails exiting the suprascapular notch portal to bring the graft inside the MSLA cannula. In a stepwise fashion, alternate pulling the other suture tails to take up any slack while traveling down the cannula into the shoulder. This will avoid any loops in the sutures from catching around the STIK knots and causing the graft to seat improperly.
- Retrieve all the sutures tails stored in the PMG cannula into the AMG cannula except for the most posterolateral STIK. Retrieve the knotted/looped end of this STIK though the PMG cannula and tie the suture ends with a sliding-locking knot and three half hitches using the non-knotted end as the post.
- Continue tying the posterior STIK sutures using the same method, one at a time, working medially, then anteriorly.

35.3.11 Tying of the Remaining Sutures from the Anchors

- With the scope in the MLSAP, retrieve both ends of the anterior anchored suture that passes though the anterolateral aspect of the graft, through the AMG portal. Cut off the knot and use the looped/knotted end as the post and tie with a sliding-locking knot.
- Repeat the process on the posterior anchor to secure the posterolateral corner of the graft.

35.3.12 Suturing the Lateral Graft to Bone

- Retrieve the medialmost remaining suture from the posterior anchor through the AMG cannula. Use the PMG cannula to pass a curved suture hook from top to bottom, 5 mm anterior to the previous suture. Retrieve the other end of the suture and store them in colored plastic suture protectors (Suture Saver, Conmed/Linvatec) outside the PMG cannula. Repeat the stitching for the anteriorly anchored suture and store it outside the AMG cannula also in a Suture Saver.

35.3.13 Insert Third/Fourth Anchors

- Most repairs only require one additional anchor at the lateral aspect of the graft. If there is more than 1 cm on each side of the centerline, two double-loaded anchors are required. Use the Revo punch to create small bone vents lateral to the anchor site.
- If only one anchor is required, place it directly lateral to the midlateral mark on the graft.
- Pass the sutures though the graft from posterior to anterior, and store each in a Suture Saver outside the PMG cannula.

35.3.14 Tying the Anchored Sutures

- Retrieve the sutures stored in the Suture Savers into the lateral cannula from an anterior-to-posterior direction using a crochet hook.
- Using sliding-locking knots, tie the sutures through the lateral portal so that the knots are on top of the graft.

35.3.15 Evaluate the Repair

- Carefully document the repair, looking for any gaps along the edges. If a gap is identified, pass additional suture with a suture hook, using the suture shuttling method.
- Once the security of the repair is verified, turn off the pump to observe bone marrow vents, which will produce the "Crimson Duvet" or super clot of red/bone marrow cells covering the graft and lateral tuberosity. These cells bring a new blood supply that will form a rich matrix replete with platelets, their growth factors, and mesenchymal stem cells (▸ Video 35.1).

35.4 Surgeon Tips and Tricks

- Patient should have good passive and active assisted motion of the shoulder with minimal arthritis. Preoperative active range of motion is the best predictor of postoperative subjective success.

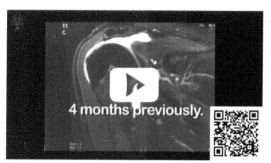

Video 35.1 Surgical demonstration of acellular human dermal allograft rotator cuff reconstruction.

- The operation should be practiced on a cadaver and ALEX model lab (Sawbones, Vashon, WA) until the steps are second nature for the surgeon and staff.
- Take care to debride tissue that might obstruct visualization and obtain good hemostasis.
- The patients should understand that, even when completely successful, this operation will never result in a "normal" shoulder. There will always be subjective weakness, especially with external rotation.
- Never suture the graft in tension. Stitch placement within the shoulder must be accurate, and closely reapproximate the position of the STIK sutures on the graft for the graft to spread out evenly. When the arm rests in the sling post-op, gravity will add some tension to the graft/cuff construct to help align the physiological stresses that will help maturation. As the graft is repopulated with host cells, it will attain a more tendon-like tone, and elasticity will decrease.
- Pay close attention to positioning the patient for surgery. Prolonged surgical time adds an increased risk for external pressure to skin and nerves.
- The operating surgeon and the assistant must be comfortable using the scope in all three subacromial portals.
- "Stay anterior": Pay close attention with each pass through though the lateral cannula to always stay anterior to the previously passed suture.
- Avoid slack in the sutures when pulling the STIK sutures into the shoulder by pulling the medial sutures first and taking up the slack in all others.
- The amount of time that goes into preoperative patient counseling is significant. Patients must understand that there will be a prolonged recovery time and that this surgery is a "salvage" operation to try to reduce pain, improve function, and avoid the need for a reverse shoulder prosthesis.
- Always direct the punch used for the vents vertically down the humerus and thus away from the subchondral bone area where the anchors will be seated and leave a 5 mm bridge of cortical bone between the vents.

35.5 Pitfalls/Complications

- Complications for this procedure are rare. The average operative time is increased approximately 1 hour when compared to standard repair of a massive rotator cuff repair, theoretically increasing the risk for transient neuropraxia and infection.
- All graft material is not alike. The rotator cuff graft must be chosen with care. Our graft of choice in symptomatic patients with chronic, nonrepairable rotator cuff

defects and minimal arthritis is a human acellular dermal matrix allograft that is 2.8 to 3.2 mm in thickness. We prefer a prehydrated product. This acellular human dermal matrix is extremely strong, free from cells, but rich in collagen, elastin, and preserved blood vessel channels as well as growth factors. We find this extracellular matrix, superior to other biologic matrices currently available.

35.6 Postoperative Care

- Immobilization sling with 15° abduction pillow (UltraSling IV ER, DJO Global, Carlsbad, CA). Immediately postoperatively, begin elbow, wrist, and hand exercises and isometric scapula shrugs. Begin small pendulum circles at 1 week postoperatively.
- Initiate formal physical therapy at 8 weeks after surgery. The program followed is intentionally slow, and progress, similar to that of a massive repairable cuff tear. We encourage pool therapy at 6–8 weeks to allow passive motion without stress on the healing graft.
- Progress activities at 2 months with active assisted lifting.

35.7 Rationale and/or Evidence for Approach

35.7.1 Methods

One hundred and six patients with 109 shoulders were treated with anacellular human dermal allograft reconstruction for a massive nonrepairable rotator cuff tear between March 4, 2003 and July 26, 2011. Many of these patients were evaluated at 3months and 1year postoperatively with an intraarticular gadolinium-enhanced magnetic resonance imaging (MRI). Two orthopedic surgeons and a musculoskeletal radiologist evaluated the MRI arthrograms to determine the status of the graft. These patients also completed a visual analog pain scale (VAS), simple shoulder test (SST), and modified University of California at Los Angeles shoulder scores preoperatively and at multiple time points postoperatively. Data were collected at 3 months, 1 year, and 2 years after the procedure. Many of the patients had late follow-up between 2 and 7 years postoperatively.

35.7.2 Results

- The 3-month postoperative MRI evaluations demonstrated that 85% (90/106) of patients had intact allografts, 15% (16/106) of patients had a tear, and three patients did not undergo the MRI.
- At 1 year postoperatively, 74% (46/62) of the previously intact reconstruction patients had intact allografts, while the other 26% (16/62) were found to have a new tear. Forty-seven did not undergo further advanced imaging.
- Preoperative outcome surveys were collected from 103 patients. Postoperative surveys were collected from 65, 53, 20, and 51 patients at the 3-month, 1-year, 2-year, and greater than 3-year follow-up, respectively. The SST significantly improved from a preoperative average of 6.2 to a postoperative score of 6.79, 9.37, 10.57, and 10.9, respectively, at 3-month, 1-year, 2-year, and greater than 3-year follow-up (all $P < 0.001$).

- UCLA scores significantly improved from 14.56 preoperatively to 23.34, 28.10, 30.4, and 28.78 at 3-month, 1-year, 2-year, and greater than 3-year follow-up, respectively (all $P < 0.001$).
- VAS scores improved from 3.3 preoperatively to 1.64, 1.01, 0.95, and 1.22 at 3-month, 1-year, 2-year, and greater than 3-year follow-up, respectively ($P < 0.001$ preoperatively compared with all postoperative time periods).
- Constant scores averaged 76 for patients at the final follow-up (> 3 years) (20).

35.7.3 Conclusion

We believe that certain types of acellular matrix allograft tissues are a viable option for surgical salvage in select cases of nonrepairable, massive, rotator cuff tears. Our evidence for this is based on our own studies, experience, as well as the research of others that have documented similar outcomes to those of our own. Of course, longer follow-up and more cases are essential to determine the longevity and viability of the graft as well as patient satisfaction. Arthroscopic techniques permit us to treat the entire joint, including biceps, subscapularis, labrum, synovium, etc., without damage to the deltoid or large skin incisions in an outpatient setting.

Suggested Readings

Adams JE, Zobitz ME, Reach JS, Jr, An KN, Steinmann SP. Rotator cuff repair using an acellular dermal matrix graft: an in vivo study in a canine model. Arthroscopy. 2006; 22(7):700–709

Aurora A, McCarron J, Iannotti JP, Derwin K. Commercially available extracellular matrix materials for rotator cuff repairs: state of the art and future trends. J Shoulder Elbow Surg. 2007; 16(5) Suppl:S171–S178

Badylak SF, Freytes DO, Gilbert TW. Reprint of: Extracellular matrix as a biological scaffold material: Structure and function. Acta Biomater. 2015; 23 Suppl:S17–S26

Bigliani LU, Cordasco FA, McIlveen SJ, Musso ES. Operative treatment of failed repairs of the rotator cuff. J Bone Joint Surg Am. 1992; 74(10):1505–1515

Bond JL, Dopirak RM, Higgins J, Burns J, Snyder SJ. Arthroscopic replacement of massive, irreparable rotator cuff tears using a GraftJacket allograft: technique and preliminary results. Arthroscopy. 2008; 24(4):403–409.e1

Burkhead WZ, Chiffern SC, Krishnan SG. Use of Graft-Jacket as an augmentation for massive rotator cuff tears. Semin Arthroplasty. 2007; 18:11–18

Clark RR, Burns JP, Snyder SJ, et al. Human dermal allograft for reconstruction of massive rotator cuff tears: Functional and MRI results of 109 patients. Presented at the Annual Meeting of the American Academy of Orthopaedic Surgeons; March 2013; Chicago, IL

Cofield RH, Parvizi J, Hoffmeyer PJ, Lanzer WL, Ilstrup DM, Rowland CM. Surgical repair of chronic rotator cuff tears. A prospective long-term study. J Bone Joint Surg Am. 2001; 83(1):71–77

Derwin KA, Codsi MJ, Milks RA, Baker AR, McCarron JA, Iannotti JP. Rotator cuff repair augmentation in a canine model with use of a woven poly-L-lactide device. J Bone Joint Surg Am. 2009; 91(5):1159–1171

Derwin KA, Badylak SF, Steinmann SP, Iannotti JP. Extracellular matrix scaffold devices for rotator cuff repair. J Shoulder Elbow Surg. 2010; 19(3):467–476

Ferguson DP, Lewington MR, Smith TD, Wong IH. Graft utilization in the augmentation of large-to-massive rotator cuff repairs: A systematic review. Am J Sports Med. 2016; 44(11):2984–2992

Galatz LM, Ball CM, Teefey SA, Middleton WD, Yamaguchi K. The outcome and repair integrity of completely arthroscopically repaired large and massive rotator cuff tears. J Bone Joint Surg Am. 2004; 86(2):219–224

Harryman DT, II, Mack LA, Wang KY, Jackins SE, Richardson ML, Matsen FA, III. Repairs of the rotator cuff. Correlation of functional results with integrity of the cuff. J Bone Joint Surg Am. 1991; 73(7):982–989

Lewington MR, Ferguson DP, Smith TD, Burks R, Coady C, Wong IH. Graft utilization in the bridging reconstruction of irreparable rotator cuff tears: A systematic review. Am J Sports Med. 2017; 45(13):3149–3157

Pandey R, Tafazal S, Shyamsundar S, Modi A, Singh HP. Outcome of partial repair of massive rotator cuff tears with and without human tissue allograft bridging repair. Shoulder Elbow. 2017; 9(1):23–30

Rockwood CA, Jr, Williams GR, Jr, Burkhead WZ, Jr. Débridement of degenerative, irreparable lesions of the rotator cuff. J Bone Joint Surg Am. 1995; 77(6):857–866

Snyder SJ, Arnoczky SP, Bond JL, Dopirak R. Histologic evaluation of a biopsy specimen obtained 3 months after rotator cuff augmentation with GraftJacket Matrix. Arthroscopy. 2009; 25(3):329–333

Snyder SJ. Reflections From a mature arthroscopic shoulder surgeon on the history and current benefits of augmentation for the revision of a massive rotator cuff tear using acellular human dermal matrix allograft. Arthroscopy. 2016; 32(9):1761–1763

Walch G, Edwards TB, Boulahia A, Nové-Josserand L, Neyton L, Szabo I. Arthroscopic tenotomy of the long head of the biceps in the treatment of rotator cuff tears: clinical and radiographic results of 307 cases. J Shoulder Elbow Surg. 2005; 14(3):238–246

36 A Comparison of the Outcomes of Two Types of Synthetic Patches for Interpositional Graft Use in Irreparable Rotator Cuff Tears

Tom Morrison, Patrick H. Lam, and George A.C. Murrell

Summary

Arthroscopic sutureanchor repair of massive rotator cuff tears has met limited success. The use of interpositional synthetic patch grafts has shown potential in recent studies with small sample sizes. The aim of this study was to evaluate the outcomes of interpositional synthetic patches for massive rotator cuff tear in a large cohort of patients. We identified 69 patients with large and irreparable rotator cuff tears who underwent arthroscopic interpositional patch repair with ePTFE (38 patients) or PTFE felt (26 patients) synthetic patches. This cohort was matched in terms of anteroposterior, mediolateral, and total area tear dimensions with 100 patients who underwent arthroscopic rotator cuff repair using direct suture-anchor repair. Strength and range of motion were recorded at 1, 6, and 12weeks and 6months postsurgery. Repair integrity was evaluated via ultrasound at 6months postsurgery. Re-tear rates in the synthetic patch groups were lower than the suture-anchor group at 6 months (PTFE felt 4%, ePTFE 3% vs. sutureanchor repair 25%, $p < 0.01$). Supraspinatus strength in the PTFE felt repair group was greater than the sutureanchor repair group at 6 weeks (22N vs. 10N, $p=0.01$). All other functional outcomes were similar between the two groups. Patients receiving synthetic patches for massive and irreparable rotator cuff tears had significantly lower re-tear rates than those repaired using sutureanchor techniques and supraspinatus strength at 6 months postsurgery.

Keywords: arthroscopy, ePTFE patch, massive rotator cuff tear, polyterafluoroethylene patch, synthetic patch

36.1 Introduction

- Rotator cuff tears can be repaired by reattaching the torn tendon back to the humeral head using suture anchors. This approach has good outcomes for patients with small-to-moderate tears; however, the reported re-tear rate for repair of massive rotator cuff tears is between 20% and 90%.[1]

- Furthermore, so-called irreparable tears cannot be repaired with this technique because of retraction of the tendon. Treatment options for these tears include debridement, partial repair, or tendon transfer; however, the outcomes of these procedures have often been unsatisfactory.[2]

- We have developed a technique for arthroscopic rotator cuff repairs using synthetic patches for massive tears not amenable to direct repair. The results have been encouraging in studies with small sample sizes.[3]

- In this study, we compare PTFE felt (Bard PTFE felt, C.R. Bard, Warwick, RI) with ePTFE (Gore-Tex Expanded PTFE Patch, W.L. Gore and Associates, Newark, DE). ePTFE differs from PTFE felt as it is stretched under high temperatures. Both devices are designed to produce micropores that allow for tissue ingrowth when implanted. No previous studies have compared results of different patch materials.

- The aim of this study, therefore, is to compare outcomes of ePTFE and PTFE felt interpositional patches with standard sutureanchor only repair for massive rotator cuff tear in a large cohort. It was hypothesized that synthetic patch repairs would have lower rates of re-tear and better functional outcomes than direct suture-anchor repairs.

36.2 Methods

36.2.1 Study Design

- Following ethics approval (HREC 12/310), a retrospective study with prospectively collected data was undertaken. Patients were considered for inclusion in the study if they had received rotator cuff repair surgery by the senior author with an ePTFE (Gore-Tex Expanded PTFE Patch) or PTFE felt (Bard Expanded PTFE felt) interpositional patch rotator cuff repair, or a direct suture-anchor repair. Patients were excluded if they had severe arthritis, lymphedema, humeral head fractures, previous shoulder arthroplasty, or did not receive an ultrasound to evaluate repair integrity 6 months postsurgery.
- Three patient groups were compared, those receiving PTFE felt interpositional synthetic patches (PTFE felt group, n=26), those receiving ePTFE patches (ePTFE group, n=39), and those receiving sutureanchor repairs (direct repair group, n=100). The direct repair group was selected to compare the efficacy of the patch procedure with suture-anchor repairs. Patients in the direct repair group were selected if they had had a suture-anchor repair performed by the senior author between the date of the first and last patch operation, with anteroposterior, mediolateral, and total area of tear size being no larger or smaller than that of patch repairs. Posthoc matching occurred, as outlined in the results section, to ensure the direct-repair group was similar to the patch groups with respect anteroposterior, mediolateral, and total area of tear size.

36.2.2 Surgical Procedures

- Prophylactic antibiotics (cephalosporin) were administered preoperatively and 4hours postoperatively.
- All patients underwent arthroscopic rotator cuff repair in the beachchair position following interscalene regional anesthesia. The shoulder, arm, and hand were prepared with iodine solution and then draped. A standard posterior portal was made to allow for the arthroscope to be positioned within the posterior glenohumeral joint capsule.
- A second lateral incision was made superior to the superior border of the supraspinatus tendon to be used for the insertion of instruments, sutures, anchors, and a patch if required. This incision was made using a spinal needle to approximate the midpoint between the anterior and posterior edges of the tear.
- Once visualized, the edges of the cuff were lightly debrided using a 4- or 5-mm soft tissue shaver (Stryker Endoscopy, San Jose, CA). Debridement allowed for visualization of tear size, and determination of tendon quality and degree of tendon retraction. Patch repairs were indicated when the tendon could not be mobilized to the footprint on the humeral head, with other tears repaired using the direct suture-anchor technique.
- For a direct suture-anchor repair, the torn edge of the rotator cuff tendon was grasped with an Opus SmartStitch suturing device. A #2 braided polyethylene suture (MagnumWire) was deployed through the tendon body in an inverted mattress

configuration, using either an Opus M-Connector or Perfect Passer (ArthroCare Sports Medicine, Sunnyvale, CA). A hole was made with a T-handle punch on the lateral margin of the rotator cuff footprint of the humeral head. The suture was passed through an Opus Magnum Knotless Implant anchor, which was secured into the hole using a single row configuration. Additional sutures and anchors were placed depending on the size of the tear.

- In the case of a patch repair, a patch was cut to a size large enough to bridge the defect while also allowing for 1.5 cm of overlap on the medial edge to account for suture overlap caused by the suture delivery device. The choice of patch material (between PTFE felt and ePTFE) was determined based upon current supplies at the surgical facility. The repair technique was the same for both patches. The medial edge of the patch was prepared first, with a Perfect Passer or M-Connector used to deliver sutures along the edge of the torn tendon in evenly dispersed 5 mm intervals. These sutures are were passed exvivo into the patch and evenly spaced using a Perfect Passer suture passer.

- The patch was secured to the torn edge of the rotator cuff using either the mattress or weave technique, as outlined by Shepherd et al[3,4] The patch was then pushed through the lateral portal until it was situated within the glenohumeral joint. A knot pusher was used to push the patch toward the tendon so that the two surfaces were carefully opposed. The free ends of the tendon edge sutures were then tied arthroscopically, and loose ends trimmed with a suture cutter. To secure the patch to the humeral head, three sutures were passed through the edge of the patch using an Opus SmartStitch device (ArthroCare, Sydney, Australia) prior to patch insertion. A T-handled punch was used to create a hole on the greater tuberosity for the anterior anchor. The suture ends were passed through an Opus Magnum 2 suture anchor (ArthroCare). The anchor was placed into the holes in the greater tuberosity, and the suture tightened to reattach the patch to the footprint. The process was repeated for the medial and posterior suture.

- Portals were closed using uninterrupted nylon sutures and steristrips.

- All patients were rehabilitated in the same manner used for a typical rotator cuff repair. The arm was placed in a sling with a small abduction pillow (UltraSling II, DJO, Normanhurst, Australia) for 6 weeks. Patients initially completed pendulum exercises and 2 weeks postoperatively were introduced to passive flexion and extension range-of-motion exercises. At a 6-week postoperative physiotherapy visit, patients initiated active range-of-motion and isometric strengthening exercises. At 12 weeks postoperation, patients proceeded to overhead activates and lifting weights < 5 kg. At 6 months postoperation, patients returned to normal activities (▶ **Video 36.1**).

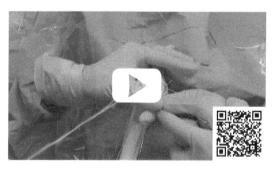

Video 36.1 Surgical demonstration of a comparison of the outcomes of two types of synthetic patches for interpositional graft use in irreparable rotator cuff tears.

36.2.3 Patient-Ranked Outcomes

All patients completed a modified L'Insalata questionnaire evaluating pain at rest, during sleep, and during specific activities as well as shoulder stiffness and sporting and work activity using a Likert scale preoperatively and postoperatively at 1, 6, and 12 weeks and 6 months.[5]

36.2.4 Examiner-Ranked Outcomes

- All patients underwent a shoulder examination consisting of passive range-of-motion and strength testing. Forward flexion, abduction, external rotation, and internal rotation were tested and determined by visual inspection.[6] Strength was tested using a handheld dynamometer upon adduction, internal rotation, lift off, external rotation, and abduction.[7]
- The integrity of the rotator cuff was determined at 6 months postoperation using a General Electric Logiq E9 ultrasound machine (GE Corporation, Sydney, Australia), with a 6-MHz and 15-MHz linear transducer by a single experienced ultrasonographer using a standardized protocol as previously described.[8]

36.2.5 Statistical Analysis

Outcomes are reported as the mean ± standard error of the mean. Nonparametric data was compared using Wilcoxon signed rank tests. Parametric data was compared using Student's t-tests.

36.3 Results

After applying initial inclusion and exclusion criteria on 2,745 patients receiving rotator cuff repairs by the senior author, 69 patients receiving synthetic patches were identified as eligible for the study—26 patients had received PTFE felt patches and 43 ePTFE patches.

36.3.1 Matching for Tear Size between Patch Groups

The intraoperatively measured tear size between the PTFE felt and ePTFE groups in mediolateral and anteroposterior planes and tear area were compared. There was a significant difference between the anteroposterior tear size (ePTFE being bigger) between the groups. To correct this, the five largest ePTFE patch patients were excluded. After these were excluded, there was no significant difference in anteroposterior tear size between the groups ($p = 0.09$).

36.3.2 Direct-Repair Comparison Group

The direct-repair group was created from all patients receiving suture-anchor repairs by the senior surgeon. Only operations occurring between the date of the first patch patient (May 25, 2010) and last patch patient (October 21, 2013) were considered. Patients also had to have tears with intraoperative measurements no larger than the maximum dimensions (80 mm anteroposterior, 70 mm mediolateral) and no smaller than the minimum dimensions (20 mm anteroposterior, 20 mm mediolateral) of the patch patients. 166 patients met these criteria.

36.3.3 Matching for Tear Size between Patch Groups and Direct-Repair Groups

- To ensure there was a similar preoperative tear size between the direct-repair and patch groups, a following posthoc matching procedure was performed.
- Tear size between all groups was compared using Student's t-tests. There was a significant difference between both PTFE felt and ePTFE and direct-repair group anteroposterior tear size, with the direct-repair group being smaller. The 48 smallest anteroposterior tears were then removed from the direct-repair group and again compared to the PTFE felt and ePTFE group, leaving no significant difference between any group for anteroposterior tear size.
- There remained a significant difference between both PTFE felt and ePTFE, and the direct-repair group in terms of mediolateral tear size, with the direct-repair group being smaller. The 26 smallest mediolateral tears were removed from the direct-repair group. After these exclusions, 80 patients remained in the direct-repair group.
- To ensure 100 patients were in the direct-repair group, the restriction on operation date was expanded. Twenty additional patients with the largest mediolateral tear size were recruited in order of most recent operation going back from the date of the earliest patch-repair operation. Patients were not included if they had mediolateral tears larger than the largest mediolateral tear size in either the ePTFE or PTFE felt groups.
- Once these additional patients were included, there was a significant difference between the direct-repair and PTFE felt and ePTFE groups in anteroposterior tear size, with the direct-repair group being larger. The 11 patients with the largest anteroposterior tear were excluded and replaced with patients with the largest anteroposterior tear that did not create a significant difference between the direct-repair group and the PTFE felt and ePTFE groups. Patients were added in order of most recent operation before the earliest operation in the PTFE felt and ePTFE groups.
- This resulted in a direct-repair group of 100 patients with comparable anteroposterior, mediolateral, and total tear area to PTFE felt and ePTFE patch groups.

36.3.4 Demographics

The three groups were similar with respect to gender, age at surgery, which shoulder was affected, or how long there had been from the initial injury to surgery between any group (▸ **Table 36.1**, ▸ **Table 36.2**).

Table 36.1 Patient demographics

Variable	Direct-repair group	PTFE felt	ePTFE patch
Number of patients	100	26	38
Male:female ratio	65:35:00	17:09	25:13:00
Left:right shoulder ratio	39:61	5:21	12:26
Age at surgery (years)	64 ± 1	63 ± 2	66 ± 2
Months from initial injury to surgery	21 ± 8	13 ± 5	8.9 ± 2

Table 36.2 Patient demographical significance

Variable	Direct repair-PTFE felt		Direct repair-ePTFE		PTFE felt-ePTFE	
	Sig	p Value	Sig	p Value	Sig	p Value
Male:female ratio	No	1	No	1	No	1
Left:right shoulder ratio	No	0.07	No	0.55	No	0.39
Age at surgery (years)	No	0.76	No	0.29	No	0.27
Months from initial injury to surgery	No	0.4	No	0.16	No	0.44

Table 36.3 Intraoperative data

Variable	Direct-repair group	PTFE felt patch	ePTFE patch
Tear size (anteroposterior)	40 mm ± 2.2	37 mm ± 1.6	35.3 mm ± 1.5
Tear size (mediolateral)	36 mm ± 1.4	33 mm ± 1.1	33.0 mm ± 2.2
Tear size (area)	1434 mm ± 104	1340 mm ± 99	1213 mm ± 132
Tissue quality (0 to 3)	1.4 ± 0.1	0.58 ± 0.2	0.73 ± 0.1
Tendon mobility (0 to 3)	1.5 ± 0.1	0.62 ± 0.2	0.54 ± 0.1
Repair quality (0 to 3)	1.9 ± 0.1	1.5 ± 0.2	1.8 ± 0.1
Operative time (minutes)	26.8 ± 1.4	58.5 ± 5.0	49.2 ± 2.0

Table 36.4 Intraoperative data significance

	PTFE felt vs. ePTFE		Direct repair vs. PTFE felt		Direct repair vs. ePTFE	
	Sig	p Value	Sig	p Value	Sig	p Value
Tear size (anteroposterior)	No	0.12	No	0.37	No	0.42
Tear size (mediolateral)	No	0.35	No	0.98	No	0.2
Tear size (area)	No	0.19	No	0.44	No	0.52
Tissue quality (0 to 3)	No	0.08	Yes	0.0001	Yes	0.0001
Tendon mobility (0 to 3)	No	0.89	Yes	0.0001	Yes	0.0001
Repair quality (0 to 3)	No	0.55	No	0.18	No	0.46
Operative time (minutes)	No	0.09	Yes	<0.0001	Yes	<0.0001

36.3.5 Intraoperative Data

- The surgeon's opinion of quality of tendon tissue and tendon mobility was significantly better in the direct-repair group than in the PTFE felt and ePTFE group (▶ Table 36.3 and ▶ Table 36.4).
- Operative time was longer for patch patients (PTFE felt 59 minutes ± 5.0, ePTFE 49 minutes ± 2.0) than for the direct-repair group (27 minutes ± 1.4); however, there was no significant difference in time for the different types of patches (▶ Table 36.3, ▶ Table 36.4).

36.3.6 Patient-Ranked Outcomes

- Overall shoulder satisfaction.
  - Patients in all groups had a significant improvement in shoulder function 1 week postoperation that was sustained at 6 months ($p > 0.001$).
  - Patients receiving a PTFE felt patch had a rated their shoulder satisfaction higher than patients receiving a direct repair at 1 week ($p=0.035$); however, there was no other significant difference between groups at any time point (▶ **Fig. 36.1**).
- Pain.
  - There was no reported difference between any group in shoulder stiffness, difficulty reaching behind back, level of pain during overhead activities, frequency of extreme pain, and current level of activity at work. ePTFE patients reported less pain than the direct-repair group preoperatively ($p=0.027$); however, this difference was not significant at future time points.
  - The direct-repair group of patients had a higher level of reported sporting activity than the ePTFE group at 6 months ($p=0.02$).
  - Patients in the ePTFE group reported significantly more pain at rest after 6 months than the direct-repair group ($p=0.031$). There was no difference in level of pain during sleep between groups; the one exception was patients at 6 weeks in the ePTFE group being worse than the PTFE felt group ($p=0.049$).
  - There was no difference reported in any group in pain during overhead activities or pain during sleep at 6 months postoperation.

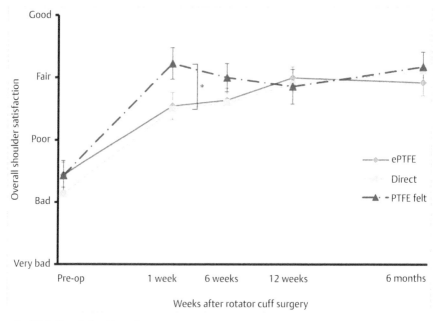

Fig. 36.1 Overall shoulder rating.

36.3.7 Strength

- Supraspinatus strength.
  - Patients in the PTFE felt group had more supraspinatus strength than the ePTFE group (p=0.043) and the direct-repair group (p=0.007) at 6 weeks postoperation. There was still a significant difference between PTFE felt and the ePTFE group at 12 weeks (p=0.024). There was no difference between any groups at 6 months (▶ **Fig. 36.2**).
- Internal rotation.
  - Patients receiving PTFE felt patches had better internal rotation strength than patients receiving ePTFE patches at 6 months postoperation (p=0.028) (▶ **Fig. 36.3**).
- External rotation.
  - The direct-repair group was significantly stronger in internal rotation than ePTFE at 12 weeks (p=0.017) and at 6 months postoperation (p=0.024) (▶ **Fig. 36.4**).
- Lift off.
  - The PTFE felt group had better lift-of-strength than the ePTFE group at 6 months postoperation (46N ± 3 vs. 38N ± 3, p=0.01) (▶ **Fig. 36.5**).
- Adduction.
  - There was no significant difference in adduction strength between groups at 6 months postsurgery (▶ **Fig. 36.6**).
- Range of motion.
  - There were no significant differences between the three groups in internal rotation, forward flexion, and abduction preoperatively and at 6 and 12 weeks postoperatively.

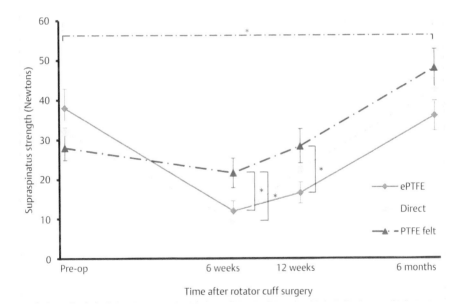

Fig. 36.2 Supraspinatus strength.

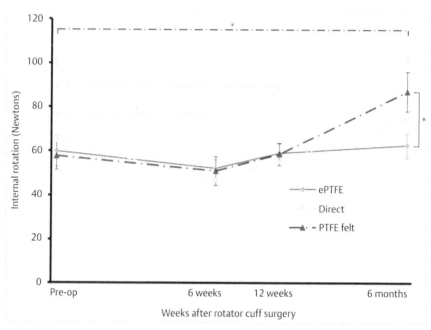

Fig. 36.3 Internal rotation strength.

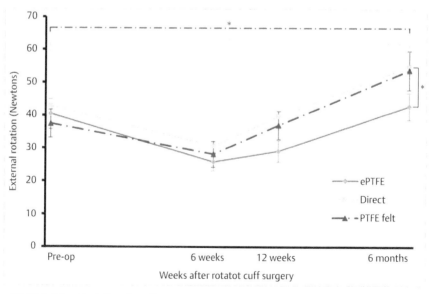

Fig. 36.4 External rotation strength.

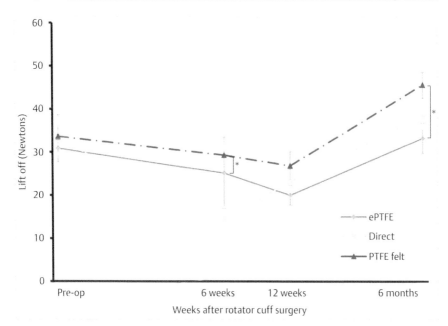

Fig. 36.5 Lift-off strength.

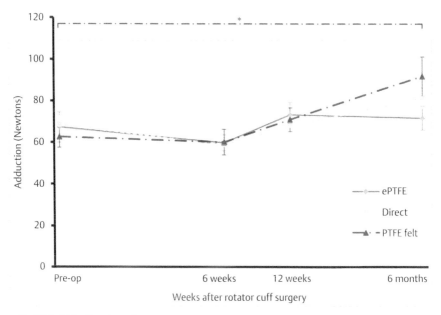

Fig. 36.6 Adduction strength.

Table 36.5 Patch re-tear rate

	Significant	P value
PTFE felt vs. ePTFE	No	1
PTFE felt vs. direct repair	Yes	0.015
ePTFE vs. direct repair	Yes	0.001

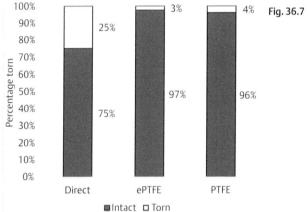

Fig. 36.7 Patch re-tear rate.

- Patients in the ePTFE group had significantly less internal rotation at 6 months than the direct-repair group ($p=0.008$).
- Patients in the PTFE felt group reported less improvement in abduction results than both the ePTFE ($p=0.01$) and direct-repair ($p > 0.001$) groups at 6 months postsurgery.
- Patients in the PTFE felt group had a greater range of external rotation than patients in the ePTFE group 6 weeks, 12 weeks, and 6 months.
- Patch re-tear rate.
  - At 6 months postsurgery, ultrasound evaluation identified 25 out of 100 re-tears in the direct-repair group. The PTFE felt group had one re-tear and the ePTFE group had one re-tear (▶ **Table 36.5**, ▶ **Fig. 36.7**).

36.4 Discussion

- We compared the short-term outcomes of patients receiving PTFE felt and ePTFE synthetic interpositional patches to direct suture-anchor repairs for large rotator cuff tears. At 6 months postsurgery, patients receiving either type of patch had significantly reduced rates of re-tear compared to those with a direct suture-anchor repair. Our hypothesis was partially confirmed with patients receiving patch repairs experiencing lower rates of re-tear; however, they did not experience superior functional outcomes at 6 months postsurgery.
- This study is unique in that it is the first to the author's knowledge to consider large groups (100 direct repair, 64 patch) of patients. Previous studies by Shepherd et al[9] (five patients), Hirooka et al[10] (27 patients), and Audenaert et al[11] (41 patients)

showed satisfying outcomes for patients; however, all had a major weakness in not having a direct-repair group with which to compare results. Hirooka's study evaluated ePTFE patches. Ronquillo et al[12] examined 16 ePTFE patch repairs compared to 21 direct repairs and found reduced re-tear rate and increased supraspinatus strength for patch repairs.

- PTFE felt and ePTFE patches are both composed of polytetrafluoroethylene; however, they differ in structure. PTFE is stretched under high temperatures to form ePTFE, producing micropores in the material that allow for tissue in growth when implanted. The expansion process also allows for a reduction in material costs. Both patch materials have previously undergone biomechanical comparison by McKeown et al,[13] finding that ePTFE had significantly greater elongation before failure when compared to PTFE felt and ovine tendon. We speculate that the lower supraspinatus strength we noted at 6 months postoperation in ePTFE patients as opposed to PTFE patients may be secondary to the more elastic nature of this material.
- When compared to the direct-repair group, the patients in the PTFE felt group had similar patient-reported outcomes 6 months postsurgery. However, the PTFE felt group showed a significant strength improvement in supraspinatus, internal rotation, external rotation, and adduction compared to the direct-repair group. The PTFE felt group also showed significant improvement in internal rotation, external rotation, and abduction range-of-motion testing compared to the direct-repair group. No patches experienced serious postoperative complications other than cuff re-tear.
- The strengths of this study included the standardized method of care from pre-op through to 6 months post-op. All patients received the same postoperative rehabilitation protocol. All operations were performed by the same surgeon, all data collection was done through standardized methods and all ultrasounds performed by the same ultrasonographer.
- There were limitations to this study. While substantial numbers of patients were recruited for each patch group, sample sizes could be greater. Similarly, the follow-up time is relatively short. Only two synthetic patch alternatives were compared. Each study cohort was also not randomized or blinded.

36.5 Conclusion

Patients with massive rotator cuff tears receiving either a PTFE felt or ePTFE synthetic patch experienced a significantly lower re-tear rate than direct suture-anchor repairs; however, they did not have corresponding improvement in functional outcomes.

References

[1] Harryman DT, II, Mack LA, Wang KY, Jackins SE, Richardson ML, Matsen FA, III. Repairs of the rotator cuff. Correlation of functional results with integrity of the cuff. J Bone Joint Surg Am. 1991; 73(7):982–989

[2] Khair MM, Gulotta LV. Treatment of irreparable rotator cuff tears. Curr Rev Musculoskelet Med. 2011; 4(4): 208–213

[3] Shepherd H, Murrell GAC. Use of synthetic patches as tendon substitutes in knotless arthroscopic repairs of massive rotator cuff tears. Tech Shoulder Elbow Surg. 2012; 13(1):32–35

[4] Shepherd HM, Lam PH, Murrell GAC. Biomechanics of synthetic patch rotator cuff repairs. Techniques Shoulder Elb Surg. 2011; 12(4):94–100

[5] L'Insalata JC, Warren RF, Cohen SB, Altchek DW, Peterson MG, L'Insalata JC. A self-administered questionnaire for assessment of symptoms and function of the shoulder. J Bone Joint Surg Am. 1997; 79(5):738–748

[6] Hayes K, Walton JR, Szomor ZR, Murrell GAC. Reliability of five methods for assessing shoulder range of motion. Aust J Physiother. 2001; 47(4):289–294

[7] Hayes K, Walton JR, Szomor ZL, Murrell GA. Reliability of 3 methods for assessing shoulder strength. J Shoulder Elbow Surg. 2002; 11(1):33–39

[8] Millar NL, Wu X, Tantau R, Silverstone E, Murrell GA. Open versus two forms of arthroscopic rotator cuff repair. Clin Orthop Relat Res. 2009; 467(4):966–978

[9] Shepherd HM, Lam PH, Murrell GAC. Synthetic patch rotator cuff repair: A 10-year follow-up. Shoulder Elbow. 2014; 6(1):35–39

[10] Hirooka A, Yoneda M, Wakaitani S, et al. Augmentation with a Gore-Tex patch for repair of large rotator cuff tears that cannot be sutured. J Orthop Sci. 2002; 7(4):451–456

[11] Audenaert E, Van Nuffel J, Schepens A, Verhelst M, Verdonk R. Reconstruction of massive rotator cuff lesions with a synthetic interposition graft: a prospective study of 41 patients. Knee Surg Sports Traumatol Arthrosc. 2006; 14(4):360–364

[12] Ronquillo JC, Lam P, Murrell GAC. Arthroscopic ePTFE patch repair for irreparable rotator cuff tears: Part II: Preliminary clinical results. Tech Shoulder Elbow Surg. 2013; 14(2):33–41

[13] McKeown ADj, Beattie RF, Murrell GA, Lam PH. Biomechanical comparison of expanded polytetrafluoroethylene (ePTFE) and PTFE interpositional patches and direct tendon-to-bone repair for massive rotator cuff tears in an ovine model. Shoulder Elbow. 2016; 8(1):22–31

37 Dermal Augmentation for Challenging Large and Massive Rotator Cuff Tears

Devon T. Brameier and Paul M. Sethi

Summary
Repairs of small and medium-sized repairs provide successful long-term functional outcomes; however, massive rotator cuff tears continue to be challenging to manage, with traditional repairs failing in 37%–94% of cases. Dermal allografts have the potential to improve these massive repairs by providing biological and mechanical support to the repair, encouraging organized recruitment of the desired tissue types while off-loading stress from the repair site. Repairs augmented with dermal allografts may exhibit superior functional outcomes and reduced repair re-tear rates, suggesting this augmented approach may be a viable option for managing massive tears. This chapter provides a modern arthroscopic surgical technique for using dermal allografts as onlay augmentations in repairing massive rotator cuff repairs and highlights relevant literature in support of dermal augmentation in challenging rotator cuff repair.

Keywords: dermal allograft, dermal augmentation, massive rotator cuff tear, onlay augmentation, rotator cuff repair, rotator cuff tear

37.1 Patient Positioning

- Patient may be positioned in beach chair or lateral position for rotator cuff repair as per surgeon preference and training.

37.2 Portal Placement

- Standard posterior, posterolateral, anterolateral, and anterior portals are traditionally used with percutaneous anchor placement portals as indicated.
- A large flexible cannula may be beneficial in the midlateral portal for graft introduction.

37.3 Surgical Technique

- Patients are brought to the operating room and a comprehensive diagnostic arthroscopy is completed.
  - In the setting of revision rotator cuff surgery, the biceps is routinely treated with tenotomy or tenodesis, depending on the patient demands and expectations.
  - The leading edge of the subscapularis is carefully examined with posterior subluxation of the humeral head. The subscapularis is repaired when torn.
  - After addressing concomitant pain generators, attention is turned to the rotator cuff.
- The rotator cuff is assessed and mobilized as required.
  - Undersurface tissue releases are carried out between capsule and rotator cuff, and up along the coracoid and glenoid.

○ We do not routinely use anterior and posterior interval releases.
- The greater tuberosity is denuded of soft tissue and the bone excoriated.
- Preexisting sutures and anchors are often removed.
- When the rotator cuff has poor mobility, the articular margin is medialized by 5 mm to enlarge the available contact area between cuff and bone.
- If the tissue cannot be mobilized, and partial repair is deemed unacceptable, superior capsule reconstruction is considered.
• When the rotator cuff has adequate excursion to the lateral tuberosity, but is significantly thinned, we will perform a dermal onlay with a transosseous equivalent repair (▶ Fig. 37.1, ▶ Fig. 37.2, ▶ Video 37.1).
- After repairing the rotator cuff tear (▶ Fig. 37.1a–c, ▶ Fig. 37.2a–b), the area to be grafted is measured. For an onlay graft, the graft size often matches the footprint area of the repair. A suture with knots tied every 10 mm, or a commercially available arthroscopic ruler (▶ Fig. 37.2c), may be used to measure the area to be patched, adding a rim of 5 mm on all but the lateral margin. These measurements are used to create a template for graft preparation (▶ Fig. 37.3a).
- The surgical author chooses to use a 20 mm × 20 mm × 1 mm Arthrex ArthroFLEX decellularized dermal allograft; however, any other equivalent decellularized dermal allograft may also be used with equivalent success. The graft is cut to size according to the intraoperative-derived template (▶ Fig. 37.3).
- Double-loaded suture anchors (from surgeon's preferred provider) are placed on the medial margin of the articular cartilage, one anterior and one posterior (▶ Fig. 37.1d).
- The sutures of the two medial double-loaded anchors are passed through the cuff in a mattress fashion.
  ○ The first pair of sutures (one from the anterior anchor and one from the posterior anchor) are tied.
  ○ The second mattress is passed through the graft and the graft is parachuted down the sutures (▶ Fig. 37.4).
  ○ The medial mattress sutures are tied down. The limbs are then crossed and placed into two lateral anchors, completing the transosseous repair (▶ Fig. 37.1e, ▶ Fig. 37.2d–f).

37.4 Surgeon Tips and Tricks

• A free suture, passed through the Nevasier portal and then through the cannula and into the dermal graft, may be used as a shuttled (or pull) switch to help draw the graft into the subacromial space (▶ Fig. 37.1d).
• As an alternative to a full-sized patch, dermal pledgets such as the Arthrex ArthroFLEX Biowashers may be used to augment the repair (▶ Fig. 37.5).[1] Full-sized dermal allografts may also be cut into smaller dermal pledgets if pre-prepared pledgets are unavailable.
- After the medial row is passed, the dermal pledget is parachuted down the suture limbs and tied into place. Sutures may be tied or bridged into a lateral row of anchors depending on the repair construct.
- Pledgets are relatively easy to use and avoid many of the technical pitfalls associated with suture tangle and graft management.
• Frequently in revision or challenging cases, the rotator cuff will not have the mobility such that a low tension repair to lateral tuberosity is feasible. In this case,

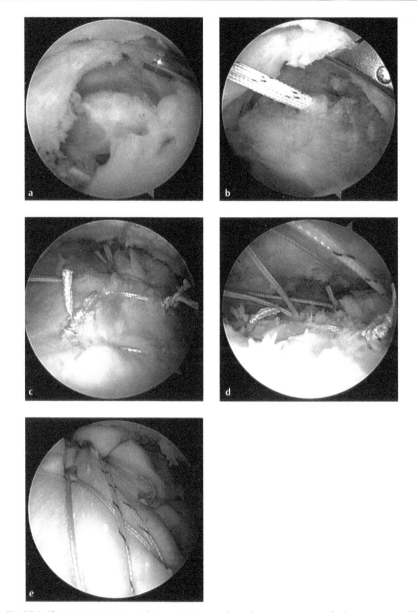

Fig. 37.1 These intraoperative arthroscopic images show the revision repair of a large rotator cuff tear with thin tissue via a single-row repair augmented with a dermal allograft. **(a)** An arthroscopic view of the tear with deficient tissue and delamination from the medial glenoid to the tuberosity. **(b)** Placement of the double-loaded anchor used to repair the tear. **(c)** The completed side-to-side and single-row repair. **(d)** The sutures from two double-loaded anchors that have not been tied and will be passed through the graft. The sutures of the double-loaded anchors (lighter blue and white/black striped) are used to create the mattress over the graft while the free suture (darker blue) is used as a shuttled stitch passed freely through Nevasier's portal to draw the graft into the repair site. **(e)** The completed augmented repair with two mattress stitches. (© Paul M. Sethi, MD.)

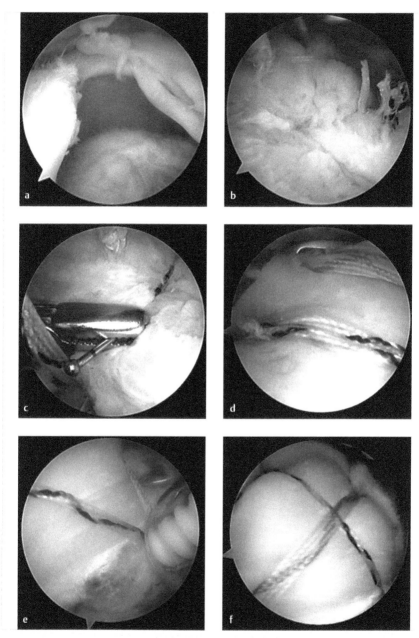

Fig. 37.2 These images show the intraoperative arthroscopic process of a revision repair of a large rotator cuff tear with thin tissue via a single-row repair augmented with a dermal allograft. **(a)** An arthroscopic view of the tear including preexisting sutures from the previous repair, which were later removed. **(b)** An arthroscopic view of the completed single-row repair. **(c)** The use of a commercially available arthroscopic ruler to measure the graft site. **(d)** The graft introduced to the repair site with the mattress sutures passed through the medial holes. **(e)** The first mattress being secured with a knotless anchor. **(f)** The completed augmented repair. (© Paul M. Sethi, MD.)

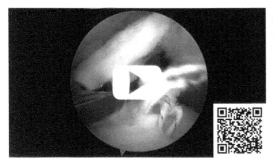

Video 37.1 Surgical demonstration of a revision repair of a large rotator cuff tear augmented with a dermal allograft.

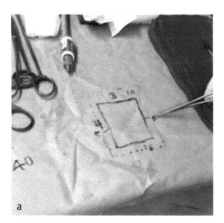

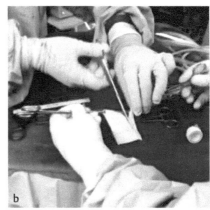

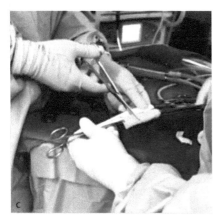

Fig. 37.3 These images show the intraoperative preparation of the acellular dermal graft. **(a)** The template created by the surgeon using intraoperative measurements of the repair site obtained arthroscopically to guide the sizing of the graft. **(b,c)** The process of sizing the graft prior to introducing it to the surgical field. (© Paul M. Sethi, MD.)

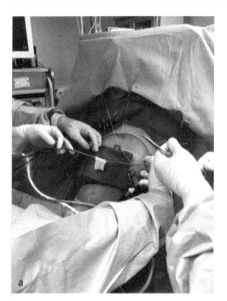

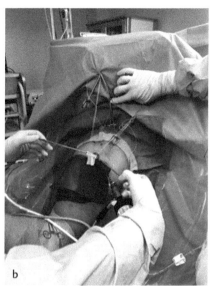

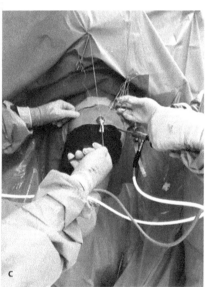

Fig. 37.4 These images show the intraoperative process of passing the sutures through the graft, which is subsequently passed into the repair site through a surgical cannula. **(a)** Shows the sized graft being introduced to the surgical field as the surgeon prepares to pass the sutures through the graft, with careful attention to avoiding suture tangles. **(b)** Shows the graft with the sutures passed through, ready for implantation. **(c)** Shows the graft being introduced to the joint through a cannula. (© Paul M. Sethi, MD.)

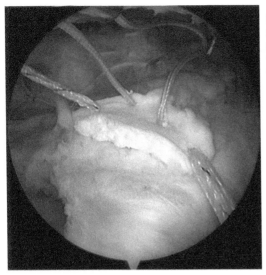

Fig. 37.5 This image shows an intraoperative arthroscopic view of a small dermal pledget being used to reinforce a deficient rotator cuff. It demonstrates the proper suture placement used to incorporate the graft into the repair. (© Paul M. Sethi, MD.)

single-row repair to the tension-free middle or medial tuberosity with a dermal onlay augment is elected.
- The articular surface of the greater tuberosity is medialized 5 mm.
- Triple-loaded suture anchors are placed on the tuberosity.
- Two mattress and one simple throw are placed through the rotator cuff. The simple suture is a Mason–Allen equivalent throw.
- After anchors are passed (2–3 typically), one mattress and one simple suture are tied. This leaves behind one untied mattress suture.
- The anteroposterior (AP) length of the tear is measured using the aforementioned methods. A mediolateral length of 15 mm is typical, and the AP length is determined by the obtained measurements.
- The two mattress sutures are passed through the dermal graft in even spaces, and the graft is parachuted down the cannula. The mattress sutures are tied but not cut. A free luggage tag suture is placed in the anterolateral and posterolateral corners of the graft. The mattress limbs are crossed and two lateral anchors are passed.
- The graft is meant to unload and augment the repair.

37.5 Pitfalls/Complications

- This is often performed as a revision or a salvage procedure; therefore, surgeon and patient must accept that complete tendon healing and restoration of completely normal function are not entirely predictable.
- Introduction of foreign grafts into the shoulder may theoretically increase risk of infection.
- These procedures do not preclude tendon transfer or subsequent arthroplasty.

37.6 Rehabilitation

- Initial focus of postoperative rehabilitation is on protecting the repair to allow for sufficient incorporation of the graft and healing of the mended tissues. This is achieved through immobilization via a sling and abduction pillow for 8 weeks.
- Pendulum exercises may be initiated immediately; however, no formal physical therapy is initiated for the first 6 weeks.
- At week 6–12, progressive passive range of motion and periscapular stabilization may commence.
- At week 12, very gentle strengthening may be incorporated into the rehabilitation program.
- At 6 months, the patient may return to previous activity level. Return to sport should be gradually introduced between week 12 and 6 months.

37.7 Rationale and/or Evidence for Approach

- Large and massive randomized controlled trials (RCTs) pose a challenge to orthopedic surgeons due to the reduced capacity for tendon-to-bone healing attributed to injuries with substantially greater tissue damage.[2,3,4,5] The poorer biological healing associated with these tears has led to reported tendon–bone fixation failure rates ranging from 37% to 94%.[2,3,6,7] This high rate of re-tear (or failure to heal) is influenced by the age of the patient, quality of the tissue, chronicity and size of the tear, degree of muscle atrophy and fatty infiltration, bone mineral density, and surgical repair technique.[7,8,9,10]
- Failed repairs of massive tears correlate with significantly inferior postoperative strength and often reduced functional shoulder outcome scores compared to successfully healed repairs, in addition to more rapidly progressed joint degeneration, in sharp contrast to functional outcomes of failed and successful small, single-tendon tear repairs in which healing yields no significant differences.[2,3,5,7,10,11,12] As such, there is a critical need for repair strategies that provide adequate strength and mechanical support while simultaneously stimulating and enhancing biological healing.
- Massive tears may be treated with nonoperative management, arthroscopic debridement, debridement with partial repair, muscle transfers, and reverse arthroplasty with a focus on reducing pain rather than regaining functional joint use.[6,13,14,15,16,17] In the growing population of young, active patients suffering from large-to-massive RCTs without signs of glenohumeral arthritis as a result of a traumatic injury, however, these methods of treatment often are less than ideal, providing suboptimal functional outcomes in relation to the patient's compatibility to return to manual labor or sporting activity.
- More recently, surgeons have used tendon transfers and nonanatomical repairs such as superior capsule repairs and the implantation of subacromial biodegradable balloons to manage massive tears in these patients; these techniques all hold promise and need to be longitudinally studied.[18,19,20,21,22,23]
- The goal of any rotator cuff repair is to restore the original biology and biomechanics of the native rotator cuff footprint through strong tendon-to-bone healing.[4,10,24] In most massive cuff tears, the poor quality of the tissue compromises the biological healing of the repair. This chapter suggests the use of acellular dermal extracellular matrices (ECMs) as scaffolds in rotator cuff repair as a potential solution for

improving tissue repair and healing with enhanced histological, mechanical, and architectural properties. ECMs may provide initial postoperative mechanical support and augmentation to repaired tissues, partially absorbing stress on the repair and protecting the sutures, and also may guide tissue healing to form tendons that mimic the original biology but with improved characteristics such as greater thickness to reduce the risk of recurrent injury.[1,9,12,13,18,25]

- There are three main forms of tendon scaffolds being investigated for augmentation of rotator cuffs: xenografts, allografts, and synthetic matrixes.
  - A variety of xenografts have been studied, including porcine small intestinal submucosa (SIS) and porcine dermal collagen; however, the current body of evidence suggests they do not enhance repairs in humans, instead inciting unfavorable inflammatory responses and resulting in similar re-tear rates when compared to nonaugmented controls.[7,8,9,10,12,13,25] Promising results using bovine Achilles xenograft matrix (▶ **Fig. 37.6**) to augment partial- and full-thickness rotator cuff tear repairs have been reported, but still are preliminary and require further investigation.[26]
  - Allografts reduce the risk of graft infection or rejection associated with xenographic matrices while demonstrating greater mean load-to-failure forces than untreated controls and exhibiting superior histological outcomes than standard repairs, including fibroblastic ingrowth at the tendon–bone interface, neovascularization of the tendon, and production of an organized collagenous ECM.[1,5,7,8,9,10,12,25,27,28,29,30,31,32,33,34,35]
  - Synthetic grafts made of biodegradable polyesters avoid the immunogenicity concerns associated with xeno- and allografts, but, as they are still relatively new to the field, few long-term studies have been conducted that explore their impact on the healing of RCTs or any side effects associated with their metabolite.[7,8,9,10,12,25]
- In light of the more extensive, successful research surrounding acellular dermal allografts, the surgical author both prefers and supports their use in augmenting repairs of torn rotator cuff tendons.[5,6,18,24,28,29,30,36]

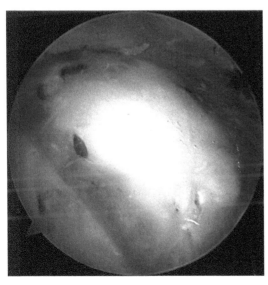

Fig. 37.6 This image shows an intraoperative view of a completed augmentation of a partial thickness rotator cuff tear using a bovine Achilles tendon xenograft and a tendon stapling method. (© Paul M. Sethi, MD.)

37.7.1 Biological Healing Rationale

- Normal bone-to-tendon interface is composed of four distinct longitudinal tissue zones: tendon, nonmineralized fibrocartilage, mineralized fibrocartilage, and bone. This interface exhibits interlocking layers of intact, oriented type I collagenous fibers leading to a strong, continuous tendon insertion on the humeral head with organized vasculature dispersed throughout the tendon.[7]
- Following a rotator cuff tear, the joint proceeds through a bone-to-tendon healing process, which joins the bone and tendon with a single layer of reactive fibroblastic scar tissue rather than recreates the histologically normal four-layer insertion site.[5,7] The healed bone-to-tendon insertion has a higher ratio of type III collagen to type I collagen than the original insertion, making it weaker.
- Additionally, the vascularity of the tendinous region typically decreases at the point of rupture, compromising the biological healing ability of the tendon tissue. The weaker tissue and reduced healing capacity at the repair site both contribute to the increased risk of failure in massive rotator cuff tear repairs.[4,7,8]

37.7.2 Mechanical Support Rationale

- Dermal grafts also may provide mechanical reinforcement between the tendon and footprint to increase repair security and load share the stress between the sutures and native tissue through their improved suture retention and mechanical properties.[8,9,12,24,25,27,31,32,33]
- Shea et al[33] estimated that the ECM graft is capable of sharing 35% of the load applied to the tendon repair.
- A cadaveric study conducted by Barber et al[31] demonstrated a 19% increase in failure load and fewer failures at suture–tissue interface in supraspinatus repairs augmented with dermal allografts when compared with nonaugmented controls. The dermal allograft was shown to significantly increase the strength of repaired tendon, augmented repairs demonstrating 324 ± 74 N average failure strength compared to 273 ± 116 N in the nonaugmented controls ($p = 0.047$).[31] These results are concurrent with those reported in biomechanical studies conducted by Ely et al,[32] Beitzel et al,[34] and Shea et al.[33]
- The studies by Ely et al, Beitzel et al, and Shea et al also demonstrated that large rotator cuff tear repairs augmented with dermal ECMs resulted in a 21%–25% decrease in gap formation.
- van der Meijden et al[37] reported that double-row repairs augmented with dermal allograft onlays result in more consistent failure loads and mechanisms of failure than nonaugmented double-row repairs.

37.7.3 Indications for Dermal Augmentation of Rotator Cuff Repairs

- The patient history, physical examination, and magnetic resonance imaging all help to guide the utilization of dermal allograft to augment repair. The decision to use a dermal graft is best made preoperatively to ensure appropriate patient consent and proper graft availability. Dermal grafts may be used in primary repair, although more frequently used for revision rotator cuff surgery.[38]

- The choice to use dermal scaffolds to repair a large or massive tear in the supraspinatus may be influenced by a short tendon stump (< 10 mm), tear at the musculotendon junction (MT rupture), > 50% thinning of the tendon, poor tissue mobility, and/or suture pull through at time of surgery.[5,11,16,38]
- Tendon tissue quality can be tested intraoperatively by passing a suture through the tissue and observing whether the suture holds or saws through the tendon when loaded (Mirzayan's test).
- Functional outcome and healing ability of rotator cuff repairs have been inversely correlated to the size and amount of retraction of tears.[6,11]

37.7.4 Clinical Evidence for the Use of Dermal Augmentation in Rotator Cuff Repair

- A summary of previous studies investigating the outcomes of dermal graft-augmented rotator cuff repairs is detailed in ▸ Table 37.1.
- Augmented repairs of massive rotator cuff tears have been shown to significantly reduce patient pain, as reported by Gupta et al,[6,13] Gilot et al,[36] Kokkalis et al,[18] and Bond et al.[28]
- They also have resulted in significantly improved joint motion and strength, as reported by Gupta et al, Kokkalis et al, and Bond et al.
- All studies of these repairs reported significant improvement in preoperative to postoperative functional outcome scores such as the American Shoulder and Elbow Surgeons (ASES), Short Form-12 (SF-12), Western Ontario Rotator Cuff (WORC), Constant, UCLA, QuickDASH, and Single Assessment Numerical Value (SANE) scores.[5,6,13,18,28,29,30,36]
- Patient satisfaction is reported at 85% to 100%.[6,13,18,28,30,36]
- In terms of repair failure, studies reported full re-tear rates of 0% to 19% and partial re-tear rates of 22% to 26%.[5,6,13,28,30,36]
- Only two of the studies reviewed included control groups. The study conducted by Gilot et al[36] suggested that improvements in visual analogue scale (VAS) pain, ASES, SF-12, and WORC scores were statistically better in the ECM group than the control group. This study found that final pain scores in the control group were reduced to 4.1 while the ECM group exhibited scores reduced to 0.9, showing a difference of 3.2, which is clinically significant.
- Barber et al[5] reported that improvements in the ASES and Constant scores of the ECM group were statistically superior to those of the control group.
- Both studies reported more favorable repair failure rates among the ECM cohort than the control cohort, Gilot et al[36] measuring 10% versus 26%, respectively, while Barber et al[5] measured 15% versus 60%.
- One of the studies measured overall patient satisfaction rates, finding that the control cohort reported 66.7% satisfaction with the outcome of their procedure while the ECM cohort reported 93.3% satisfaction.[36] Greater postoperative function and satisfaction has been related to the presence of an intact repair.[2,3,5,12]

Table 37.1 Clinical outcomes of rotator cuff tears repaired with dermal graft augmentation

Study	No. of subjects	Procedure	Control? (Y/N)	Retear rate	Functional outcomes	Patient satisfaction
Gupta et al 2012[3]	24 patients	Augmented mini-open repair of massive irreparable rotator cuff tear using human dermal allografts to bridge the retracted cuff and the native anatomic footprint	N	19 patients returned for follow-up ultrasound: 74% fully intact repairs No full re-tears 1 of 5 partial tears caused by patient noncompliance	VAS pain decreased from 5.4 to 0.9 ($p = 0.0002$) Active forward flexion improved from 111.7° to 157.3° ($p = 0.0002$) ER improved from 46.2° to 65.1° ($p = 0.001$) Abduction improved from 105.0° to 151.7° ($p = 0.0001$) Supraspinatus strength improved from 7.2 to 9.4 ($p = 0.0003$) Infraspinatus strength improved from 7.8 to 9.3 ($p = 0.002$) ASES score improved from 66.6 to 88.7 ($p = 0.0003$) SF-12 score improved from 48.8 to 56.8 ($p = 0.03$)	All patients were satisfied
Gupta et al 2013[13]	26 patients (27 shoulders)	Augmented mini-open repair of massive irreparable rotator cuff tear using porcine dermal tissue matrix xenografts to bridge the retracted cuff and the native anatomic footprint	N	22 shoulders returned for follow-up ultrasound: 73% fully intact repairs 22% partially intact repair, 1 of 5 caused by patient noncompliance 5% complete re-tear, caused by fall	VAS pain decreased from 5.1 to 0.4 ($p = 0.002$) Active forward flexion improved from 138.8° to 167.3° ($p = 0.024$) Abduction improved from 117.9° to 149.3° ($p = 0.001$) ER strength improved from 7.4 to 9.5 ($p = 0.001$) Supraspinatus strength improved from 7.2 to 9.4 ($p = 0.001$) ASES score improved from 62.7 to 91.8 ($p = 0.0007$) SF-12 score improved from 48.4 to 56.6 ($p = 0.044$)	25 of 26 patients were satisfied

(Continued)

Table 37.1 (Continued) Clinical outcomes of rotator cuff tears repaired with dermal graft augmentation

Study	No. of subjects	Procedure	Control? (Y/N)	Retear rate	Functional outcomes	Patient satisfaction
Gilot et al 2015[36]	35 patients	Augmented arthroscopic repair of massive rotator cuff tear using human dermal allografts	Y, 15 repaired via standard methods, 20 via ECM graft augmentation	Control group: 4 re-tears (26%) ECM group: 2 re-tears (10%) Verified via ultrasound	VAS pain decreased from 6.9 to 4.1 in control group and from 6.8 to 0.9 in ECM group (ECM group statistically better, p = 0.024) ASES score improved from 62.1 to 72.6 in control group and from 63.8 to 88.9 in ECM group (ECM group statistically better, p = 0.02) SF-12 and WORC scores improved in both groups, statistic differences significantly favoring graft augmentation (p = 0.031 and p = 0.0412)	Patient satisfaction rate of 66.7% in control group Patient satis-faction rate of 93.3% in ECM group
Kokkalis et al 2014[18]	21 patients	Augmented mini-open repair of massive rotator cuff tears using human dermal allografts	N	No observed re-tears as assessed by physical exam No structural evalua-tion via ultrasound or MRI	VAS pain decreased from 7.6 to 1.8 (p = 0.001) Forward flexion improved from 77° to 139° (p = 0.001) ER improved from 9° to 47° (p = 0.001) Abduction improved from 67° to 126° (p = 0.001) ASES score improved from 25.2 to 74.3 (p = 0.001)	18 of 21 patients were very satisfied or satisfied
Barber et al 2012[5]	42 patients	Augmented arthroscopic repair of massive rotator cuff using GraftJacket acellular human dermal matrix	Y, 22 repaired with aug-mentation, 20 repairs without	35 patients returned for gadolinium-en-hanced MRI: 6 of 15 (40%) in control group had intact repairs 17 of 20 (85%) in augment group had intact repairs	ASES score improved from 46.0 to 94.8 in control and from 48.5 to 98.9 in augment group (augment group statistically better, p = 0.035) Constant score improved from 45.9 to 85.3 in control group and from 41.0 to 91.9 in augment group (augment group statistically better, p = 0.008)	Not reported

(Continued)

Table 37.1 (Continued) Clinical outcomes of rotator cuff tears repaired with dermal graft augmentation

Study	No. of subjects	Procedure	Control? (Y/N)	Retear rate	Functional outcomes	Patient satisfaction
Wong et al 2010[29]	45 patients	Augmented arthroscopic repair of massive rotator cuff using GraftJacket dermal matrix allograft	N	Not reported	UCLA score increased from 18.4 to 27.5 ($p < 0.001$) Final post-op WORC score was 75.2 Final post-op ASES score was 94.1	Not reported
Petri et al 2016[30]	12 patients (13 shoulders)	Augmented open repair of massive rotator cuff tears using human dermal allografts	N	5 patients returned for follow-up MRI: 5 of 6 (83.3%) showed intact repairs 1 of 6 (16.7%) showed a failed repair, history of 4 prior cuff repairs	No significant improvement to total ASES and pain component of ASES scores ASES function score improved from 25.0 to 41.7 ($p = 0.008$) SF-12 score improved from 44.5 to 52.9 ($p = 0.005$) QuickDASH score improved from 36.5 to 11.3 ($p = 0.006$) SANE score improved from 54.3 to 74.8 ($p = 0.011$)	Average patient satisfaction recorded as 9 out of a maximum score 10
Bond et al 2008[28]	16 patients	Augmented arthroscopic repair of massive rotator cuff using GraftJacket acellular human dermal matrix	N	All patients returned for follow-up MRI: 13 of 16 (81%) had full incorporation of graft into native tissue 3 of 16 (19%) had clinical and radiographic failure of graft	Pain improved from 4.6 to 9.8 ($p = 0.0001$) Forward flexion increased from 106° to 142° ($p = 0.0001$) Forward flexion strength improved from 2.5 to 4.2 ($p = 0.0001$) ER improved from 43° to 47.2° ER strength improved from 2.5 to 4.4 ($p = 0.001$) Constant score improved from 53.8 to 84 ($p = 0.0001$) UCLA score improved from 18.4 to 30.4 ($p = 0.0001$)	15 of 16 patients were satisfied

References

[1] Acevedo DC, Shore B, Mirzayan R. Orthopedic applications of acellular human dermal allograft for shoulder and elbow surgery. Orthop Clin North Am. 2015; 46(3):377–388, x

[2] Gerber C, Fuchs B, Hodler J. The results of repair of massive tears of the rotator cuff. J Bone Joint Surg Am. 2000; 82(4):505–515

[3] Zumstein MA, Jost B, Hempel J, Hodler J, Gerber C. The clinical and structural long-term results of open repair of massive tears of the rotator cuff. J Bone Joint Surg Am. 2008; 90(11):2423–2431

[4] Nho SJ, Delos D, Yadav H, et al. Biomechanical and biologic augmentation for the treatment of massive rotator cuff tears. Am J Sports Med. 2010; 38(3):619–629

[5] Barber FA, Burns JP, Deutsch A, Labbé MR, Litchfield RB. A prospective, randomized evaluation of acellular human dermal matrix augmentation for arthroscopic rotator cuff repair. Arthroscopy. 2012; 28(1):8–15

[6] Gupta AK, Hug K, Berkoff DJ, et al. Dermal tissue allograft for the repair of massive irreparable rotator cuff tears. Am J Sports Med. 2012; 40(1):141–147

[7] Cheung EV, Silverio L, Sperling JW. Strategies in biologic augmentation of rotator cuff repair: a review. Clin Orthop Relat Res. 2010; 468(6):1476–1484

[8] Thangarajah T, Pendegrass CJ, Shahbazi S, Lambert S, Alexander S, Blunn GW. Augmentation of rotator cuff repair with soft tissue scaffolds. Orthop J Sports Med. 2015; 3(6):2325967115587495

[9] Derwin KA, Badylak SF, Steinmann SP, Iannotti JP. Extracellular matrix scaffold devices for rotator cuff repair. J Shoulder Elbow Surg. 2010; 19(3):467–476

[10] Papalia R, Franceschi F, Zampogna B, D'Adamio S, Maffulli N, Denaro V. Augmentation techniques for rotator cuff repair. Br Med Bull. 2013; 105:107–138

[11] Meyer DC, Farshad M, Amacker NA, Gerber C, Wieser K. Quantitative analysis of muscle and tendon retraction in chronic rotator cuff tears. Am J Sports Med. 2012; 40(3):606–610

[12] Longo UG, Lamberti A, Maffulli N, Denaro V. Tendon augmentation grafts: a systematic review. Br Med Bull. 2010; 94:165–188

[13] Gupta AK, Hug K, Boggess B, Gavigan M, Toth AP. Massive or 2-tendon rotator cuff tears in active patients with minimal glenohumeral arthritis: clinical and radiographic outcomes of reconstruction using dermal tissue matrix xenograft. Am J Sports Med. 2013; 41(4):872–879

[14] Moser M, Jablonski MV, Horodyski M, Wright TW. Functional outcome of surgically treated massive rotator cuff tears: a comparison of complete repair, partial repair, and debridement. Orthopedics. 2007; 30 (6):479–482

[15] Nobuhara K, Hata Y, Komai M. Surgical procedure and results of repair of massive tears of the rotator cuff. Clin Orthop Relat Res. 1994(304):54–59

[16] Millett PJ, Hussain ZB, Fritz EM, Warth RJ, Katthagen JC, Pogorzelski J. Rotator cuff tears at the musculotendinous junction classification and surgical options for repair and reconstruction. Arthrosc Tech. 2017; 6(4): e1075–e1085

[17] Mulieri P, Dunning P, Klein S, Pupello D, Frankle M. Reverse shoulder arthroplasty for the treatment of irreparable rotator cuff tear without glenohumeral arthritis. J Bone Joint Surg Am. 2010; 92(15):2544–2556

[18] Kokkalis ZT, Mavrogenis AF, Scarlat M, et al. Human dermal allograft for massive rotator cuff tears. Orthopedics. 2014; 37(12):e1108–e1116

[19] Warner JJP. Management of massive irreparable rotator cuff tears: the role of tendon transfer. Instr Course Lect. 2001; 50:63–71

[20] Petri M, Greenspoon JA, Moulton SG, Millett PJ. Patch-augmented rotator cuff repair and superior capsule reconstruction. Open Orthop J. 2016; 10:315–323

[21] Longo UG, Franceschetti E, Petrillo S, Maffulli N, Denaro V. Latissimus dorsi tendon transfer for massive irreparable rotator cuff tears: a systematic review. Sports Med Arthrosc Rev. 2011; 19(4):428–437

[22] Savarese E, Romeo R. New solution for massive, irreparable rotator cuff tears: the subacromial "biodegradable spacer". Arthrosc Tech. 2012; 1(1):e69–e74

[23] Rosa D, Balato G, Ciaramella G, Di Donato S, Auletta N, Andolfi C. Treatment of massive irreparable rotator cuff tears through biodegradable subacromial InSpace balloon. BMC Surg. 2013; 13 Suppl 1:A43

[24] Rotini R, Marinelli A, Guerra E, et al. Human dermal matrix scaffold augmentation for large and massive rotator cuff repairs: preliminary clinical and MRI results at 1-year follow-up. Musculoskelet Surg. 2011; 95 Suppl 1:S13–S23

[25] Derwin KA, Baker AR, Spragg RK, Leigh DR, Iannotti JP. Commercial extracellular matrix scaffolds for rotator cuff tendon repair. Biomechanical, biochemical, and cellular properties. J Bone Joint Surg Am. 2006; 88(12): 2665–2672

[26] Washburn R, III, Anderson TM, Tokish JM. Arthroscopic rotator cuff augmentation: Surgical technique using bovine collagen bioinductive implant. Arthrosc Tech. 2017; 6(2):e297–e301

[27] Mirzayan R, Moore MA, May J, Dorfman A, Trapani T. Augmenting rotator cuff repairs with ArthroFLEX can improve clinical outcomes. LifeNet Health. Available at https://www.lifenethealth.org/healthcare-professionals/clinical-resources

[28] Bond JL, Dopirak RM, Higgins J, Burns J, Snyder SJ. Arthroscopic replacement of massive, irreparable rotator cuff tears using a GraftJacket allograft: technique and preliminary results. Arthroscopy. 2008; 24(4):403–409.e1 LL

[29] Wong I, Burns J, Snyder S. Arthroscopic GraftJacket repair of rotator cuff tears. J Shoulder Elbow Surg. 2010; 19(2) Suppl:104–109

[30] Petri M, Warth RJ, Horan MP, Greenspoon JA, Millett PJ. Outcomes after open revision repair of massive rotator cuff tears with biologic patch augmentation. Arthroscopy. 2016; 32(9):1752–1760

[31] Barber FA, Herbert MA, Boothby MH. Ultimate tensile failure loads of a human dermal allograft rotator cuff augmentation. Arthroscopy. 2008; 24(1):20–24

[32] Ely EE, Figueroa NM, Gilot GJ. Biomechanical analysis of rotator cuff repairs with extracellular matrix graft augmentation. Orthopedics. 2014; 37(9):608–614

[33] Shea KP, Obopilwe E, Sperling JW, Iannotti JP. A biomechanical analysis of gap formation and failure mechanics of a xenograft-reinforced rotator cuff repair in a cadaveric model. J Shoulder Elbow Surg. 2012; 21(8): 1072–1079

[34] Beitzel K, Chowaniec DM, McCarthy MB, et al. Stability of double-row rotator cuff repair is not adversely affected by scaffold interposition between tendon and bone. Am J Sports Med. 2012; 40(5):1148–1154

[35] Snyder SJ, Arnoczky SP, Bond JL, Dopirak R. Histologic evaluation of a biopsy specimen obtained 3 months after rotator cuff augmentation with GraftJacket Matrix. Arthroscopy. 2009; 25(3):329–333

[36] Gilot GJ, Alvarez-Pinzon AM, Barcksdale L, Westerdahl D, Krill M, Peck E. Outcome of large to massive rotator cuff tears repaired with and without extracellular matrix augmentation: A prospective comparative study. Arthroscopy. 2015; 31(8):1459–1465

[37] van der Meijden OA, Wijdicks CA, Gaskill TR, Jansson KS, Millett PJ. Biomechanical analysis of two-tendon posterosuperior rotator cuff tear repairs: extended linked repairs and augmented repairs. Arthroscopy. 2013; 29(1):37–45

[38] Gilot GJ, Attia AK, Alvarez AM. Arthroscopic repair of rotator cuff tears using extracellular matrix graft. Arthrosc Tech. 2014; 3(4):e487–e489

38 Case Discussions on Surgical Decision Making for Massive Rotator Cuff Tears: Repair, Reconstruction, or Reverse Shoulder Replacement?

Mark Frankle and Mark Mighell

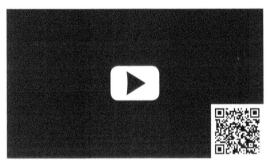

Video 38.1 Case discussion and surgical demonstration of reverse shoulder arthroplasty in an 80 year old male with a large superior, retracted rotator cuff tear.

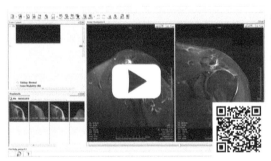

Video 38.2 Case discussion and surgical demonstration of arthroscopic rotator cuff repair in a 68 year old male with a large posterior superior rotator cuff tear.

Index

Note: Page numbers set **bold** or *italic* indicate headings or figures, respectively.